Dermatopathology

Eduardo Zappi • Eduardo A. Zappi

Dermatopathology

Classification of Cutaneous Lesions

Springer

Eduardo Zappi
Zappi Dermatopathology
New York, NY
USA

Eduardo A. Zappi
Ryerson Avenue
Caldwell, NJ
USA

ISBN 978-1-4471-2893-9 ISBN 978-1-4471-2894-6 (eBook)
DOI 10.1007/978-1-4471-2894-6
Springer London Heidelberg New York Dordrecht

Library of Congress Control Number: 2012950002

Printed on acid-free paper

Springer is part of Springer Science+Business Media (www.springer.com)

To Elda and Marta

The primary object of classification is to arrange the facts so that we can acquire the greatest possible command over them with the least possible effort.

Joseph William Mellor
Modern Inorganic Chemistry, p. 806
Longman, Green and Co.
London

Preface

The author's ideas with respect to dermatopathology have already been presented in the Spanish edition of this book and have been translated into English for this edition.

Chapter 1 of this book covers basic concepts of cutaneous embryology, anatomy, and biochemistry. A short introduction to topics of immunology is more conveniently placed at the beginning of Chapter 6, in which the lesions of inflammatory nature are discussed.

Chapter 2 deals with the taxonomic criteria that were applied for developing the classification of cutaneous lesions used in this text.

In Chapters 3, 4, 5, 6 and 7, a histopathologic analysis is conducted of the lesions of hereditary, malformative, inflammatory, proliferative, and miscellaneous nature, respectively.

Along with lesions pertaining to the most common dermatologic conditions, coverage of unusual lesions is also provided. The latter are discussed for didactic or illustrative purposes or for the sake of completion of the topics under discussion.

Throughout the text brief descriptions of the external aspects of lesions under discussion are offered. Pertinent clinical information which may yield clues leading to more precise diagnosis of the lesions is also provided when warranted.

The reader's efforts are further supported with abundant tabulated material, along with drawings and photomicrographs of mainly hematoxylin and eosin (H&E) stained sections. This book endorses the use of the H&E staining technique, often maligned but irreplaceable as a standard procedure in a diagnostic histopathology laboratory. The original magnification (o m) of the photomicrographs is stated in each case.

Ancillary tests that may help in the diagnosis of certain lesions are also mentioned, although in-depth technical detail on these techniques is not provided. These may be found by the interested reader within a list of pertinent references located at the end of the book.

Acknowledgments

The senior author would like to pay tribute to Dr. Walter F. Lever. Dr. Lever was a pioneer and a leader in dermatopathology. He combined his extensive knowledge and vast experience in this field with great modesty as well as exemplary respect and tolerance toward the ideas of others. These traits are constantly reflected in his admirable opus, *Histopathology of the Skin*, whose seventh edition constitutes a milestone which will be difficult to surpass. Dr. Lever's personal qualities made it a pleasure to interact with.

The authors gratefully acknowledge the expert assistance of Daniel Esparza and the invaluable support of Dany K. Menuau, manager of our office, during this endeavor.

Prologue to the Spanish Edition

Dermatopathology is a branch of general pathology. It should, therefore, follow its guidelines, observe its rules and criteria, as well as use its nomenclature. This, however, is not the case. This situation may be due to two reasons. The first is that during the formative years of dermatopathology, pathologists immersed in the study of the dramatic and spectacular processes of the internal organs, overlooked events occurring in the skin. This fact was bluntly pointed out by W. Lever, who in 1949, in the preface to the first edition of his well-known book stated, "...dermatopathology is not given much attention in pathology texts." The second reason that leads to this situation is that, since the nosologic processes in dermatology occur at the level of the skin, lesions can be easily removed and subjected to microscopic examination by dermatologists functioning as pathologists.

Hence, dermatopathology grew under the leading influence of clinical dermatology. This discipline imposed upon its nomenclature, its schemes and dogmas, and even its prejudices, transforming it into a science only understandable to dermatologists, as the author of this book – a pathologist converted into a dermatopathologist after many years of effort – could attest.

To enhance communication between clinicians and pathologists, as well as to facilitate their mutual understanding in this field, the senior author developed a classification system of cutaneous lesions previously presented as a succinct guide [1] which was favorably received among its targeted audience. That guide, with expanded discussions on diverse topics, abundant tabulated material, and a large number of original, mostly black and white photomicrographs and drawings, is introduced here as a book of dermatopathology [2].

Its basic science contents were reviewed and updated by the junior author.

The authors strive to maintain the balanced character of the previous guide, integrating knowledge from both dermatology and pathology. Since advances in these fields are supported by ever-evolving techniques in biochemistry, molecular biology, genetics, etc., the authors felt compelled to incorporate material derived from these sources. They did so but in a way commensurate to the character of the book, devoid of encyclopedic pretense and, on the contrary, of an eminent practical character. The interested reader may find details on these techniques in a list of authoritative sources at the end of the book.

If the practicing pathologist and dermatologist find this book helpful in their daily activities, the authors feel that they have been successful in their efforts.

Woodside, N.Y.

References

1. Zappi E. Guide for the classification and microscopic diagnosis of cutaneous lesions. New York: Automation Graphics; 1991.
2. Zappi E, Zappi EA. Dermatopatología. Clasificación y estudio razonado de las lesiones cutáneas. Buenos Aires: Editorial Ascune Hnos; 2007.

Contents

Elements of Cutaneous Embryology, Anatomy, and Biochemistry

1

Cutaneous Embryology

Embryology of the Skin

The youngest human embryos in which cutaneous development was observed were about 4–5 weeks old. At that point, the embryo's external surface is covered by the ectoderm, a monolayer of cells stretching over a mesenchymal mantle. It is partially overlaid by the "periderm," a second layer of bulky elements endowed with microvilli. This situation and ensuing events are presented in Fig. 1.1.

The ectodermal layer develops into the stratum germinativum, a permanent element which evolves into the germinal layer of postnatal life, whereas the periderm, a decidual layer, flattens and is ultimately shed into the amniotic cavity. By the tenth week of gestation, when the embryo turns into a fetus, an intermediate layer of cells develops from the stratum germinativum beneath the periderm. This is known as the "stratum intermedium." This layer, which corresponds to the stratum spinosum of postuterine life, proliferates and, by week 23, undergoes keratinization. This event is evidenced by the appearance of keratohyalin granules; the development of the granular layer is coincident with the loss of the periderm into the amniotic cavity.

By week 6–7, a basement membrane appears and soon attains considerable thickness. Melanocytes reach the epidermis by the 12th week of gestation, remaining from that point on in the stratum germinativum. The origin of the Merkel cells is not well established, but the presence of desmosomes among them and the surrounding keratinocytes suggests that they may differentiate from the latter. Langerhans cells, the fourth cellular component of the epidermis, are generated in the bone marrow, from where they migrate and colonize the epidermis.

Embryology of the Cutaneous Adnexa

Toward the 12th week of gestation, primary epithelial germs develop as condensations on the underface of the stratum germinativum. Some of these, which then give rise to the pilosebaceous/apocrine complex, protrude into the dermis as pilar germs, as part of a process induced by mesenchymal cells beneath. Later, when the pilar papilla – of mesenchymal origin – intrudes into the basis of the pilar germs, they are transformed into bulbopilar germs. As the bulbopilar germs keep growing downward, two bulges emerge from their exterior: a superior one corresponding to the origin of the sebaceous gland and an inferior one linked to the insertion of the *arrector pilorum*. In certain areas of the body, the bulbopilar germs exhibit a top third bulge corresponding to the origin of the apocrine gland. The central part of the bulbopilar germ is transformed into the hair shaft and the peripheral part into the inner radicular sheath, later to be surrounded by the outer radicular sheath, of epidermal origin.

The eccrine glands originate from primary epithelial germs, independently from the bulbopilar ones. The ungual complex appears upon the 12th week of gestation as epidermal thickenings at the dorsum of the fingertips, being laterally limited by two folds, and at the base by the proximal fold, from beneath which the nail matrix develops.

Cutaneous Anatomy and Biochemistry

Disregarding major regional differences, it may be stated that the skin is formed by a highly specialized epithelium connected by a thin, acellular layer to a mesenchymal base, which offers to it support and other vital functions.

E. Zappi, E.A. Zappi, *Dermatopathology*,
DOI 10.1007/978-1-4471-2894-6_1, © Springer-Verlag London 2013

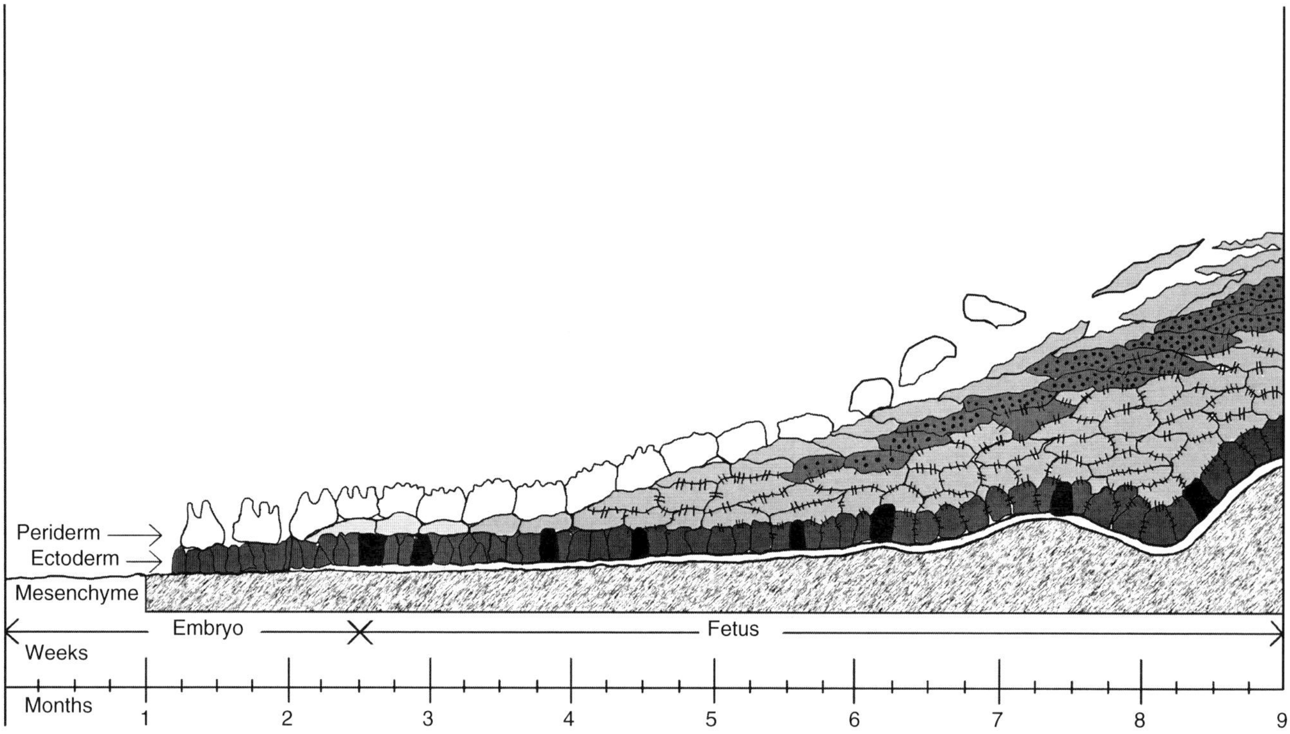

Fig. 1.1 Diagrammatic representation of the development of human skin. The germinal layer is depicted in *heavy gray*, and the melanocytes interspersed in it are shown in *black*. The granular layer is represented as a *dark gray dotted band* while desmosomes are pictured as *faint interstitial lines*. The basement membrane appears as a *heavy double line*. For the sake of simplicity, Langerhans and Merkel cells, as well as nuclear contours, are omitted from the drawing. The time of gestation in weeks and months is indicated along the horizontal axis of the figure

As a primary approach to the study of the skin, the cellular components of the epithelium that covers it – that is, the epidermis – will be examined. Secondarily, the mesenchymal structures underneath shall be discussed. Lastly, a review will be made of the cutaneous adnexa, as well as of the irrigation and innervation systems of the skin.

Epidermis

The epidermis is constituted by four cellular elements [1–5]. The keratinocytes, which amount to about 90 % of the epidermal cell population, do not have dendritic projections and are tightly apposed, leaving just, under normal conditions, virtual intercellular spaces between them. The three other epidermal components, the melanocytes, the Merkel, and the Langerhans cells, are furnished with dendritic projections (Fig. 1.2). These cells are not in contact with each other but are scattered throughout this layer and surrounded by the keratinocytic population.

The four cellular components of the epidermis are shown in Fig. 1.3, a schematic rendering of this layer and the underlying dermis, viewed under light microscopic (LM) examination.

Non dendritic	Keratinocytes
Dendritic	Melanocytes
	Merkel cells
	Langherhans cells

Fig. 1.2 Cellular components of the epidermis

Keratinocytes: Keratinocytes derive directly from the embryonal ectoderm. Early microscopists noted that these cells were surrounded by thorn-like structures, which they named "prickles." Over time, this designation tended to be substituted by the term "intercellular bridges." Through these, it was first assumed that intracellular fibers were able to spread from one cell to neighboring ones, forming a continuous network which would hold together the epidermis. This idea turned out to be wrong since it was proven by electron microscopy (EM) that intracellular fibers never abandon their own keratinocytes [6].

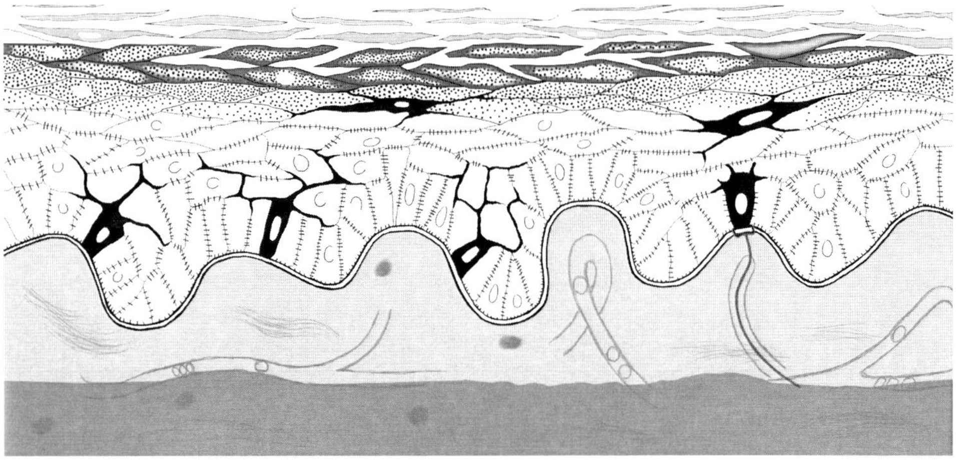

Fig. 1.3 Schematic drawing of a vertical section of the skin under light microscopy. The epidermal surface appears covered by loose keratin scales. The lower epidermal boundary is outlined by a *double line* corresponding to the basal membrane. This one appears irregularly woven due to the epidermal ridges projected downward. The dermis is molded by these, forming intervening mounds known as dermal papillae. Keratinocytes, the only nondendritic elements of the epidermis are represented in *white*, with the plasma membrane (*PM*) surrounded by intercellular bridges. Note the variability in size and shape of the keratinocytes, from small, low cylindrical in the basal layer to bulkier and progressively flattened at upper layers. Also note the progressive decrease of intercellular bridges to the point that at the upper epidermal layer, the cellular interstitia appear devoid of these. Simultaneously, within the keratinocytes at the midepidermal level appear keratohyalin granules, characteristic of the granular layer. Also, at this level, the PM of the keratinocytes begins to thicken by apposition of involucrin to the inside of the plasma membrane. The buildup of tonofilaments within keratinocytes and the thickening of their walls end up obliterating the cavity of keratinocytes, which terminate as homogeneous keratin plaques ready to be desquamated. Melanocytes, Merkel cells, and Langerhans cells, the three dendritic elements of the epidermis, are represented in *black*. At the epidermal basal layer in the figure, there are, from left to right, three melanocytes with profuse cellular projections. To their right appears an isolated Merkel cell with blunt dendritic projections, sitting on a synaptic plaque connected to a nervous fiber. In contrast to melanocytes, Merkel cells appear joined by intercellular bridges to neighboring keratinocytes. Beneath the granular layer are seen two Langerhans cells, endowed with long dendritic projections but devoid of intercellular bridges. The superficial or papillary dermis just below the basement membrane is depicted *faintly gray*. The deep or reticular dermis underneath may be distinguished from the papillary dermis by its *deeper gray tone*. Between the superficial and the deep dermis run the vessels of the subpapillary plexus. Additional details are found in the text

Fig. 1.4 Keratin filament. Note the modular, head to tail attachment of the tetramers (**a**) to form a keratin filament (**b**)

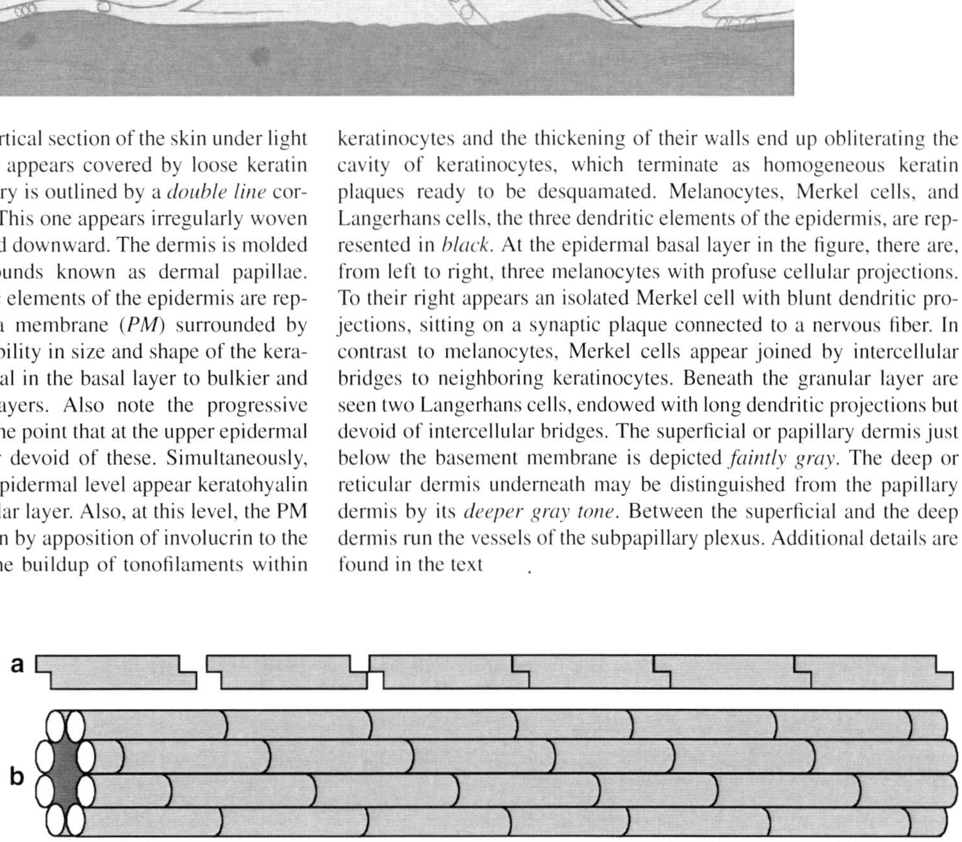

Over the years, the name "prickle cell" lost its appeal in favor of the terms "squamous cell" and "keratinocyte." The latter name was given to this type of cell on account of its important, although by no means its only property (!) of generating keratin (*keras* [G] horn). The production of this substance is the basis for the epidermal keratinization or cornification.

Keratin is a fibrous intracellular protein which gives stability and mechanical resistance to the various epithelia. The complicated molecular composition of keratin explains the variety of forms under which this substance may appear [7]. From a practical viewpoint, it is not so important to study the molecular composition of keratin, as recognizing the existence in the various types of epithelia of two forms of this substance, soft and hard keratin [2].

Keratin is formed, in both cases, starting from intermediate filaments, integrants of the cytoskeleton (p. 193). These filaments were initially described as "tonofilaments," an old-fashioned term today, although still convenient as a shorthand term for "intermediate keratin filaments."

The primary component of tonofilaments are cytokeratins, that is, seven amino acid polypeptides coded by several genes, dispersed along various chromosomes. Cytokeratin monomers are paired off into dimers. The dimers in turn are laterally adjoined into tetramers. Tetramers are attached to each other in a modular fashion forming protofilaments. Eight protofilaments are laterally attached in a tubular fashion to form a keratin filament [8] (Fig. 1.4).

Keratin filaments are steadily produced by keratinocytes during their upward progression through the epidermis until the cytoplasmic spaces are almost totally filled with them. The type of keratin they will ultimately produce depends on the fact that keratinocytes *may* or *may not* generate filaggrin [9]. Filaggrin is a glycoprotein of the family of the ligand proteins, whose name indicates precisely their capacity to aggregate filaments (p. 193).

Soft Keratin: As tonofilaments are being produced, the cell simultaneously generates profilaggrin. This substance joins the tonofilaments in their upward progression. Upon reaching the granular layer, profilaggrin breaks down into many filaggrin fragments. These join with tonofilaments forming basophilic keratohyalin granules [10]. This process is called fast keratinization on account of the speed of profilaggrin breakdown and keratohyalin granule buildup [11]. Keratohyalin granules, the hallmark of soft keratinization, can be easily observed by LM.

Hard Keratin: Tonofilaments are produced here without a simultaneous synthesis of profilaggrin. In the absence of any intervening substance, tonofilaments attach side by side to each other, establishing disulfide bridges. This process, called "slow keratinization," proceeds *without forming keratohyalin granules* in contrast to the former, lending to its final products, hair and nail, their characteristic hardness [12].

During the process of epidermal keratinization, other important events take place as well [9]. These include the production of a sulfur-rich protein, involucrin (*involucrum* [L] envelope), which is deposited on the inside of the keratinocytes' plasma membrane (PM) at the upper level of the epidermis, thus thickening and strengthening it. Upon their arrival at the upper epidermal levels, keratinocytes also release Odland bodies into the interstitial spaces. These are granules around 300 nm in diameter, which contain cholesterol and other lipids, along with inactive lipases. Spread through the interstitial spaces, the lipids promote epidermal cohesion and contribute to the buildup of a barrier which prevents water loss from the body [13].

Through progressive dissolution of intercellular bridges and loss of the nucleus, mitochondria, and other organelles, keratinocytes are transformed over a period of time slightly longer than two months from living cells into inert keratin scales ready to be desquamated. Activation of the previously secreted lipases, which hydrolize cholesterol and loosen intercellular attachments, contributes to this process in a decisive manner.

The above-stated successive changes impress characteristic features on the epidermal layers, as reflected by their current nomenclature: basal or germinative layer (*stratum germinativum*), the only featuring mitotic activity under normal conditions; squamous or prickle cell layer (*stratum spinosum*); granular layer (*stratum granulosum*) and horny layer (*stratum corneum*). The terms "layer" and "stratum" are equivalent and may be used interchangeably.

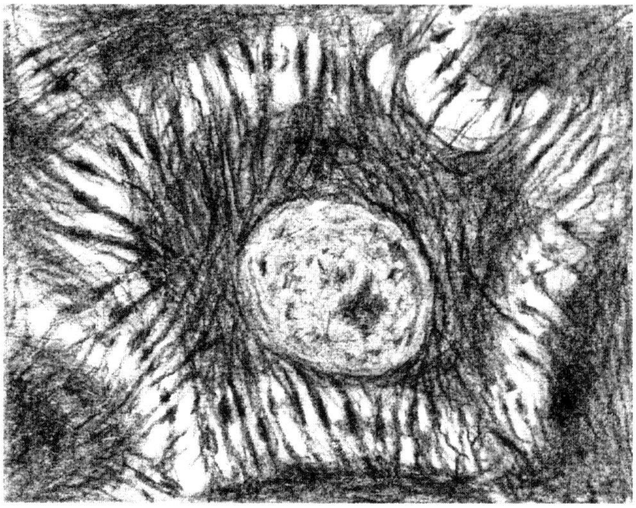

Fig. 1.5 Drawing from a high-resolution EM picture of a keratinocyte. Observe the fibrillar network in the keratinocyte and the rows of parallel desmosomes spanned between it and the surrounding ones. Note the central thickening in the desmosomes, corresponding to Bizzozero nodules

In areas of intense keratinization of the body such as the palms and soles, an additional, acellular and faintly eosinophilic layer, the stratum lucidum, is present in the epidermis, located between the horny and granular layers.

At the end of the seventeenth century, the Italian anatomist M. Malpighi made the observation that the epidermis was formed by an external layer of dead, cornified elements and an inner one of living cells. He called these "stratum corneum" and "stratum mucosum," respectively. The term "stratum malpighii," frequently used in dermatology, is derived from this observation and refers to the three layers of living cells of the epidermis together, the germinative, the prickle cell, and the granular layer [14].

At the point of mucosal transformation of the epidermis in order to line up the external recesses of the body (such as the oral or vaginal cavity), keratinocytes lose their keratinizing capacity, being transformed into large clear cells, with a high content of glycogen. During their upward migration, these cells undergo a combined microbial/ traumatic degenerative process and are finally eliminated as straps or isolated elements.

An EM image of a keratinocyte (Fig. 1.5) reveals their fibrous network, as well as the intercellular bridges spanning between them. Each intercellular bridge is formed by two bundles of tonofilaments which, projected from opposite keratinocytes, meet in the intercellular space in a thickening named "Bizzozero's nodule," [15] which actually corresponds to a desmosome.

Desmosomes (*desmos* + *soma* [G] bind + body) are numberless structures located between keratinocytes [16]. These play a fundamental role in the cohesion and mechanical resistance of the epidermis. Their framework can be appreciated in Fig. 1.6 (left), an artistic rendering of the vertical section of a desmosome viewed by EM. Prior to its discussion, it should be stated that dark lines in EM images represent "electron-dense" or "high electron density bands," whereas clear lines correspond to "electron-lucent" or "low electron density bands."

In summary, the desmosome shows eight alternating electron-dense and electron-lucent lines, located four on each side of a central electron-dense line, adding up to a total of nine lines [18] (nine, as the number of Beethoven's symphonies). This is shown in Fig. 1.7 which is a high-resolution EM image of one of these structures.

Melanocytes: The existence of melanocytes in the human epidermis was reported in 1926 by P. Masson [19]. He initially called them "clear cells" because of the contrast they offered against the well-stained keratinocytes of the germinal layer in skin sections to which the current staining procedures had been applied: in contrast to the much more abundant keratinocytes, melanocytes appeared as pale, vacuolated elements along the germinal layer, at a rate of 1 melanocyte to about 10/20 keratinocytes (Fig. 1.8).

Upon in vitro application of Bloch's reaction, clear cells were shown to produce melanin. As a result of this discovery, their name was changed to "melanocytes."

Bloch's reaction is based on the presence of tyrosinase in determined cells. This enzyme is responsible for the transformation of the amino acid tyrosine into melanin (*melas* [G] dark or black) via dioxyphenylalanine (DOPA) and other intermediate compounds. Upon incubating tissues in a DOPA solution, the cells which possess tyrosinase develop the brown color of melanin (melanin is actually not one but a mixture of substances of closely similar chemical structure whose color varies within a wide spectrum).

Through the distribution of melanin in the epidermis, melanocytes play a fundamental defensive role against harmful solar radiation, absorbing UV radiation and preventing it from reaching deeper levels of the skin.

In response to the specific stimulus of solar radiation, tyrosine is transformed into melanin within special organelles of the melanocytes, the melanosomes. This process takes place during the migration of the melanosomes along the dendritic projections of the melanocytes so that when they reach their tips, they are converted into solid melanin granules. After a process of apoptosis (p. 193), the dendritic tips are incorporated and dispersed into the cytoplasm of neighboring keratinocytes, where the granules are ultimately dissolved and the melanin is liberated in order to exert its protective action.

The process of pigment production and transfer does not occur diffusely on the epidermal surface but within discrete units called "epidermal melanin units" [20]. Each of these is formed by a central melanocyte surrounded by keratinocytes in a circular territory, marked by the radial reach of its dendrites. In a panoramic view, the natural waviness of the epidermis prevents the simultaneous focusing of all the units in the field. Nevertheless, when seen from above, a clear idea about the regular distribution of the epidermal melanin units in the epidermis is conveyed (Fig. 1.9).

In conclusion of this section, a discussion about the relationship between nevocytes and melanocytes is in order. The term "nevocyte" derives from "nevus." This word, whose origin may be found in Sanskrit [21], has been of common usage since ancient times. It has a range of distinct and extravagant meanings, having been used to describe such things as "a beauty spot," "a birthmark," and "a liver spot" to "a pregnant woman's craving" and even "a stork's bite" but always with the connotation of a *defective*, *pigmented*, and *congenital* lesion. Over time, the term "*nevus*" became a favorite of dermatologists, who applied it in liberal fashion, coupled to graphic and picturesque descriptions, although always with the implication of *defective*, *pigmented*, and *congenital*. At the end of the nineteenth century, P. G. Unna, the renowned dermatologist from Hamburg, Germany, examining under LM lesions designated as "*nevi*," found in these certain cells which, in obvious reference to their site of origin, he called "nevus cells" or "nevocytes" [22]. Due to their morphologic features, Unna concluded that *nevocytes were of epithelial nature*, although he made the explicit reservation that, in contrast to epidermal cells, nevocytes lacked filaments and "prickles." This observation contributed decisively to dismiss Unna's interpretation that the cells he was referring to were keratinocytes since keratinocytes *do have* "prickles"!

Due to the common origin of melanocytes and nevocytes in the neural crest and to the fact that both were DOPA positive, it was assumed that these were identical and that they should bear the same denomination as indicated by the careless expression "if nevocytes and melanocytes are the same (*assuming that the identity of melanocytes and nevocytes has been settled*!), let us give them the same name" [23]. The word "nevomelanocyte" was even coined to designate them conjointly. Table 1.1, although pointing out to common features between melanocytes and nevocytes, also presents other features that prevent from accepting them as identical elements.

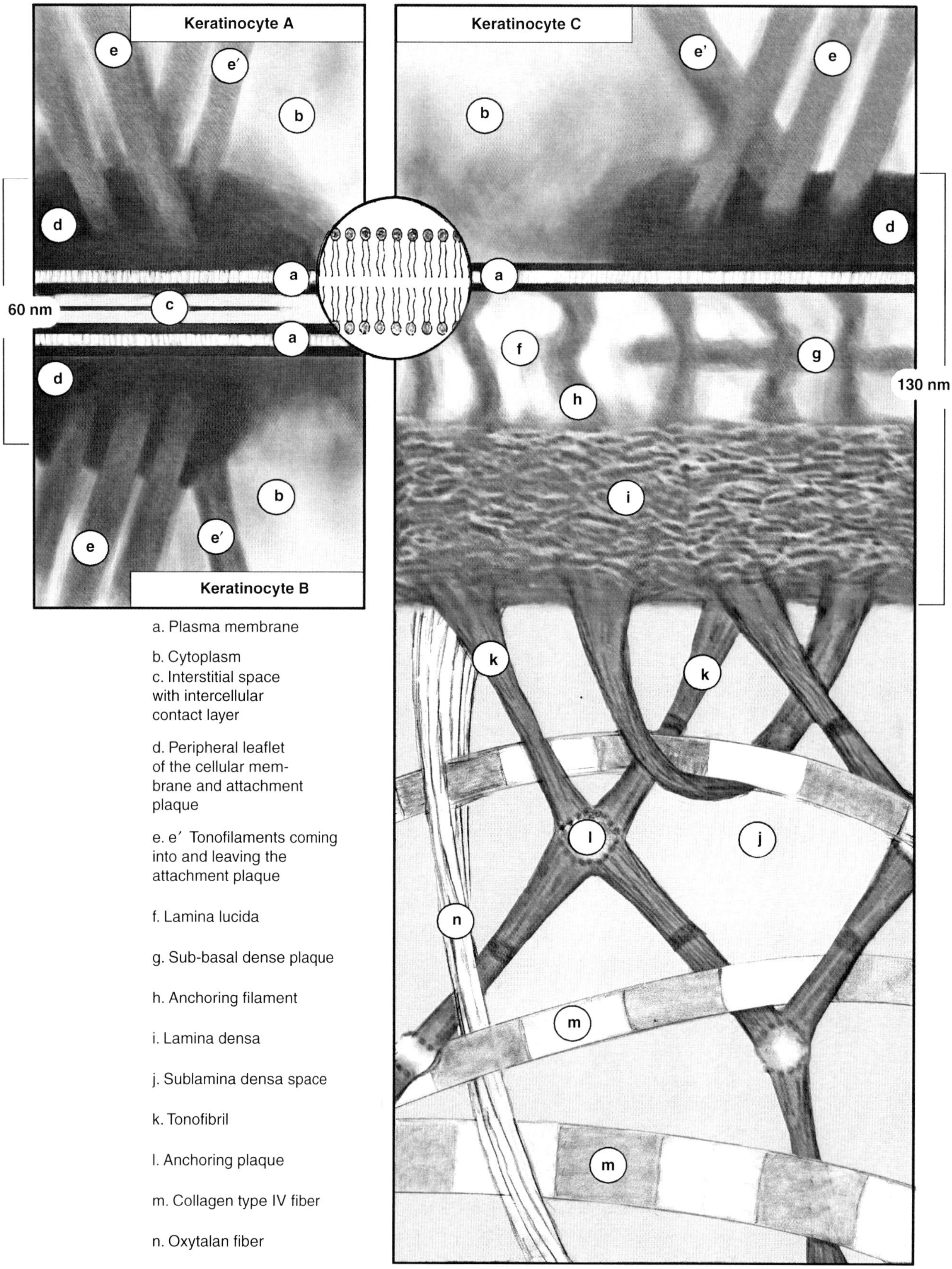

a. Plasma membrane

b. Cytoplasm

c. Interstitial space with intercellular contact layer

d. Peripheral leaflet of the cellular membrane and attachment plaque

e. e′ Tonofilaments coming into and leaving the attachment plaque

f. Lamina lucida

g. Sub-basal dense plaque

h. Anchoring filament

i. Lamina densa

j. Sublamina densa space

k. Tonofibril

l. Anchoring plaque

m. Collagen type IV fiber

n. Oxytalan fiber

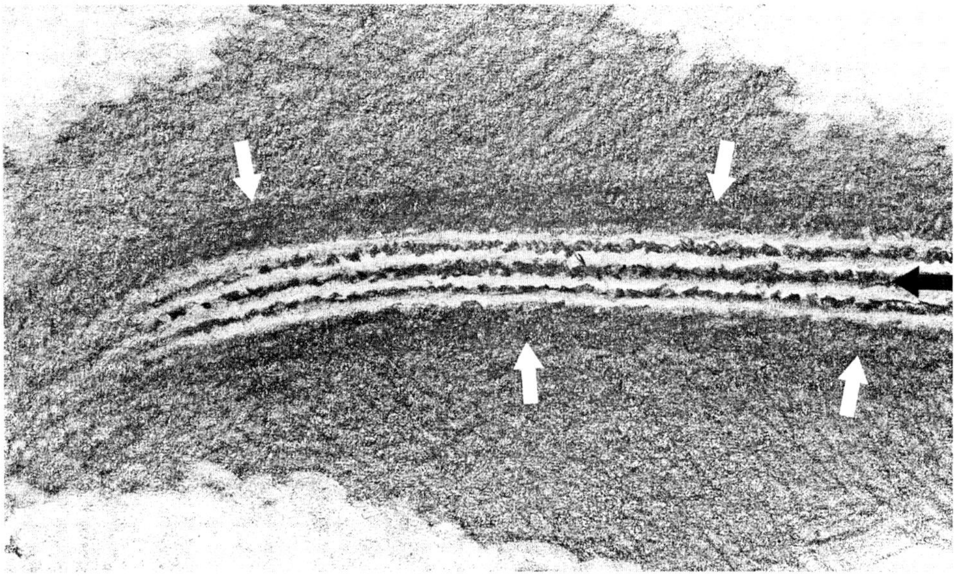

Fig. 1.7 Desmosome at high EM magnification showing its nine component lines. The barely visible pair of external electron-dense lines obscured by the ingoing and outgoing tonofilaments is highlighted by *white arrows*. The *black arrow* indicates the intercellular contact layer

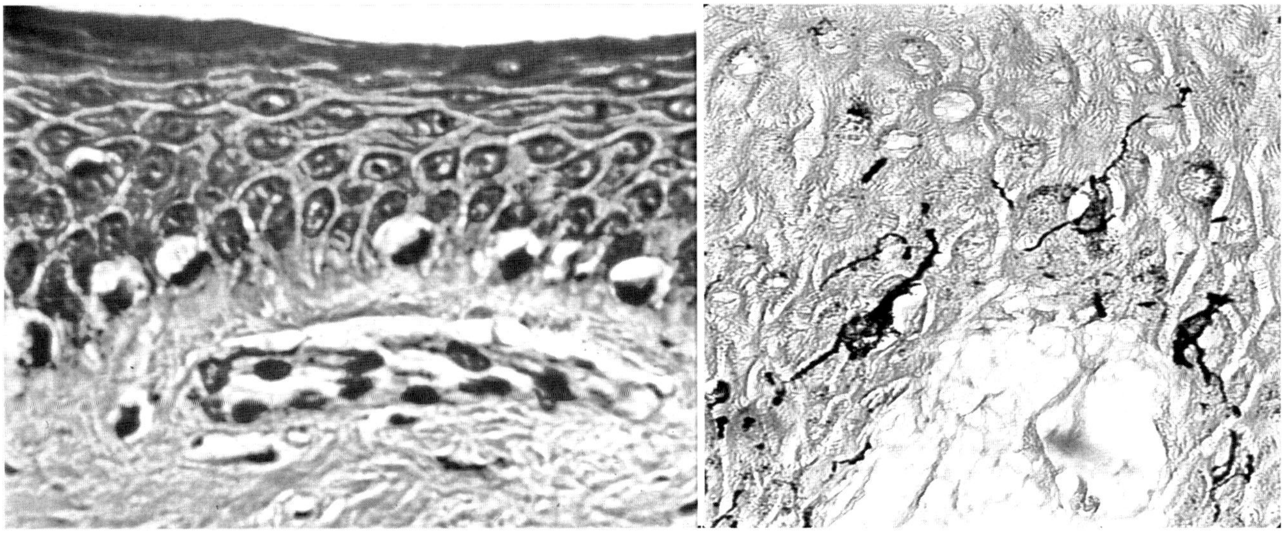

Fig. 1.8 Skin section with epidermal melanocytes. On the *left half* of the figure, melanocytes appear as a succession of clear cells along the germinal layer. On the *right half* of the figure, melanocytes appear black stained, featuring their dendritic projections. H&E ×100; DOPA ×100, o m

Fig. 1.6 Artistic rendering comparing the vertical section of a desmosome and a hemidesmosome, viewed by EM. The desmosome hereby analyzed (*left*) is found between keratinocytes A, above, and B, below. The section of the two cells shown in the picture is delimited by their cell membrane or "plasma membrane" (*PM*) (*a*): within the PM is the cytoplasm or "cytosol" (*b*) and, on the outside, the interstitial space with the intercellular contact layer (*c*). The PM has a trilaminar fabric homologous to the trilaminar membrane, a phospholipid bilayer of 8–10 nm in thickness, ubiquitous in living cells. In the *central circle* of the figure, the phospholipid bilayer of the PM is seen at higher magnification: the two outer layers of the PM composed of the phosphatidic heads are represented as *black dots*, whereas the central layer formed by the lipid tails of these molecules fused together is symbolized by parallel lines turned to the inside. These layers are called the "peripheral" and "central leaflets" of the PM, respectively. Located on the surface of the peripheral leaflet of the PM facing the inside of the cell is a structure about 20 nm in thickness called the "attachment" or "fixation plaque." (*d*) The peripheral leaflet and the attachment plaque sitting on it are fused together and form the outermost and heaviest pair of bands of the desmosome. Tonofilament bundles (*e*) converge at various angles from the nuclear vicinity toward the attachment plaques. They are then reflected back into the cell's cytoplasm (*e´*). From the face of the fixation plaque oriented toward the outside of the cell, cadherins emerge from the cell to meet their analogs from the opposite keratinocyte in the interstitial space. These transmembranous glycoproteins are invisible under EM inspection. The pair of electron-lucent lines, which follows the first electron-dense line, is just the central leaflet of both PMs. The following pair of electron-dense lines represent the external leaflet of the PM. This one, in fact, represents the external boundary of each of the participating keratinocytes. The external surface of the keratinocytes is covered by an electrolucent layer of glycocalyx, which is a mixture of glycolipids and glycoproteins: the glycocalyx bands overlap, forming the central electron-dense line of the desmosome, that is, the intercellular contact layer (*c*) [17]

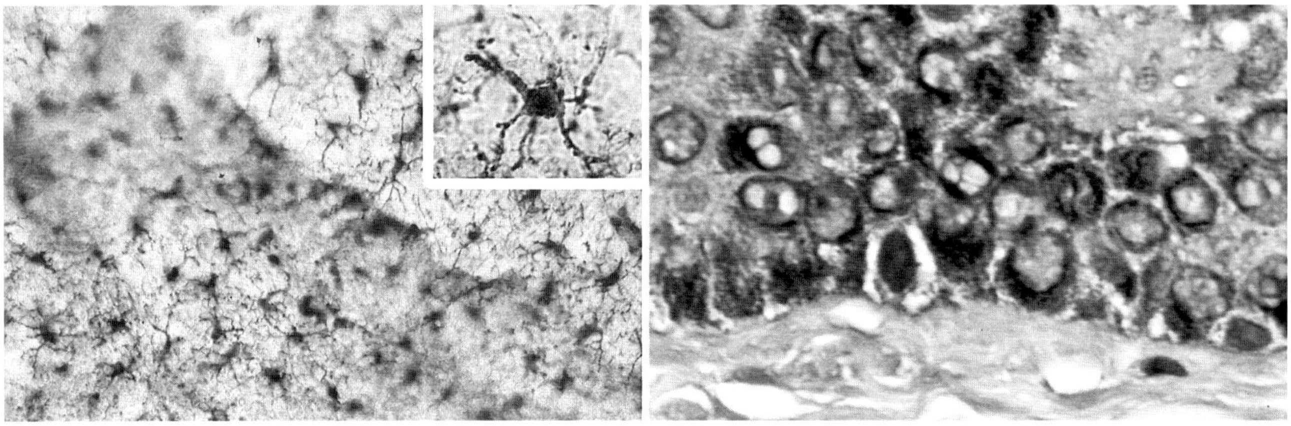

Fig. 1.9 Epidermal melanin units in a panoramic view and in a vertical section. *Left*: after artifactual separation of the epidermis from the skin, melanocytes in the germinal layer appear black stained by means of a Bloch reaction. In the *inset*, a melanocyte is seen at higher magnification. *Right*: vertical section of an incidentally found epidermal melanin unit seen under immersion oil. A central melanocyte with a clear cytoplasm is found, surrounded by melanin-loaded keratinocytes. DOPA ×40; ×100; H&E ×1,000, o m

Table 1.1 Similarities and differences between melanocytes and nevocytes

	Melanocytes	Nevocytes
Similarities		
Origin	Neural crest	Neural crest
Tonofilaments and desmosomes	Absent	Absent
Tyrosinase	Present	Present
Melanin production	Yes	Yes
Differences – under normal conditions		
Presence in the epidermis	Constant	Not found
Presence in the dermis	No	Yes
Shape	Dendritic	Epithelioid
Association with keratinocytes	Yes	No
Melanin production	Physiologically regulated	Erratic
Integration of the melanin production with any physiologic process	Yes	No

For instance, in contrast to melanocytes, which play a fundamental role in the protection of the organism against solar radiation, nevocytes *do not have any known function.* The latter are endowed with the capacity for melanin production but only in erratic fashion, without integrating the pigment into any physiological process. Thus, the melanin produced by nevocytes is stored within them. When the storage capacity of these cells is exceeded, the pigment spills over into the interstitial spaces where it is phagocytized by macrophages, which are thus transformed into melanophages (Fig. 1.10).

A rhetoric, although plausible argument against the purported identity of melanocytes and nevocytes, is that, if it had been accepted, it would be a common use to designate alternatively the normal epidermal melanogenic cell, that is, the *melanocyte*, as "*nevocyte*." This, however, does not occur, at least as evidenced by the bibliographic search [1–5] where the normal epidermal melanogenic element is called without exception "*melanocyte*" without even mentioning the terms "*nevocyte*" or "*nevomelanocyte*." Ultimately, the categoric opinion of the most distinguished dermatopathologist H. Pinkus has to be taken into account. He states unequivocally that "The nevus cells are abnormal cells, not a normal tissue component" [24].

Although, based on their common features, nevus cells and melanocytes may be considered closely related, a clear differentiation is warranted insofar as their lesions are concerned. This is not just an academic matter but an issue of great practical importance: melanocytic and nevocytic lesions differ significantly in their behavior, in their response to various therapeutic approaches, and in their prognosis. For this reason, the microscopist must attempt to the best of his or her ability to state the *melanocytic* or *nevocytic* progeny of the melanogenic lesion under study. More about the question "melanocytes versus nevocytes" may be found in Chap. 4.

Merkel Cells

Merkel cells are the third cellular component of the epidermis [25] (Fig. 1.3). These cells are found in the germinal layer. Since they are furnished with desmosomes, it has been speculated that they may represent modified keratinocytes. Merkel cells are connected to synaptic ends of terminal nerve filaments called "Merkel disks." These cells belong to the cutaneous neuroendocrine system and are believed to secrete chemical neurotransmitters in response to mechanical stimuli.

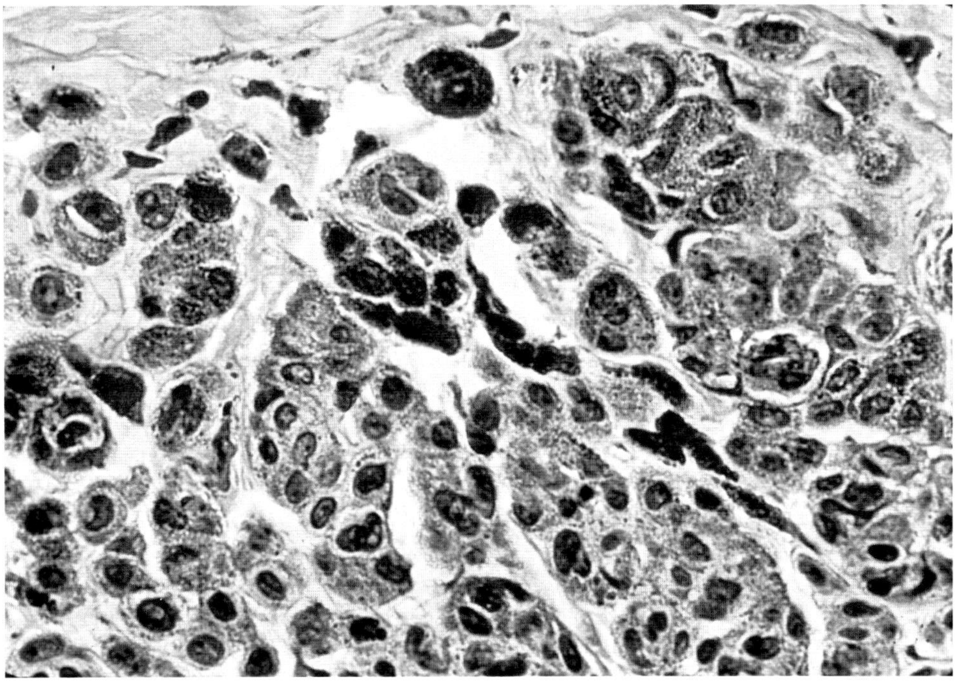

Fig. 1.10 Nevocytes and melanophages in the dermis. Nevocytes have a rounded, regular contour and are found in a nestiform arrangement, whereas melanophages show an angular shape, a *solid black discoloration* due to their melanin load, and appear disposed in disarray. H&E ×100, o m

Langerhans Cells

Langerhans cells (LC), the fourth cellular component of the epidermis [26], are dendritic histiocytes, which begin migrating from their point of origin in the bone marrow toward the epidermis, reaching it on the seventh week of gestation. In Fig. 1.3, they appear in their usual position at midepidermal level. If sections of digested skin are stained by a technique appropriate for LCs, an epidermal distribution of these cells is noted [27] closely similar to the one displayed by the melanocytes in Fig. 1.9. LCs resemble melanocytes in that they lack intercellular bridges but differ from them in not belonging to the fixed epidermal cellular population. In their capacity as antigen-presenting cells, LCs migrate from the skin to the regional lymph nodes. Upon EM observation, LCs exhibit their characteristic detail, tennis racquet-shaped organelles called "Birbeck's granules."

Biochemistry of the Subepidermal Components of the Skin

The space beneath the epidermis, that is, the subepidermal space (SES) is filled by an amorphous gel – the ground substance – in which amorphous and fibrillar components are found. Before these are separately analyzed, a brief reference should be made to the proteins, the main component of the ground substance.

Proteins

Proteins may be hereby distinguished as *simple* and *conjugated*. Simple proteins are just formed by amino acids joined by peptide bonds. Conjugated proteins are *hybrid* compounds which contain, in addition to their proteic moiety, a LARGE prosthetic – *nonproteic* – component.

Proteoglycans (PG) are proteins with a small carbohydrate component. Because of the large proportion of their proteic moiety, PGs display a physicochemical behavior close to that of simple proteins. Glycoproteins (GP) are also hybrid compounds but with a predominantly nonproteic component of glycosaminoglycans, which imparts to them physicochemical properties far different from those of proteins and proteoglycans.

Glycosaminoglycans (GAG) are polysaccharides formed by repetitive units of disaccharides. One of the monosaccharides involved is either uronic or iduronic acid or galactose. The other is an amino sugar such as *N*-acetylglucosamine or *N*-acetylgalactosamine. The large number of acidic groups bestows GAGs a marked anionic character. Table 1.2 presents a group of GAGs of importance in cutaneous biology.

All the GAGs featured on Table 1.2, with the exception of hyaluronic acid, contain sulfate groups. Likewise, all of them, except hyaluronic acid, may combine to a proteic core to build glycoproteins.

Glycoproteins: GPs are made of slender proteic cores onto which GAGs are covalently bound and perpendicularly inserted, forming structures comparable, because of their

Table 1.2 Glycosaminoglycans of importance in cutaneous biology

Trivial name	Disaccharide units
Hyaluronic acid	Glucuronic acid/*N*-acetylglucosamine
Heparan sulfate	Iduronic acid/*N*-acetyl-glucosamine-sulfate
Chondroitin sulfate	Glucuronic acid/*N*-acetyl-glucosamine-sulfate
Dermatan sulfate	Iduronic acid/*N*-acetyl-glucosamine-sulfate
Keratan sulfate	Galactose/*N*-acetylglucosamine sulfate

shape, to "bottle brushes." Due to the predominance of GAGs in their molecule, GPs have a strongly acidic character and a great capacity to accumulate water.

The terms "mucopolysaccharides" and "acid mucopolysaccharides" were assigned years ago to PGs and GAGs when their chemical composition was still undetermined, on account of the viscous or mucilaginous appearance and the strongly acidic character they displayed. Once their chemical composition was deciphered, those names lost acceptance, and today, they are only used in a descriptive way, without any precise chemical connotation.

Ground Substance: The ground substance has an overwhelming aqueous character due to the highly hydrated condition of its two main components, GAGs and PGs. It also features a minor component of nutrients and minerals.

Fibrillar Components

The fibrillar components in the SES are either *structural* and *accessory* or *auxiliary* (p. 193). The main structural component is collagen, which amounts to 70 % of its dry weight. Collagen type I is the prototypic and most abundant member of this family of proteins.

Collagen: The synthesis of collagen type I [28] begins with the ribosomal assemblage of long linear polypeptides, the prepro-alpha chains. Upon their transfer to the cisternae of the rough endoplasmic reticulum, they undergo modifications which transform them into pro-alpha chains and then into alpha chains. Alpha chains are polypeptides with an MW of 97 kD, each consisting of about 1,000 amino acids. They are arranged in repeated sequences – Gly-X-Y – (Gly = glycine) in which the position X is very frequently occupied by proline or hydroxyproline and the position Y by any other amino acid.

After further modifications, alpha chains are able to associate into triplets with a helical shape, giving rise to procollagen molecules. Subsequently, these are exported to the extracellular space where, at the end of the process, they are transformed into collagen molecules with an MW of 94 kD and about 300 × 10 nm in size.

In the cytoplasm, collagen molecules assemble spontaneously into fibrils. In the particular case of collagen type I, the fibrils are arranged in a staggered, partially overlapping fashion. Due to this arrangement, fibrils display a regular cross striation with a 67-nm periodicity (Fig. 1.11). The molecular arrangement of other types of collagen fibrils leads to different types of cross striations or to none at all [29].

The human genome contains over thirty genes related to the biosynthesis of collagen. These genes are dispersed through several chromosomes, opening the possibility for a wide variety of fibril types and, consequently, of even more collagen types to occur. That possibility has not materialized, however: at present, only as many as 20 collagen types have been identified, designated by Roman numerals I to XX.

Collagen type I, the most frequent member of the family, is found in large amounts in bone and cartilage, as well as in the dermis. Other collagens of interest in dermatology are type III collagen formerly called "embryonal collagen" from which reticulin fibers are made; collagen type IV, which gives rise to the basement membrane; and collagen VII, the component of anchoring fibrils. In contrast to most of the collagen types, which appear in a linear arrangement, type IV is found in a planar arrangement.

Elastic fibers are the second of the structural fibrillar component of the dermis [30]. They are formed by elastin, an 830-amino-acid-long protein rich in proline and glycine. After its secretion in the dermis, elastin fibers are assembled into a stretchable mat of fibers. Elastin features a strong plexus in the middermis. From it derives a secondary plexus, the elaunin plexus in the papillary dermis. This secondary plexus in turn emits microfibrils of oxytalan, which end up in close proximity to the LD (Fig. 1.12; see also Fig. 1.6).

Reticulin fibers are a third fibrillar component of the dermis. Their distinctive property "argyrophilia" (p. 193) is probably related to the presence in it of collagen type III.

Basement Membrane Zone

The interphase between the epidermis and the papillary dermis is called "basement membrane zone" (BMZ) [31]. This area appears as a faintly eosinophilic, acellular band of undefined limits under LM inspection of H&E-stained sections. It measures between 500 and 1,000 nm in thickness. Due to its predominant composition in GPs and PGs, the BMZ yields a strongly positive PAS reaction. Under this circumstance, it appears as a tightly folded purple band located between the epidermis and the dermis (Fig. 1.13).

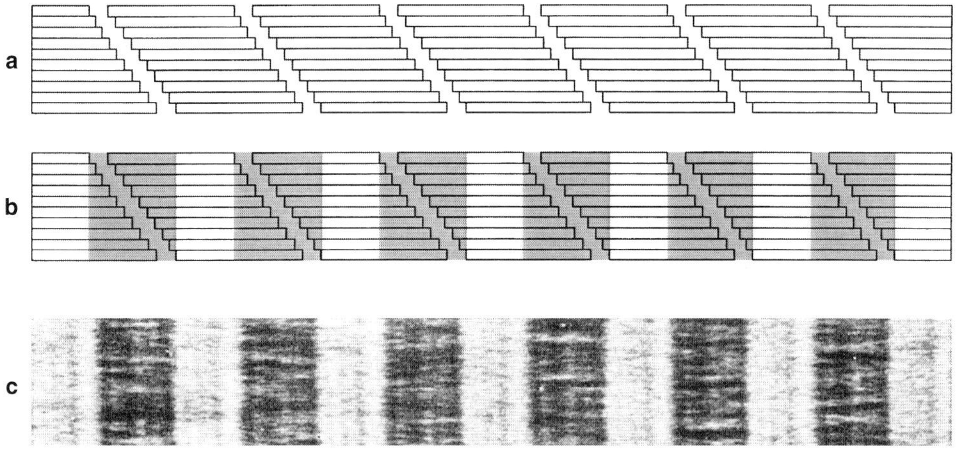

Fig. 1.11 Diagrammatic representation of a collagen type I fiber. (**a**) The collagen molecules are arbitrarily depicted as flat, empty boxes staggered and partially overlapping each other (*overlapping areas*), leaving half-empty spaces (*lacunar area*) alternating with the former (**b**). The same fiber treated with osmium tetroxide prior to EM examination: osmium tetroxide has been deposited into the half-empty lacunar areas, skipping the solid overlapping areas (**c**). Actual EM image of a collagen I fiber treated with osmium tetroxide. Note the periodic cross striation of the fibers, given by the succession of lacunar and overlapping areas

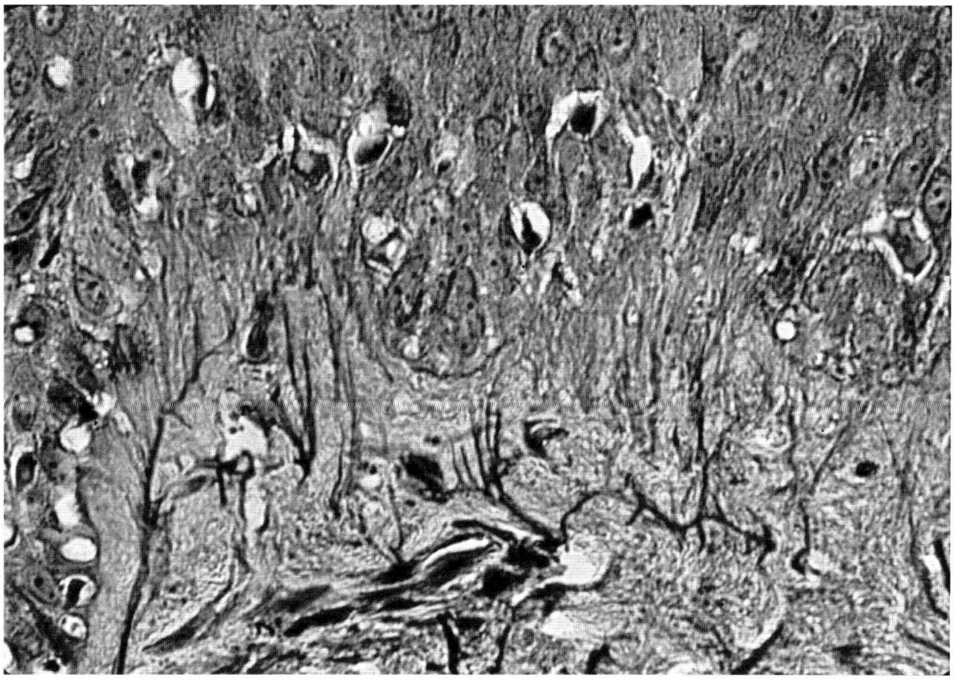

Fig. 1.12 Normal skin stained by an elastic tissue technique. Note the oxytalan fibers rising perpendicularly from the elaunin fibers. EvG ×400, o m

Basement Membrane and Hemidesmosome

Located within the BMZ and running roughly parallel to it can be found the actual basal membrane (BM). This structure, measuring about 130 nm in thickness, is intimately integrated with the hemidesmosomes and can only be studied by EM and in combination with the BM (Fig. 1.6).

The upper part of the hemidesmosome, depicted to the right in Fig. 1.6, has a composition identical to the corresponding upper half of the desmosome shown to the left. Therefore, there is no need for further descriptions. The lettering also applies to both cases.

The mentioned upper part of the hemidesmosome is positioned upon the lamina lucida (LL) (f). This is an electron-lucent layer about 40 nm in thickness, formed by an amorphous gel mostly composed of PGs and GAGs. In this context, it is particularly worth mentioning *heparan sulfate* due to its important role in the control of water displacement

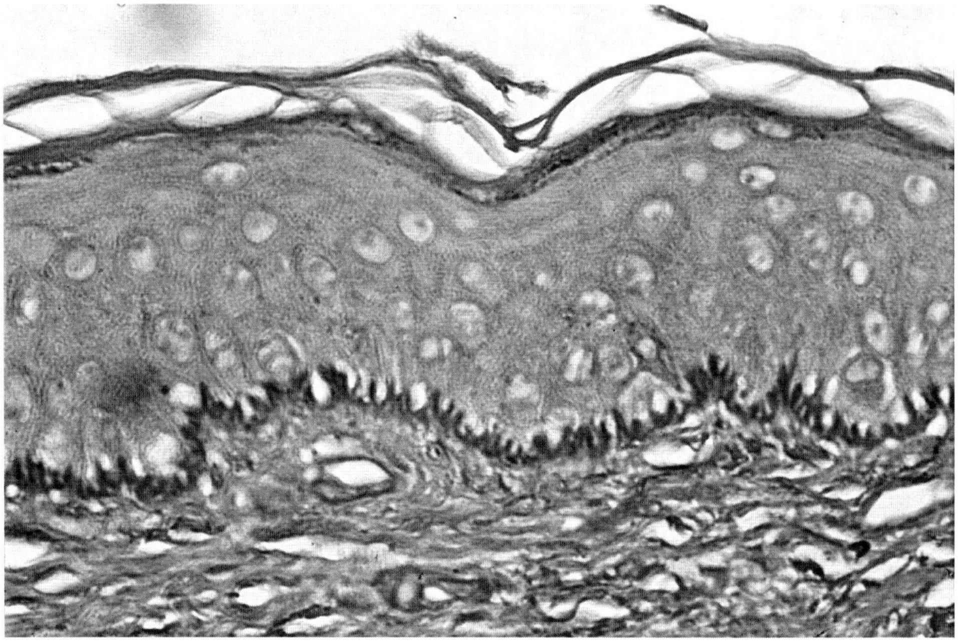

Fig. 1.13 Normal skin featuring the basement membrane zone. This preparation has been stained by the PAS technique in order to make the basement membrane zone stand out. PAS ×100, o m

in the skin. Transmembrane GPs integrin and laminin (p. 194) are also present in the LL, as well as other GPs, such as antigen 1 and antigen 2 of bullous pemphigoid, BPAg1 and BPAg2, respectively.

Within the LL, tenuous anchoring filaments (h) run from the overlying keratinocytes into the lamina densa, directly or through an interposed structure known as the "subbasal dense plaque" (g).

The lamina densa (LD) (i) is a meshwork of about 60 nm in thickness, representing the lower part of the BM. It is made of tightly interwoven collagen type IV fibrils.

From the lower face of the LD (i), threads of anchoring fibrils spread down into the sublamina densa space (SLDS) (j). Anchoring fibrils (k) – not to be mistaken with the previously mentioned "anchoring filaments" – are collagen VII fibers 20–60 nm in thickness, featuring an irregular cross striation. They either end up directly in the dense collagenous framework of the papillary dermis or, after following a recurrent trajectory, reach back to it, either directly or after joining anchorage plaques (l), small collagen IV structures. In some cases, anchoring fibrils loop around the most superficial collagen fibers of the papillary dermis before returning to the LD. Note incidentally in the figure the variable thickness and the constant periodicity of the collagen I fibers. In the SLDS are found other fibrillar elements, including collagen type III (n), belonging to oxytalan fibers derived from the elaunin plexus of the dermis.

The above description emphasizes the pivotal role of the LD in dermoepidermal cohesion: the keratinocytes are tightly attached to it by the adhesive force of the gelatinous LL, reinforced by anchoring filaments running down from the keratinocytes into it. The LD, in turn, is firmly "sewn" to the dermis by anchoring fibrils attached to the collagen fibers of the SLDS or the papillary dermis. The pathology of the congenital epidermolysis bullosa and the blistering conditions offers an example of the problems faced by patients and doctors when the above-mentioned adhesive system built around the LD fails.

Hypodermis

The hypodermis, also known as the "subcutaneous tissue," is formed by adipocytes of mesenchymal origin. They show a lobular structure and are surrounded by sheets of connective tissue with embedded vascular elements and thin nerve branches.

Cutaneous Adnexa

The cutaneous adnexa are the hair follicle, the sebaceous gland, the tubular glands, and the ungual complex.

The hair follicle with the hair shall be first examined. In this discussion, a large hair follicle in the anagen phase will serve as a model (Fig. 1.14). Keeping differences in mind, its features apply to the small hair follicle of the vellus hair, which covers the majority of the body.

A hemicross section of the hair follicle at its midlevel (Fig. 1.15) offers additional details of the just-mentioned structures.

The follicle in Fig. 1.14 is divided by two horizontal dotted lines, which run at the level of entrance of the sebaceous gland into the follicle and of the bulge of the *arrector pilorum*,

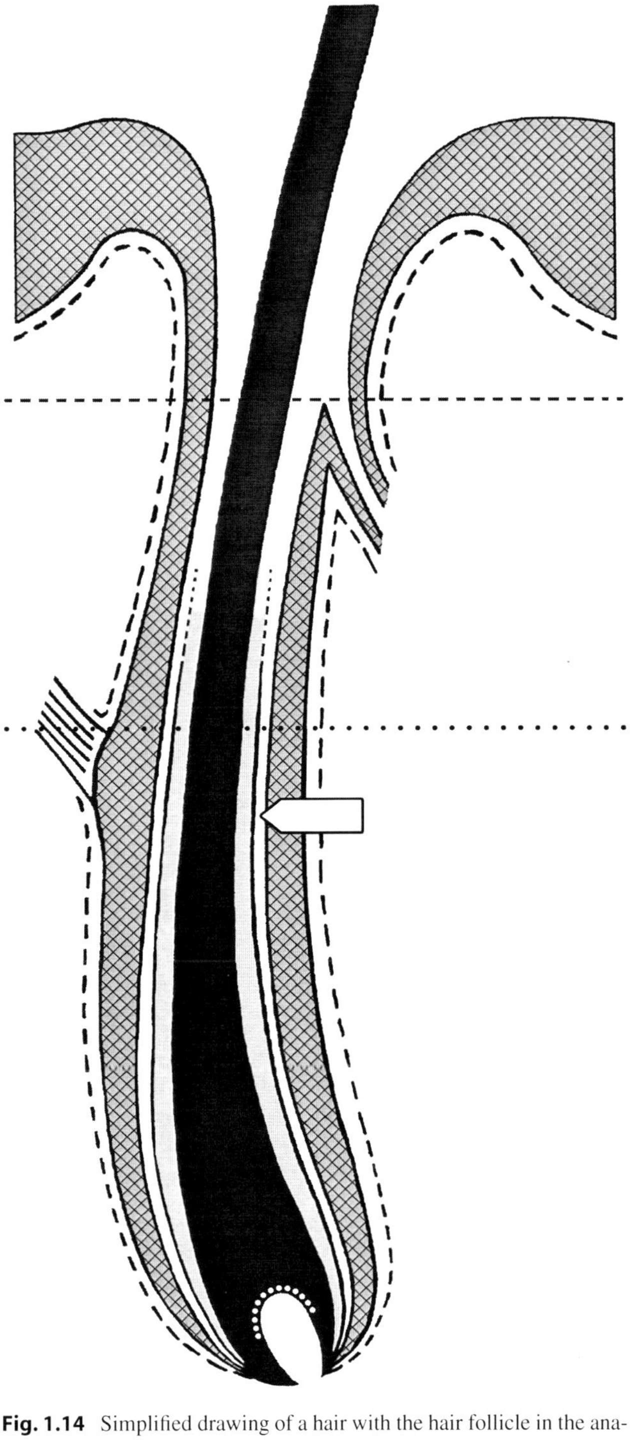

Fig. 1.14 Simplified drawing of a hair with the hair follicle in the anagen phase. The hair with its three elements, medulla, hair cortex, and inner cuticle – from the center on outward – are depicted together in solid black. The free portion of the hair shaft is rising above the surface of the skin, whereas its root is buried in the dermis, within the hair follicle (*folliculus* [L] a little leather bag). The three elements of the inner sheath of the hair follicle (outer cuticle, Huxley, and Henle's layer), always going outward and represented together by a *light-gray band*, are surrounded by the outer sheath of the hair follicle, formed by the trichilemma, presented in *crosshatched gray*, and the vitreous or glassy membrane featured as a hyphenated line running on its exterior. The dermal papilla is at the bottom of the follicle, covered by the hair matrix, indicated by a *line of white dots*

into three parts: the infundibulum above, the isthmus in the center, and the inferior part at the bottom, mnemotechnically associated as "*the three Is*" of the hair follicle.

The hair with its three elements and the inner sheath of the hair root with its three other elements, thus six elements in total, are produced simultaneously and differentially by the hair matrix. The trichilemma and the glassy membrane *are not produced* by the hair matrix but are *derivatives from the surrounding epidermis*. This is indicated in Fig. 1.14 by the continuation of the gray cross-hatching and the hyphenated line of the hair follicle with corresponding elements of the epidermis. Moreover, the different origin of the hair and inner root sheath, on one side, and the outer root sheath, on the other, is emphasized by the artifactual separation of these structures in that figure (arrow).

The hair and the root sheath grow together, sliding along the static trichilemma.

Upon reaching the entrance of the sebaceous gland, the inner root sheath suffers a combined enzymatic/microbial aggression and disintegrates, thus disappearing from the follicle.

Keratinization occurs in the hair follicle via two different pathways: in the hair medulla and cortex, it happens *without production* of keratohyalin granules and with *hard keratin* as an end product. In both cuticles, as well as in Huxley's and Henle's layers, keratinization proceeds *with participation of keratin granules* and final production of *soft keratin*. As an interesting observation, it may be mentioned that contrary to the basophilic keratohyalin granules of the epidermis, those related to hair keratinization are eosinophilic [32].

Since the trichilemma is derived from the epidermis, it would be expected to keratinize as in this layer, with accompanied production of keratohyalin granules and soft keratin as a final product. However, the opposite occurs via a special process called "trichilemmal keratinization" [33]; this layer yields hard keratin as a final product. The glassy membrane, an equivalent of the epidermal BMZ, is an amorphous structure which does not keratinize.

The hair follicle is not a dead structure but rather a living one, which presents a unique life cycle [34]: its activity is regulated by the dermal papilla. The hair follicle in Fig. 1.14 is in the anagenic phase or anagen (*ana* + *gen* [G] renovated + growth), which lasts for years. During this period, the dermal papilla sticks to the matrix and the hair grows actively.

At the end of anagen, the dermal papilla loses its turgor and its PG content, becoming detached from the matrix. In this fashion, the hair follicle enters the catagenic phase or catagen (*cata* + *gen* [G] downgrowth). This phase, the shortest one, lasts weeks, at most, and is characterized under LM by a fibrous cord, representing the collapsed inferior part of the follicle. This cord stretches down from the follicle to the papillary remnants. Another characteristic of catagen hair is

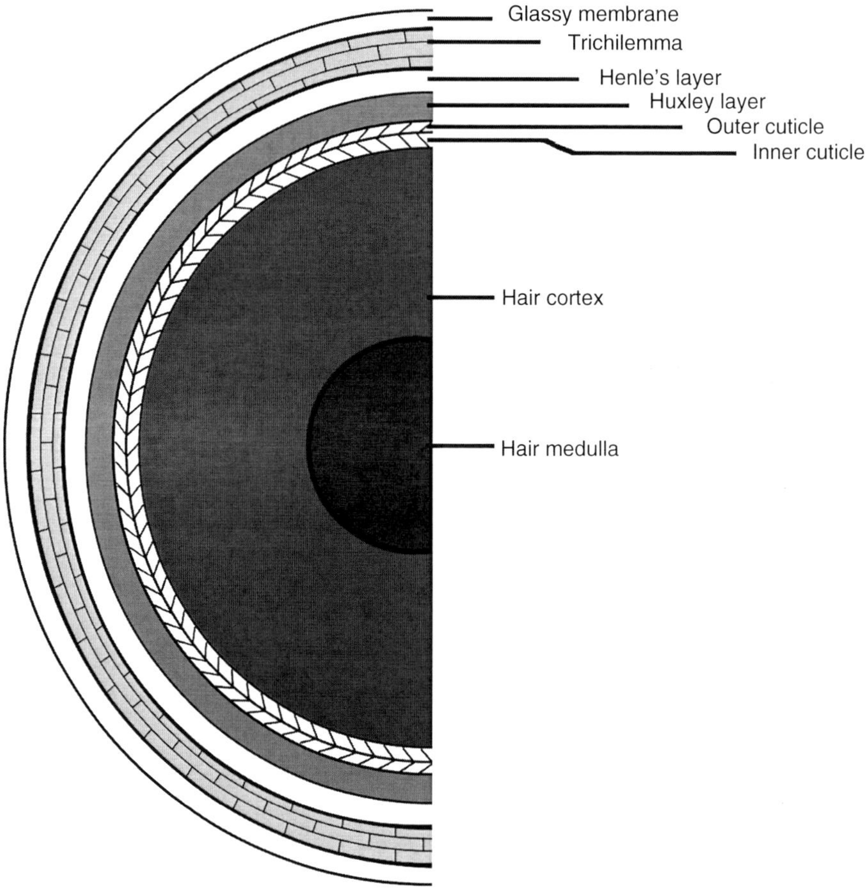

Fig. 1.15 Hemicross section of the hair follicle at its midlevel

a thickening of the inferior pole of the hair shaft, which appears "club shaped" (Fig. 1.16).

Catagen phase is followed by the telogenic phase or telogen (*telo + gen* [G] end of growing), considered to be *the resting phase* of the hair follicle. During this time, the bottom of the follicle retracts upward to the level of the bulge and remains inactive for a few months until the dermal papilla again moves upward and once more contacts the matrix to recommence the cycle.

Adnexal Glands: Figure 1.17 features the adnexal glands, making special reference to the way they pour out their secretion.

The sebaceous gland (a) is a frequent companion of the hair follicle. This is a gland of holocrine type (*holos + krinos* [G] total + separate, segregate). Its secretion is fully liberated upon bursting of the gland and passes through a short duct (b) into the infundibulum of the hair follicle (d).

Tubular Glands: Regarding the tubular glands, the eccrine ones (e), *which are the actual sweat-secreting glands*, have a generalized distribution and are found throughout the skin. Apocrine glands (c), *which do not secrete sweat but rather a scent* – eventually associated with sexual attraction [35] – are mainly restricted in distribution to the face, axillae, and genitoperineal areas.

Both tubular types of glands have a comparable general structure. They are formed by a secretory tuft or "adenomere" (*adeno + mere* [G] gland + part) located between the dermis and the subcutaneous tissue and have an excretory duct. The duct of the apocrine gland, as the one of the sebaceous gland, opens into the infundibulum of the hair follicle, whereas the one of the eccrine gland ends directly onto the surface of the skin by means of its terminal portion, the "acrosyringium" (f) (*acro + syrinx* [G] distal + tube).

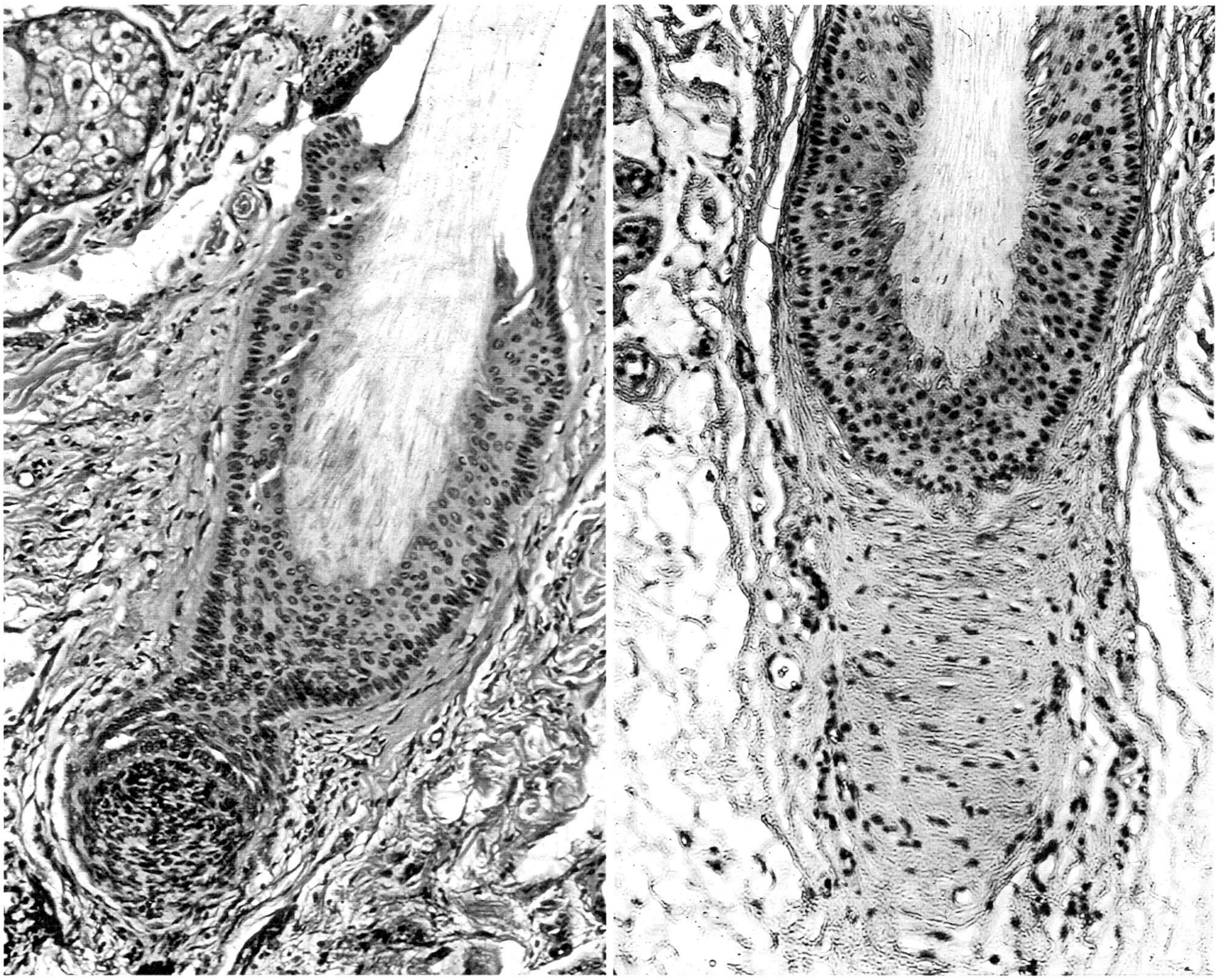

Fig. 1.16 Hair in the catagen phase. The picture to the left captions a hair follicle in early catagen. The hair papilla has just been disconnected from the follicle, and the lower pole of the hair shows the typical "club shape." The figure to the right visualizes the fibrous cord left by the retracting hair. H&E ×100; ×400, o m

The eccrine gland's adenomere (up, in Fig. 1.18) shows two types of secretory cells, clear and dark, easily distinguishable under LM of H&E-stained sections. They secrete a watery and a viscous material (*serous* and *mucous*), respectively. The apocrine gland's adenomere (down, in the same figure) is considerably wider than that of the eccrine gland, being lined by a single row of cylindrical, eosinophilic cells, which display secretion droplets attached to their apices. These droplets are "pinched off" from the cells by a process nicknamed "decapitation" in order to fall into the gland's lumen.

Ungual Complex: The ungual complex (Fig. 1.19) is located on the dorsal area of the distal part of the finger, between the two lateral nail folds and the transversal, proximal one at the base.

The nail matrix located beneath the proximal fold generates the nail plaque, which moves forward along the longitudinal ridges of the nail bed and in between the lateral folds. The nail plaque keratinizes through the before-mentioned *trichilemmal process* (p. 13) with hard keratin as an end product. Since the nail plaque does not desquamate spontaneously, its

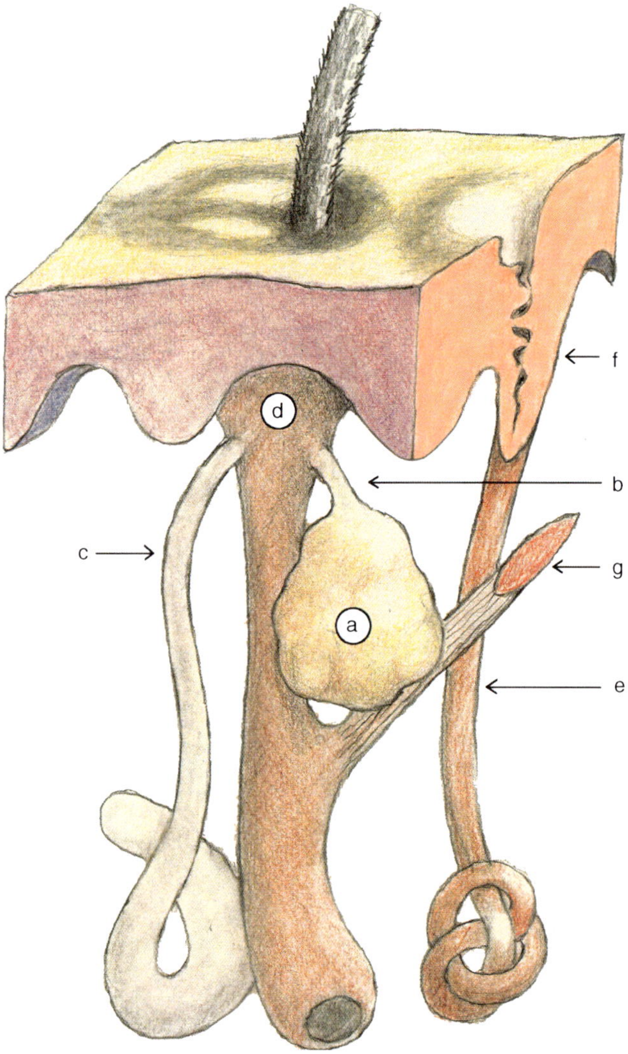

Fig. 1.17 Hair follicle with the three adnexal glands. The sebaceous gland (*a*) is partially overlapping the hair follicle; the apocrine gland is at its left and the eccrine gland at its right. Note the entrance of the sebaceous (*b*) and the apocrine duct (*c*) into the infundibulum (*d*). Observe the eccrine gland (*e*) and the vertical section of its terminal part, the acrosyringium (*f*). *g* arrector pilorum

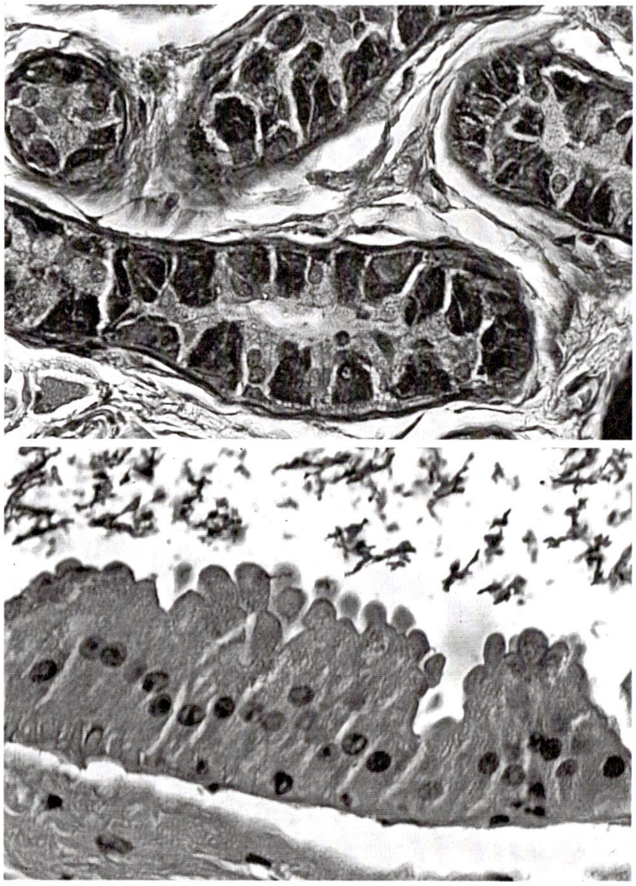

Fig. 1.18 Secretory epithelium of the apocrine and eccrine adenomere. The epithelium of the eccrine gland (*up*) is formed by alternating serous- and mucous-secreting cuboidal cells. Although they were named "clear" and "dark cells" based on the aspect they presented upon LM observation of H&E-stained sections, the PAS stain used in the present preparation produced the opposite result, imparting a dark stain to the serous cells, while leaving the mucous cells unstained. The epithelium of the apocrine gland (*down*) is formed by tall cylindrical cells featuring the characteristic "decapitation." H&E ×400; PAS ×400

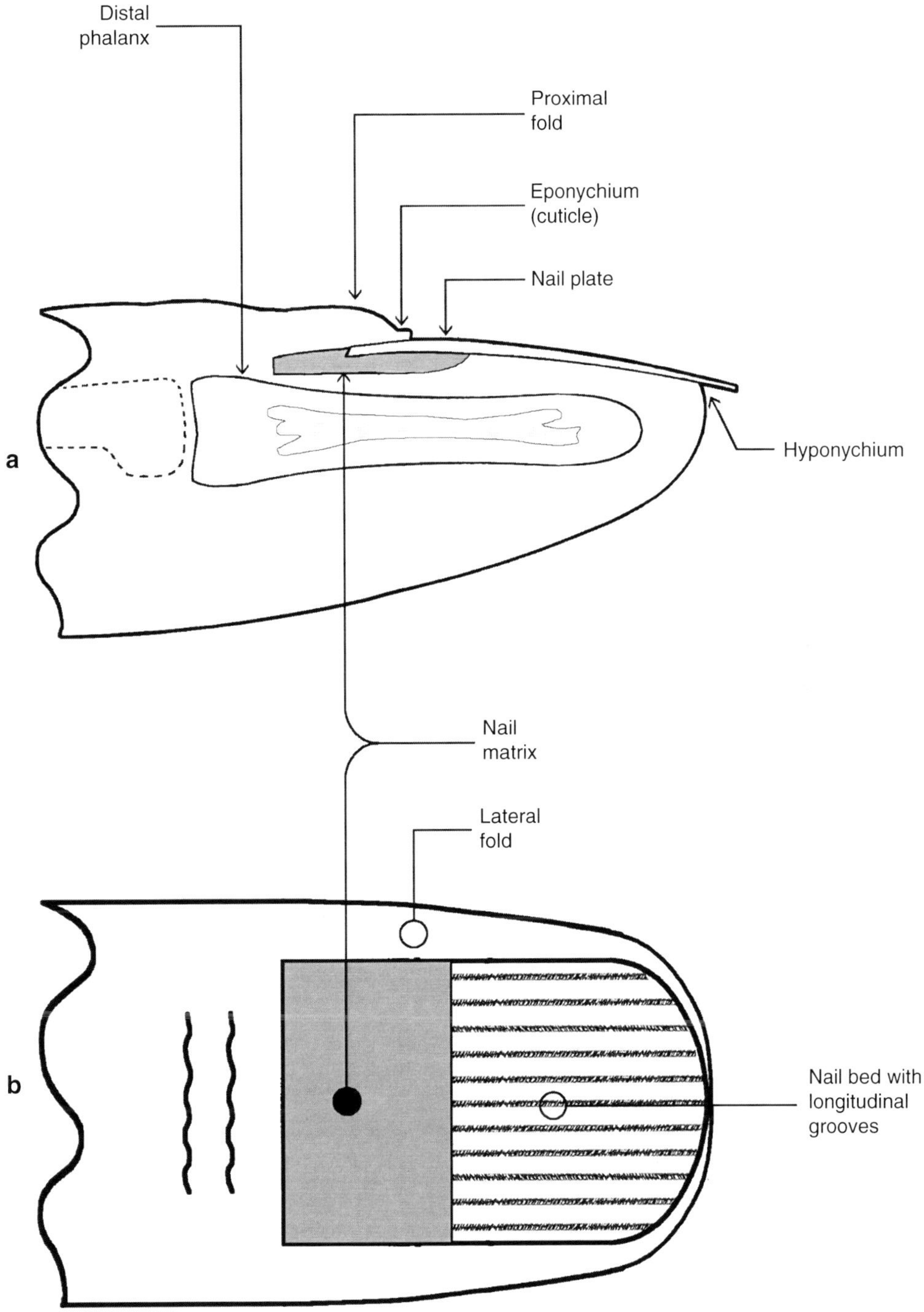

Fig. 1.19 Ungual complex, schematic. View of a vertical section along the distal phalanx (**a**) and a panoramic view from above after removing the nail plate (**b**). The diverse structures are indicated

free edge is customarily submitted to periodic trimmings in order to prevent its indefinite growth.

Cutaneous Irrigation

The skin presents a main vascular plexus between the deep dermis and the adipose panniculus (Fig. 1.3). Blood vessels ascend from here into the reticular dermis where they build up a secondary subpapillary plexus. This irrigates adnexal structures present at this level and projects capillaries into the dermal papillae. Blood returns through channels of corresponding caliber to be conducted to the subcutaneous tissue, the deep fasciae and beyond.

At this point, it is important to mention the vascular structure known as "glomus body" since it, not infrequently, is the source of painful vascular tumors. Glomus bodies (Fig. 1.20) are arteriovenous shunts with a thermoregulatory function, described by P. Masson in 1924 [36]. These organs develop from arterioles branching in the deep dermis. They are

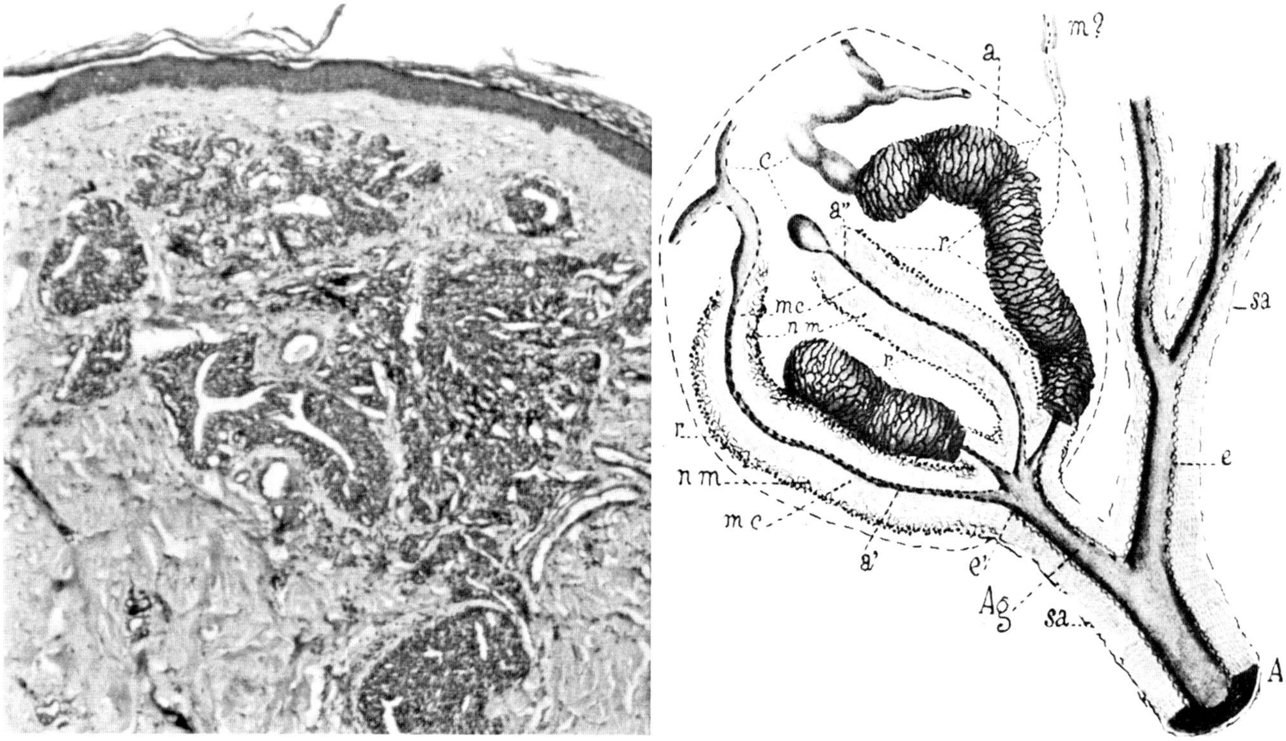

Fig. 1.20 Glomus body. (*left*) Note the intricate appearance of the organ and the well-developed Sucquet-Hoyer channels. H&E ×40, o m. Compare with P. Masson's original illustration in Lyon Chir 21:257, 1924, *right*

mainly located in hands and fingers. The branching vessels become surrounded by myoepithelial cells, forming perivascular cuffs called "Sucquet-Hoyer channels." These are the structures actually responsible for the thermoregulatory function of the organs. After passing through the channels, blood enters the labyrinthic venous plexuses, from where it returns to general circulation.

Cutaneous Innervation

Peripheral nerves exiting the spinal cord are formed by bundles of nerve fascicles held together by a fibroadipose, nonspecific structure, the epineurium. The nerve fascicles in the peripheral nerves are formed by motor, sensorial, and autonomic fibers found either isolated or in groups in spaces filled with a proteinaceous fluid – the endoneurium – and ensheathed by a specialized membrane, the perineurium [37], actually a continuation of the pia-arachnoid of the central nervous organs (Fig. 1.21). As the fibers abandon the nerve fascicle, they spread out providing the skin with ample sensorial and autonomic innervation.

Sensorial fibers may end up freely in the dermis or even in the epidermis or, otherwise, as sensorial pressure receptors such as Merkel touch corpuscles or as the encapsulated Vater-Paccini's and Meissner's organs and other structures (Fig. 1.22).

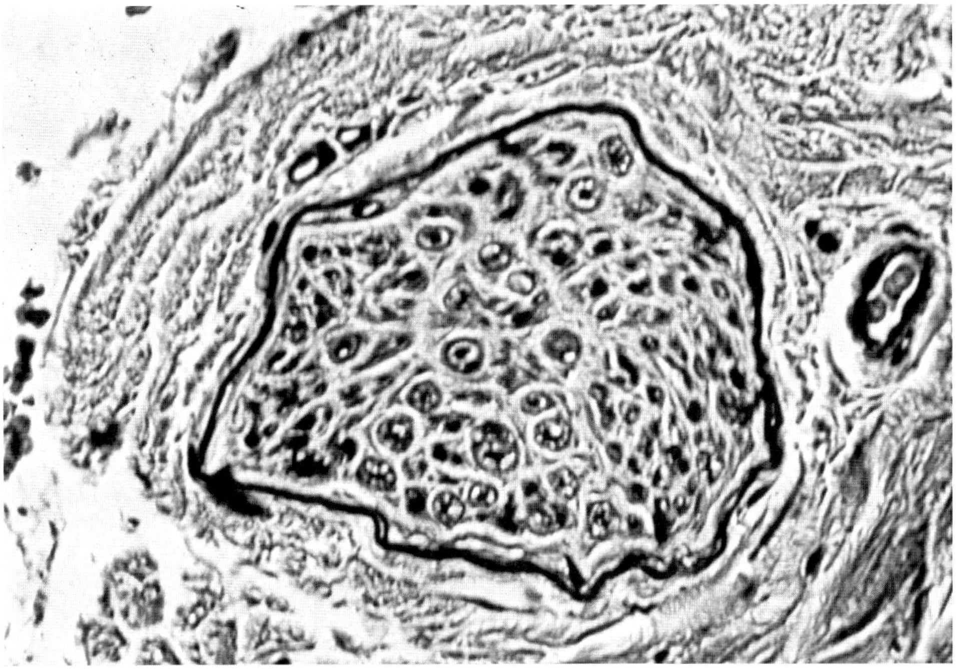

Fig. 1.21 Cross section of a nerve fascicle. Note the presence of myelinated and amyelinated nerve fibers in the endoneurium, surrounded by the perineurium. H&E ×400, o m

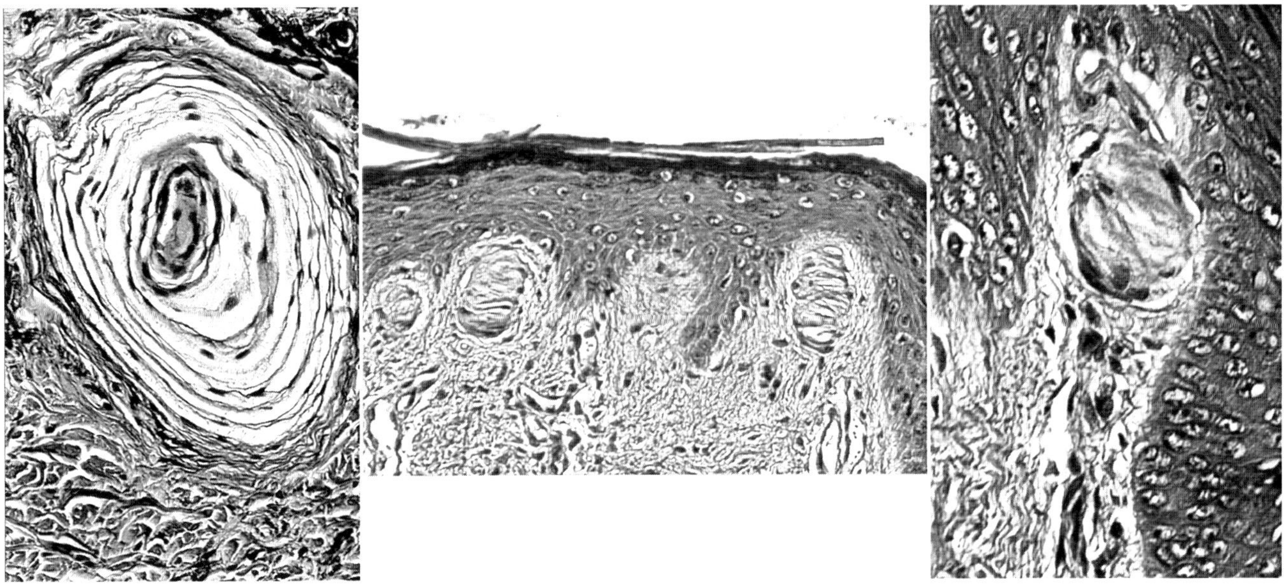

Fig. 1.22 Vater-Paccini's and Meissner's organs. (*left*) Vater-Paccini organ displaying its typical "onion-layer" shape. (*center*) Four Meissner's organs in an intrapapillary position. (*right*) A Meissner organ occupying a dermal papilla. The Vater-Paccini organ to the left and the Meissner corpuscles in the center are presented at the same magnification (×40) for the purpose of comparing their size. The isolated Meissner corpuscle to the right is shown at higher magnification – ×400 – to make its structural details more visible. H&E

References

1. Montagna W, Parakkal PF. The structure and function of skin. 3rd ed. New York: Academic; 1974. p. 75–95.
2. Lever WF, Schaumburg-Lever G. Histopathology of the skin. 7th ed. Philadelphia: J.B. Lippincott; 1990. p. 9–21.
3. Odland GF. In: Goldsmith LA, editors. Physiology, biochemistry, and molecular biology of the skin, 2nd ed. New York: Oxford University Press; 1991. p. 3–5.
4. Hib J. Histologia de Di Fiore. Buenos Aires: El Ateneo; 2001. p. 171.
5. James WD, Berger TG, Elston DM, editors. Andrews' diseases of the skin. 10th ed. Philadelphia: W.B. Saunders Elsevier; 2006. p. 1.
6. Montagna W, Parakkal PF. The structure and function of skin. 3rd ed. New York: Academic; 1974. p. 48.
7. Steinert PM, Freedberg IM. In: Goldsmith LA, editors. Physiology, biochemistry, and molecular biology of the skin, 2nd ed. New York: Oxford University Press; 1991. p. 113–41.
8. De Robertis EMF, Hib J. Fundamentos de biologia celular y molecular de De Robertis. 3rd ed. Buenos Aires: El Ateneo; 2001. p. 80–1.
9. James WD, Berger TG, Elston DM, editors. Andrews' diseases of the skin. 10th ed. Philadelphia: W.B. Saunders Elsevier; 2006. p. 3.
10. Resing KA, Dale Ba. In: Goldsmith LA, editors. Physiology, biochemistry, and molecular biology of the skin, 2nd ed. Oxford: Oxford University Press; 1991. p. 148–62.
11. Lever WF, Schaumburg-Lever G. Histopathology of the skin. 7th ed. Philadelphia: J.B. Lippincott; 1990. p. 851.
12. Lever WF, Schaumburg-Lever G. Histopathology of the skin. 7th ed. Philadelphia: J.B. Lippincott; 1990. p. 30.
13. Lever WF, Schaumburg-Lever G. Histopathology of the skin. 7th ed. Philadelphia: J.B. Lippincott; 1990. p. 15.
14. Montagna W, Parakkal PF. The structure and function of skin. 3rd ed. New York: Academic; 1974. p. 18.
15. Montagna W, Parakkal PF. The structure and function of skin. 3rd ed. New York: Academic; 1974. p. 24.
16. De Robertis EMF, Hib J, Ponzio R. Biologia celular y molecular de De Robertis. 15th ed. Buenos Aires: El Ateneo; 2010. p. 162–3.
17. Elder DE, et al., editors. Lever's histopathology of the skin, 9th ed. Philadelphia: Lippincott Williams & Wilkins; 2005. p. 9.
18. Lever WF, Schaumburg-Lever G. Histopathology of the skin. 7th ed. Philadelphia: J.B. Lippincott; 1990. p. 858.
19. Zelickson AS. In: Zelickson AS, editors. Ultrastructure or normal and abnormal skin. Philadelphia: Lea & Febiger; 1967, p. 163.
20. Rosai J. Rosai and Ackerman's surgical pathology. 9th ed. Edinburgh: Mosby; 2006. p. 154.
21. Leider M, Rosenblum MA. A dictionary of medical words, terms and phrases. West Haven: Dome Laboratory; 1976. p. 297.
22. Unna PG. Histopathologie der Hautkrankheiten. Berlin: A. Hirschwald Verlag; 1894. p. 1148.
23. Magana Garcia M, Ackerman AB. Naming acquired melanocytic nevi. Am J Dermatopathol. 1990;12(1):193–209.
24. Mehregan AH, Hashimoto K, editors. Pinkus's guide to dermatohistopathology. 5th ed. Norwalk: Appleton-Lange; 1991. p. 444.
25. Montagna W, Parakkal PF. The structure and function of skin. 3rd ed. New York: Academic; 1974. p. 89.
26. Mehregan AH, Hashimoto K, editors. Pinkus's guide to dermatohistopathology. 5th ed. Norwalk: Appleton-Lange; 1991. p. 39.
27. Mescher AL, editor. Junqueira's basic histology. 12th ed. New York: McGraw Hill; 2010. p. 233.
28. De Robertis EMF, Hib J. Fundamentos de biologia celular y molecular de De Robertis. 3rd ed. Buenos Aires: El Ateneo; 2001. p. 113–4.
29. Mescher AL, editor. Junqueira's basic histology. 12th ed. New York: McGraw Hill; 2010. p. 96.
30. Uitto J, Fazio H, Bashir H, Rosenbloon J. In: Goldsmith LA, editor. Physiology, biochemistry, and molecular biology of the skin, 2nd ed. New York: Oxford University Press; 1991, p. 530.
31. Lever WF, Schaumburg-Lever G. Histopathology of the skin. 7th ed. Philadelphia: J.B. Lippincott; 1990. p. 11.
32. Lever WF, Schaumburg-Lever G. Histopathology of the skin. 7th ed. Philadelphia: J.B. Lippincott; 1990. p. 28.
33. Mehregan AH, Hashimoto K, editors. Pinkus's guide to dermatohistopathology. 5th ed. Norwalk: Appleton-Lange; 1991. p. 27.
34. Lever WF, Schaumburg-Lever G. Histopathology of the skin. 7th ed. Philadelphia: J.B. Lippincott; 1990. p. 27.
35. Lever WF, Schaumburg-Lever G. Histopathology of the skin. 7th ed. Philadelphia: J.B. Lippincott; 1990. p. 24.
36. Enzinger FM, Weiss SW. Soft tissue tumors. 3rd ed. St. Louis: Mosby; 1995. p. 703–4.
37. Scheithauer BW, Woodruff JM, Erlandson RA. In: Rosai J, editors. Atlas of tumor pathology, 3rd series, Fascicle 24. Washington, D.C.: Armed Forces Institute of Pathology; 1999, p. 1–15.

2 Classification of Cutaneous Lesions

The adjective "cutaneous" hereby refers to the skin and external mucosae, to its adnexa, and to the subcutaneous panniculus. Cutaneous lesions are those that involve the mentioned elements, although they may also comprise cartilage, salivary glands, synovial remnants, and even other elements which may appear incidentally on the external surface of the body. The classification of these lesions would be highly desirable in order to approach the study of dermatopathology in a rational way. However, given the frequently poorly defined histopathologic character of the cutaneous lesion, their often mixed and overlapping features, and, furthermore, the continuous change of the lesions throughout their evolution, that classification may turn out to be a difficult task.

The challenges encountered in attempting to classify cutaneous lesions can only be met by using ample and yielding guidelines and parameters, a tolerant attitude upon their application, and a readiness to modify or change these when the results of their application do not satisfy the expectations of the author. In fact, the objective of such classification should not be to obtain a rigid and immutable taxonomic structure but rather to provide a dynamic tool which facilitates the introduction to and further study of dermatopathology to the interested person.

After this cautionary note, it may be stated that skin lesions, either solitary or multiple, associated to any concomitant process or not, may be considered either the expression of hereditary problems or instead, of sheer malformative, inflammatory, or proliferative conditions. These lesions may therefore be placed in any of the four Divisions of hereditary, malformative, inflammatory, or proliferative nature. If the features of a lesion do not justify its inclusion into any of these four Divisions, it may be placed into a fifth Division of lesions of miscellaneous nature (Table 2.1). This is a more rational approach than skipping or ignoring that "problem lesion" or forcing it into a position where it does not belong and where it may constitute a continuous irritant prone to alter the logic of the entire taxonomic system.

The lesions comprised in the five postulated Divisions are discussed in Chapters 3, 4, 5, 6, and 7, in the second part of this work. A leading distinctive color assigned to each division (see Table 2.1) is displayed on the running titles, and the background of legends of tables and figures of the corresponding chapter highlights the nature of the lesions dealt with in each of the chapters.

The lesions in each Division are progressively segregated into Subdivisions, Classes, Subclasses, Groups, and Subgroups until finally reaching sets of lesions with resemblances to the ones in the same set but varying significantly from those in other sets. The variable, pragmatic character of the criteria applied for the initial separation of the lesions in the five divisions may be appreciated in Fig. 2.1.

In the Division of hereditary lesions, the separation is based on clinical criteria which allow the identification of four Subdivisions of this type of lesions. In the second Division, an evaluative criterion is applied which permits the separation of the lesions into two Subdivisions, as occurring in the early and late ontogenesis. Regarding the lesions in the third and fourth Divisions, microscopic criteria are preferred. These lead to the identification of three Subdivisions of inflammatory lesions, that is, evolutive, postevolutive, and transitional, and two Subdivisions of proliferative lesions, that is, reactive and neoplastic, respectively. The highly dissimilar character of the lesions enclosed in the fifth division prevents their systematic separation as in the previous subdivisions, and only classes of lesions are presented, based on their most prominent features.

The process of segregation of the lesions is graphically explained in the particular case of the Division of inflammatory

Table 2.1 Divisions of the cutaneous lesions according to their primary nature – distinctive color for each division

Division	Distinctive color
Hereditary	Orange
Malformative	Blue
Inflammatory	Red
Proliferative	Gray
Miscellaneous	Green

E. Zappi, E.A. Zappi, *Dermatopathology*,
DOI 10.1007/978-1-4471-2894-6_2, © Springer-Verlag London 2013

Divisions / **Subdivisions**

- Cutaneous lesions
  - Hereditary
    - Genodermatoses.
    - Multisystemic disorders with cutaneous participation
    - Multisystemic disorders with cutaneous repercussion
    - Failure of control Repair and surveillance, with cutaneous repercussion
  - Malformative
    - Early
    - Late
  - Inflammatory
    - Evolutive
    - Post–evolutive
    - Transitional
  - Proliferative
    - Reactive
    - Neoplastic
  - Miscellaneous

Fig. 2.1 Criteria applied for the initial separation of the cutaneous lesions in the five divisions

lesions – which is the most numerous and complicated of the ones of cutaneous lesions (Fig. 2.2). After the initial characterization of the lesions contained in the top central circle of the figure as "inflammatory" – by the red color used for that purpose – the lesions fan out into three beams: the broadest one in bright red, the next in dull red, and the narrowest one in port-wine red. They represent the *evolutive*, the *postevolutive*, and the *transitional* inflammatory lesions respectively (Fig. 2.2).

Upon applying the chosen taxonomic criteria stated to the left of the figure to the three mentioned, Subdivisions, Classes, Subclasses, Groups, and Subgroups of lesions are progressively generated, as indicated on the right side of the figure. The dots at the base of the figure represent sets of evolutive, postevolutive, and transitional lesions resulting from the working out of the division. Although the number under which the sets are purported is arbitrary, they somehow reflect the proportion in which the three types of lesions are found in practice: the evolutive are the most numerous, whereas the transitional are the scantest.

The nomenclature applied in this work uses mostly precise histopathologic terms combined whenever possible to current and traditional names used in clinical dermatology. The employed vocabulary attempts to avoid confusing terms or those with an excessively clinical accent.

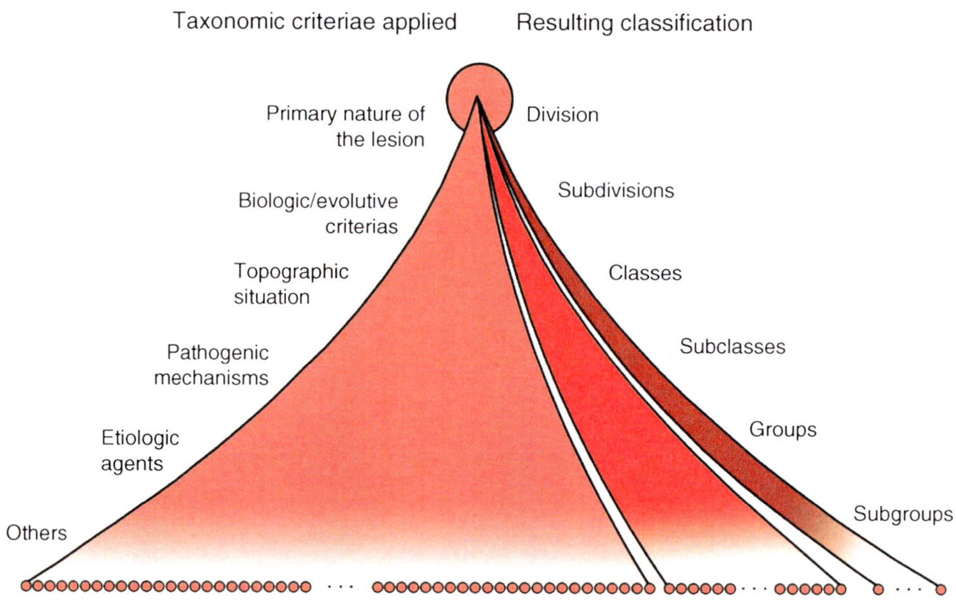

Fig. 2.2 Graphic representation of the taxonomic workout of the lesions of inflammatory nature

3 Hereditary Lesions

The malformative, inflammatory, or proliferative nature of cutaneous lesions may be confidently ascertained by their histopathologic picture. However, in the case of hereditary lesions, external examination is far more valuable. The external examination enables the practitioner to recognize at a glance, without recurring to ancillary studies, the probable hereditary nature of the disorder and hence the genetic background of the patient's cutaneous lesions. Valuable clues for this purpose are the multiplicity of the lesions, their disseminated and variegated character, and their frequent association to metabolic problems and often to mental deficiency. The clinical impression is confirmed if the malady happens to run in the patient's family and is transmitted according to Mendelian patterns of inheritance.

Four types of genetic defects may disfavorably affect the skin: (a) genetic defect of material selectively involved in the epidermopoiesis, (b) defects of genetic material involved in the development of the skin and extracutaneous systems, (c) defects of genetic material resulting into abnormal metabolic cycles, and (d) defects of genetic material implicated in the control, repair, and defense of the organism. To these genotypic defects correspond, as phenotypic manifestations, the following four types of hereditary conditions: (A) disorders with permanent faulty epidermopoiesis, (B) combined cutaneous and extracutaneous defects, (C) skin of abnormal quality or the outpouring of abnormal metabolites which would indirectly affect the skin, and (D) sporadic triggering of adverse reactions, unrepaired damage of genetic material, and ineffective surveillance activity, with the eventual emergence of neoplastic clones on the skin.

The term "*genodermatosis*," which may be literally translated as "a *cutaneous condition of genetic nature*," is casually used to designate these four types of hereditary disorders with cutaneous involvement in a general and conjoint way. However, although the first term of the definition, the genetic, is obvious by the Mendelian patterns through which these disorders are transmitted, that is not the case with the second term of the definition, the cutaneous character. The cutaneous character is only constant and of utmost significance in disorders of the first type: in these conditions, cutaneous manifestations are *constant and obligatory*, that is, *if there are no cutaneous manifestations, there is* no *disease*. In the three other types of disorders, the cutaneous component is not of such significance: in disorders of the second type, although the cutaneous component is *constant*, it is only one and often not even the most important in the symptomatologic picture of the disorder. In the third type of disorders, the cutaneous manifestations *are not constant* and may even disappear after their apparition. In the fourth type of disorders, the cutaneous manifestations eventually appear as sporadic episodes during the patient's life.

For the exposed reasons, in this text the term "*genodermatosis*" is restricted to those inherited conditions exclusively manifested through epidermal defects. The three other types of conditions are designated "*hereditary polysystemic disorders with cutaneous participation*" (HPDwCP), "*hereditary metabolic errors with cutaneous repercussion*" (HMEwCR), and "*hereditary defects of control and defense with sporadic repercussion*" (HDCwCR) (Table 3.1).

The lesions associated with genodermatoses display pathognomonic details which often enable the microscopist to recognize the ongoing condition. In contrast, the lesions

Table 3.1 Cutaneous expression (phenotypic) of genetic defects

Genotypic defect	Phenotypic expression
(a) Of genetic material selectively involved in the epidermogenesis	(A) Genodermatoses
(b) Of genetic material involved in the morphogenesis of the skin and other organs	(B) Hereditary polysystemic disorders with cutaneous participation
(c) Of genetic material involved in cycles of intermediary metabolism	(C) Hereditary metabolic errors with cutaneous repercussion
(d) Of genetic material involved in mechanisms of control and defense of the organism	(D) Hereditary defects of control and defense with sporadic manifestations

E. Zappi, E.A. Zappi, *Dermatopathology*,
DOI 10.1007/978-1-4471-2894-6_3, © Springer-Verlag London 2013

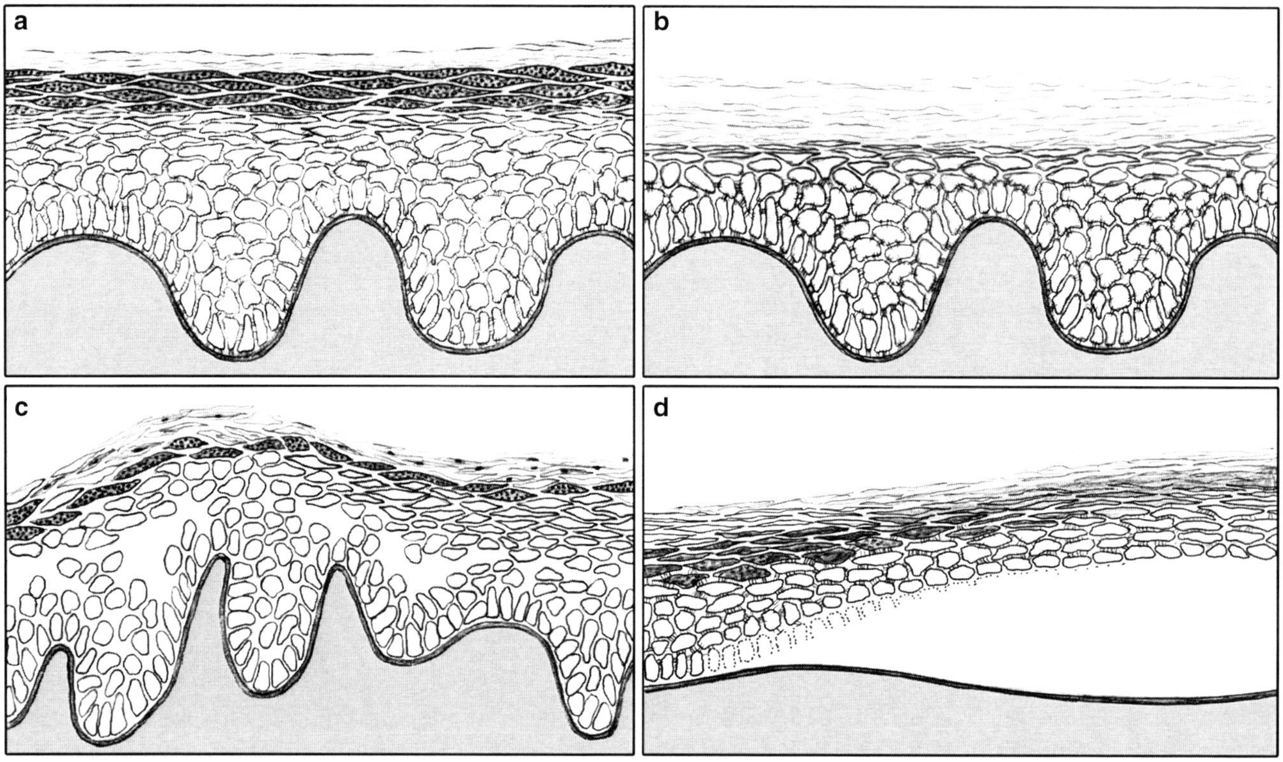

Fig. 3.1 Comparison of the levels at which lesions occurs in genodermatosis of upper, mid, or low epidermal level of expression. (**a**) Normal epidermis. (**b**) Lesion in ichthyosis vulgaris, paradigm of a genodermatosis of upper epidermal type, illustrates the absence of a granular layer. (**c**) Lesion in Hailey-Hailey's disease prototypic example of a genodermatosis of mid epidermal level of expression features disintegration of the *stratum spinosum*. (**d**) Lesion in EB simplex, a recognized type of genodermatosis of *low epidermal* level of expression, displays dermoepidermal separation. More details in the text

associated with the three other types of hereditary conditions lack distinctive histopathologic features, and their microscopic examination reveals pictures comparable to the ones of lesions devoid of any hereditary background, such as those presented in Chaps. 3, 4, 5, 6, and 7.

In anticipation of the analysis of cutaneous lesions which follows in the next chapters, it is convenient to comment on two microscopic features often found in these: *dyskeratosis* and *acantholysis*.

Dyskeratosis (*dys* + *keratos* [G] defective keratin) is manifested by alterations of the horny and granular layer. The thickening or thinning of the horny layer, "hyper-" or "hypokeratosis," and the presence of nuclei in the horny layer – from which they should have already disappeared – "parakeratosis," are the simplest manifestations of dyskeratosis. The successive thickening and thinning of the granular layer, *that is*, the "beading of the granular layer" in lichen planus (p. 94), is another manifestation of dyskeratosis, as is the presence of "*corps rondes*" and "*grains*" in the lesion of Darier's disease (p. 30). "Squamous eddies" and their counterpart "keratin pearls," respectively, characterizing the "benign" and "malignant types" of dyskeratosis in irritated seborrheic keratosis and squamous cell carcinoma (p. 124) are also manifestations of this condition.

"Acantholysis" and related terms have their root in the Greek language (*acanthos* = a thorn) and refers to the prickles surrounding keratinocytes. For instance "acanthosis" means an increase in thickness of the prickle cell layer, and "acanthoma" is a tumoral increase of that layer; "acantholysis" is the destruction of the keratinocyte after disappearing of the desmosomes, and by extension, "acantholytic cells" are keratinocytes devoid of desmosomes.

Genodermatoses

According to the position of the epidermis in which their defect resides, genodermatoses may be classified as, of upper, mid, and low epidermal level of expression. Following the same topographic approach, cutaneous lesions associated to genodermatoses may be classified as of upper, mid, and low epidermal level. Figure 3.1 presents a diagrammatic comparison of the level at which the lesion occur in the three types of genodermatosis.

The lesions in the genodermatoses show a particular histopathologic feature at each epidermal level: dyskeratosis at upper epidermal level, acantholysis at mid epidermal level, and dermoepidermal separation at low epidermal level (Table 3.2).

Table 3.2 Genodermatoses: clinical examples, level of epidermal expression, dominant histopathologic detail of the lesions, and hereditary transmission

Clinical entity	Dominant histopathologic feature	Hereditary transmission
Of upper epidermal level of expression		
Ichthyosis vulgaris	Dyskeratosis	Aut.dom.
Ichthyosis X-linked	Dyskeratosis	X-link.rec.
Bullous congenital ichthyosiform erythroderma	Dyskeratosis	Aut.dom.
Lamellar ichthyosis	Dyskeratosis	Aut.rec.
Porokeratosis of Mibelli	Dyskeratosis	Aut.dom.
Acrokeratosis verruciformis	Dyskeratosis	Aut.dom.
Of mid epidermal level of expression		
Darier's disease	Acantholysis	Aut.irreg.dom.
Hailey-Hailey's disease	Acantholysis	Aut.irreg.dom.
Of low epidermal level of expression		
Epidermolysis bullosa simplex	Dermo	Aut.dom.
Epidermolysis letalis	Epidermal	Aut.rec.
Epidermolysis bullosa dystrophic, recessive	Separation	Aut.rec.

Lesions Associated to Genodermatoses of Upper Epidermal Level of Expression

Upon examining the class of genodermatoses of upper epidermal level of expression, the frequency with which "ichthyosis" and related terms are used appears remarkable. The term ichthyosis was originally and aptly applied since immemorial times to a disorder which affected some individuals whose skin presented horny formations resembling fish scales (*ichthys+osis* [G] fish+condition). In regard to this term, Pinkus insisted since the original edition of his textbook in 1962 [1] that "ichthyosis" is one of those diagnostic terms which covers disorders not related to each other (Fig. 3.2), and that it is a purely clinical designation for chronic hyperkeratotic skin. Pinkus' remarks were not listened to by the dermatologic community which instead of restricting its use, expanded it, creating a picturesque zoomorphic nomenclature which includes, in addition to fish and lizards, porcupines as well as other creatures. Instead of facilitating the understanding of these disorders, this nomenclature made it more difficult.

The pathogenesis of hyperkeratosis in the ichthyosiform disorders is in a continuous process of study and revision which has not yet reached definitive results in all cases. Nevertheless, in light of the present knowledge, it is accepted that these disorders may be of *retentive* or *hyperproductive nature*, or otherwise of a mixed nature [2] (Table 3.3).

Ichthyosis vulgaris, the condition at the top of the list in Table 3.3, was the first of these disorders to be identified and is the most frequent. This disorder, of autonomic dominant transmission and relatively benign evolution, tends to improve over the years and is characterized by a scaly and cracked skin featuring the characteristic "scales," which are particularly noticeable on the extension surface of the inferior limbs. The microscopy of ichthyosis vulgaris discloses a fragment of skin with a horny layer that is thick and dehiscent, with frequent dilated follicular infundibula plugged with keratin scales. The pathognomonic detail of the lesion is the absence of the granular layer from the epidermis (Figs. 3.1 and 3.2 left).

X-linked ichthyosis, the second disorder mentioned in Table 3.3, was recognized in the second half of the last century and is also known as "sex-linked ichthyosis" because of its propensity to appear in male patients, in which the more severe forms are also seen. The distribution of the lesions in the flexural folds and the "dirty" character of their scales along with its characteristic hereditary transmission and its evolution without remission contribute to distinguish it from ichthyosis vulgaris. X-linked ichthyosis is a retentive condition caused by the lack of cholesterol sulphatase. This enzyme is normally activated in the late phase of evolution of keratinocytes, hydrolyzing interstitial cholesterol and contributing to the desquamative process of these (p. 4). LM examination of X-linked ichthyosis reveals a nonspecific picture in which an orthokeratotic thickening of the horny layer is evident.

Subsequent to the two ichthyoses exposed in Table 3.3, the two congenital ichthyosiform erytrodermas should be considered.

Bullous congenital ichthyosiform erythroderma (BCIE), a condition of autonomic dominant transmission, was described by J. L. Brocq at the beginning of the nineteenth century. It is today considered a type of hyperproductive hyperkeratosis due to the mutation of one of the keratin genes, which causes excessive production of tonofilaments and keratohyaline granules: this prevents the normal desquamation of keratin scales. The initial bullous erythroderma of newborns resolves into a chronic warty condition with spiny plaques mainly found on the nape of neck, axillae, groin, and other flexural folds, which may eventually regress by puberty.

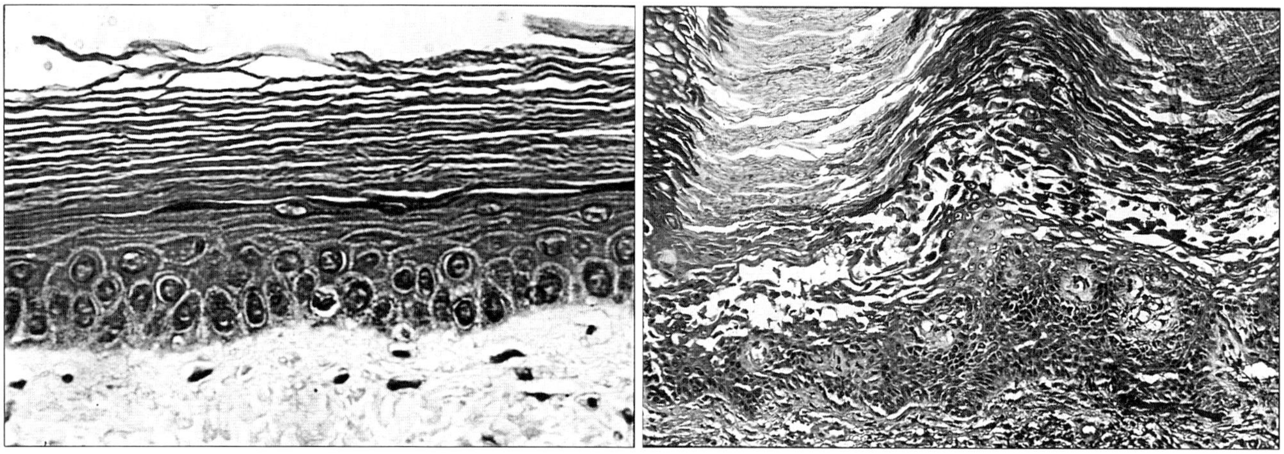

Fig. 3.2 Ichthyosis vulgaris and bullous congenital ichthyosiform erythroderma. Judging from the comparative examination of the microscopic image of ichthyosis vulgaris and bullous congenital ichthyosiform erythroderma, it must be conceded that Pinkus was correct when he stated that "ichthyosis" is a term which covers dyskeratotic disorders of widely different nature: whereas ichthyosis vulgaris (*left*) shows an inconspicuous picture in which the only noticeable abnormality is the lack of the granular layer, bullous congenital ichthyosiform erythroderma (*right*) presents a dramatic alteration of the epidermis in which all its layers, except for the germinal one, have been replaced by a dehiscent horny material with keratohyaline granules. H&E ×100; ×40, o m

Table 3.3 Hereditary ichthyosiform disorders: type of hyperkeratosis – responsible defect and hereditary transmission

Nosologic entity	Type of hyperkeratosis	Responsible defect	Hereditary transmission
Ichthyosis vulgaris	Retentive	Defective filaggrin	Aut.dom.
X-linked ichthyosis	Retentive	Lack of cholesterol sulfatase	X-link.rec.
Bullous congenital ichthyosiform erythroderma	Retentive/hyperproductive	Excessive production of tonofilaments and keratohyaline granules	Aut.rec.
Nonbullous congenital ichthyosiform erythroderma	Under study	Undetermined	Aut.rec.

Its concise and objective name, "bullous congenital ichthyosiform erythroderma," which clearly indicates its main clinical characteristics, now tends to be replaced by "epidermolytic hyperkeratosis." However, epidermolytic hyperkeratosis is a *histopathologic* term whose microscopic details may be observed in Fig. 3.2(right). On account of its histopathologic character, the term "*epidermolytic hyperkeratosis*" does not match with the clinical nomenclature applied to the other ichthyoses. The purported microscopic picture in BCIE is also observed in the more restricted form of this condition, the so-called ichthyosis hystrix [3] (*hystrix* [G] porcupine), named after the same trend "sauriosis" (*sauros*+*osis* [G] lizard+condition), and even in other disorders unrelated to BCIE. For these reasons, it is not advisable to use the term "epidermolytic hyperkeratosis" in replacement of BCIE. The term "bullous ichthyosiform erythroderma" could be accepted as a shortened alternative for BCIE since at least, it indirectly implies that contrary to the "bullous type" of ichthyosiform erythroderma, a nonbullous type of this condition exists in which no bullae are featured on the skin of the newborn.

Nonbullous congenital ichthyosiform erythroderma (NBCIE), the counterpart of BCIE, is an entity not as clearly defined as BCIE. It is a condition of retentive/hyperproductive nature and autosomal recessive transmission. At birth, the condition is manifested, not by bullae (as in BCIE), but by a horny membrane encasing the newborn and transforming it into a so-called collodion baby (Fig. 3.3).

The horny membrane tends to be shed after a few days, disclosing a reddened epidermis with whitish scales. In the most favorable cases, the manifestations of NBCIE tend to regress, freeing the patient of this nuisance upon reaching puberty. It must be remembered that "collodion baby" is not indefectively tantamount of NBCIE, since it may also appear as the sporadic component of other entities and then disappear without major consequences. However, under unfavorable conditions which have not yet been clarified, NBCIE tends to be transformed into "lamellar ichthyosis."

Lamellar ichthyosis is the most deforming of all the ichthyosiform conditions. Hyperkeratosis tends to increase over the years, transforming its lesions, in spite of their inconspicuous microscopic aspect, into thick plaques and keratinous

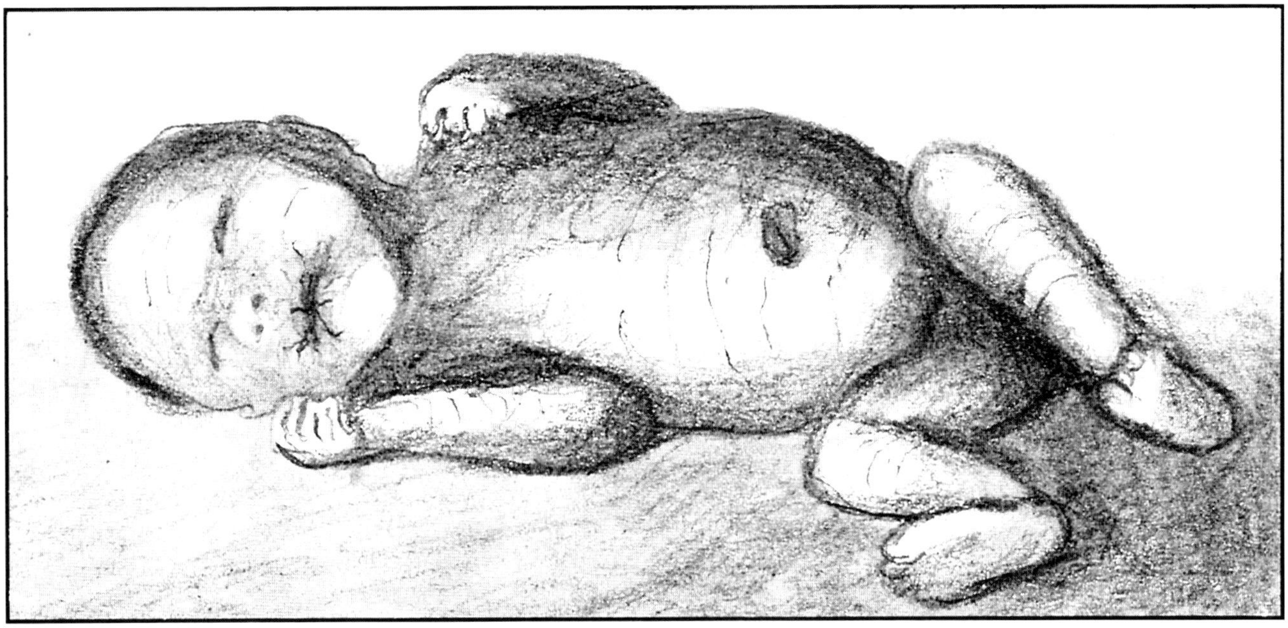

Fig. 3.3 Collodion baby. This newborn is covered by a shiny membrane but otherwise does not show external abnormalities (Compare with the harlequin fetus in Fig. 3.5)

excretions which deform the patient's aspect to such an extent that some faced the sad destiny of exposure to public amazement under such titles as "*the batrachian man*" or the "*lizard woman*" (Fig. 3.4).

Harlequin fetus: It is pertinent to state that harlequin fetus despite its vague resemblance to the collodion baby is not related to the former. Harlequin fetus is usually an unexpected condition of extraordinary appearance and of very low incidence. It appears as a dead or unviable fetus (Fig. 3.5).

Following this discussion, the existence of a group of hereditary multisystemic disorders with cutaneous participation should be mentioned, whose cutaneous component is an ichthyosiform rash (Table 3.5).

It may lastly be added that the sudden and unexpected appearance of ichthyosis may be the first indication of an ongoing sarcoidosis or even of an internal malignancy in a patient, particularly Hodgkin's disease, reason for which extemporary ichthyosis may be eventually appraised as the cutaneous marker of an internal malignancy.

In continuing the discussion of genodermatoses of upper epidermal level (Table 3.2), the porokeratoses should be examined next. These disorders also represent a group of genodermatoses of upper epidermal level of expression and autosomal dominant hereditary transmission, but totally different from the precedent group. It includes, in addition to porokeratosis

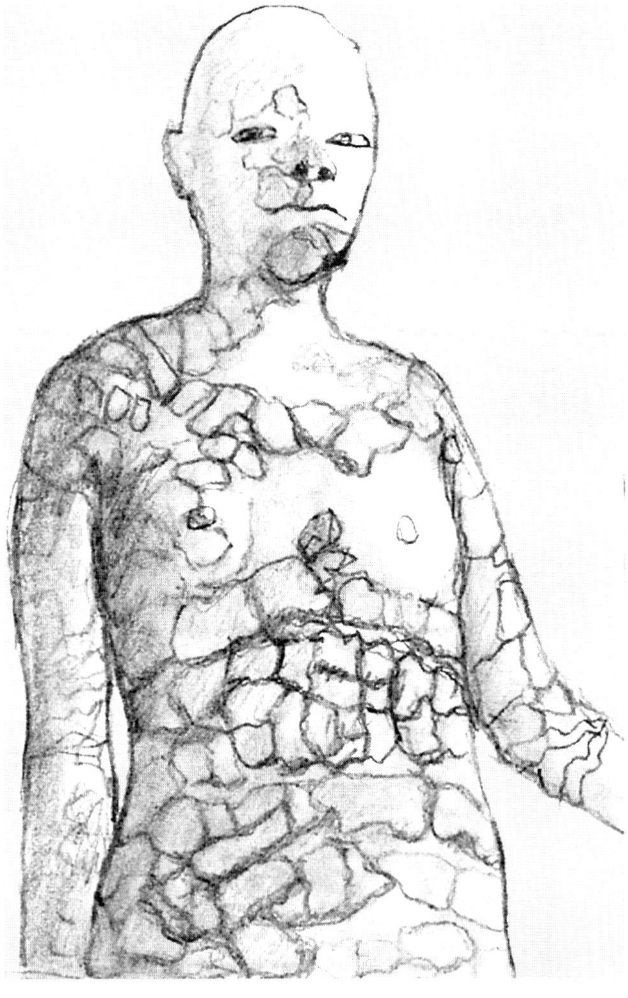

Fig. 3.4 Lamellar ichthyosis. Note the strange expression of the patient, with her eyelids transformed into rigid curtains, while the face as well as the rest of her body is deformed by the presence of course, irregular plaques of keratin

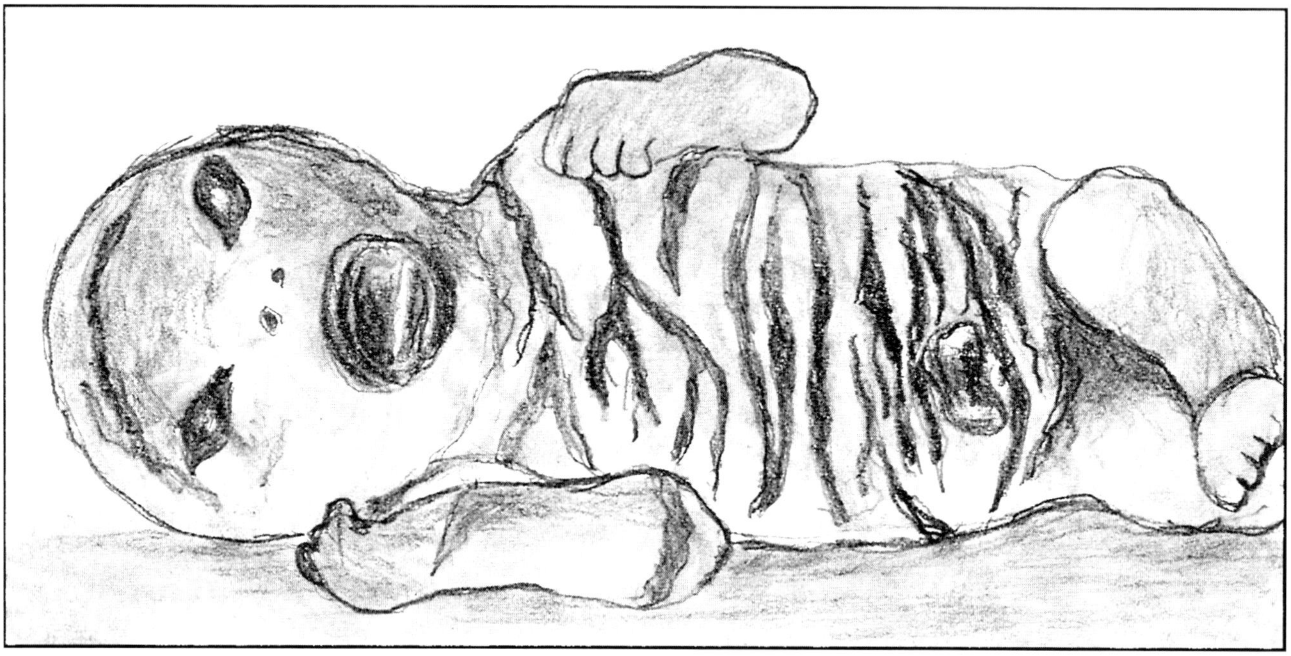

Fig. 3.5 Harlequin fetus. The body of the fetus appears covered by keratin plaques separated from each other by deep creases. Marked ectropion and eclabium are also noticeable. In addition to the severe external alterations, abnormalities of lipid and protein metabolism are present in these patients

Mibelli's, the entity originally described by this author, "superficial disseminated actinic porokeratosis," the most frequent of all of these, linear porokeratosis, and some other entities. It is arguably assumed that the lesions originate in abnormal clones of perifollicular keratinocytes, which tend to propagate on the skin surface in a centrifugal manner (Fig. 3.6).

Acrokeratosis verruciformis of Hopf: The last integrant of the list of genodermatoses of upper epidermal level of expression is acrokeratosis verruciformis Hopf (Table 3.2), a disorder manifested by multiple papules on the dorsum of hands and feet. Due to the frequent coexistence of these lesions with Darier's disease, it was speculated that acrokeratosis was a special form of the former. However, LM examination does not support that assumption, since acrokeratosis is characterized by hyperkeratosis and papillomatosis, without featuring suprabasal acantholysis, the distinctive sign of Darier's disease.

Lesions Associated to Genodermatoses of Mid Epidermal Level of Expression

As was already mentioned, the lesions associated to genodermatoses of mid epidermal level of expression display acantholysis as the dominant histopathologic feature (Table 3.2). Acantholysis may also occur under other circumstances too, compromising the cohesion among keratinocytes, as it happens in inflammatory (p. 77) and neoplastic (p. 131) conditions. For this reason, acantholysis should not be appraised as an invariable sign of genodermatosis.

Darier's disease: Darier's disease is a chronic condition of irregular dominant hereditary transmission, caused by defects in the desmosomal/tonofilament complex. The fact that the cutaneous alteration appeared to be related to hair follicles induced its initial reporter, J. Darier, to call it "keratosis follicularis." However, as it was later recognized, such association is not constant nor necessary for the diagnosis of Darier's disease, whose lesions may also appear on areas devoid of hair follicles, such as palms and soles, and even more important from a differential diagnostic viewpoint, in the bucal mucosa, as in pemphigus vulgaris!

LM examination of Darier's disease (Fig. 3.7) reveals a conspicuous histopathologic picture characterized by irregular epidermal folds deepening into the dermis, giving to the base of the lesion a papillomatous profile. The germinal layer appears firmly attached to the BM but separated from the rest of the epidermis by confluent clefts running above basal keratinocytes, configurating a clear example of suprabasal acantholysis. The resulting irregular space spreading above the germinal layer, the so-called "lacuna", is filled with keratotic material, in which "corps rondes" and "grains" are frequent and characteristic elements. The marked acantholysis and parakeratosis imparts a disorganized appearance to the overlying epidermis. The dermis surrounding the lesion presents a diffuse infiltration by mononuclear elements.

Characteristic details of the lesion may be better appraised at higher magnification. Figure 3.8 shows, on the left, suprabasal acantholysis with clean dermoepidermal separation and two corps rondes in the overlying epidermis. On the right

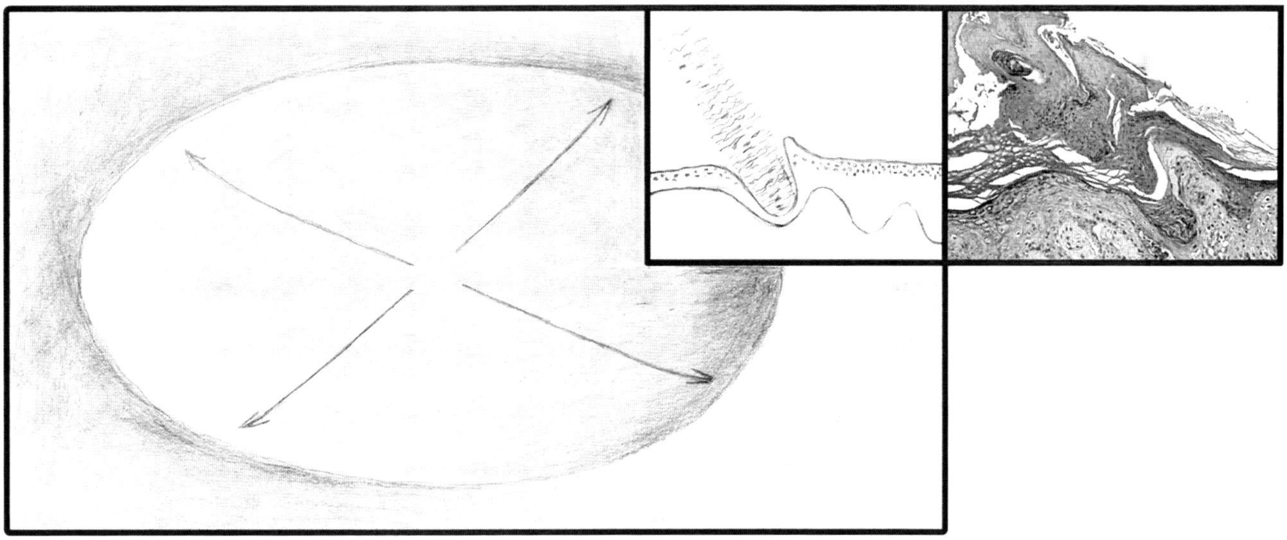

Fig. 3.6 Mibelli's porokeratosis. The figure presents a panoramic view of the lesion showing its circular contour. The *arrows* indicate the peripheral expansion of the lesion, and the *right upper inset* shows a simplified drawing of the advance front of the lesion. It features a tall formation of parakeratin, the "cornoid lamella" pointing out of the center. To the *right of the inset* is an actual photomicrograph of the same area, including the cornoid lamella. H&E ×100, o m

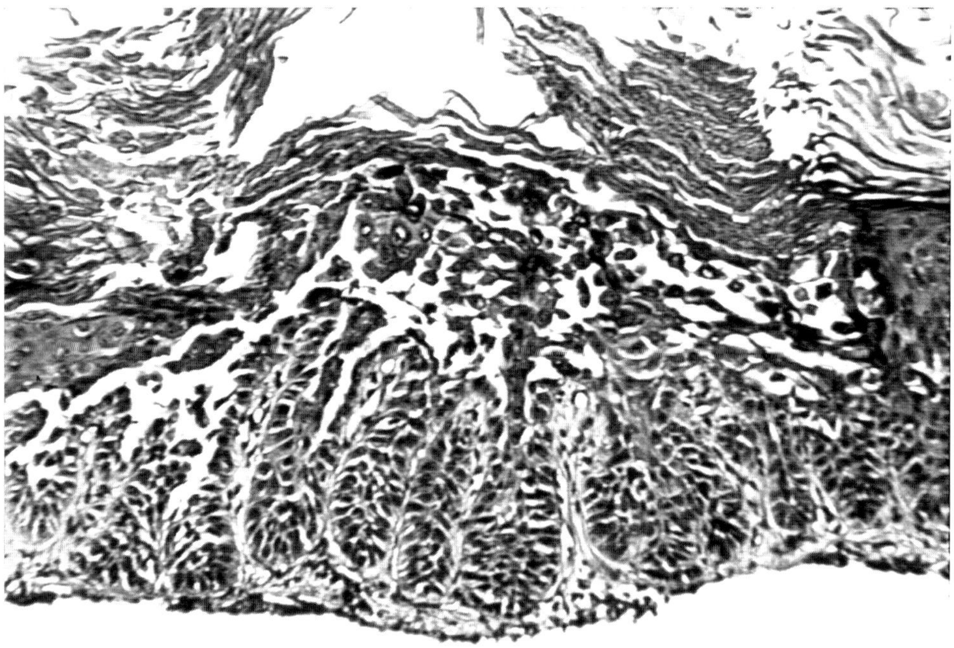

Fig. 3.7 Darier's disease. See details in the text. H&E ×40, o m

can be seen details of the benign dyskeratotic mass within the lacuna, in which corps rondes, grains, and parakeratotic scales are found.

Hailey-Hailey's disease: This condition was reported in 1939 by the brothers H. and W. Hailey as "benign familial pemphigus." This discovery was welcomed by dermatologists, since it enabled them to microscopically recognize and tell apart from pemphigus – a disease of almost invariable fatal outcome these days – a hereditary condition which in spite of its unpleasant chronic course, was not of a lethal character.

The pathogenesis of Hailey-Hailey's disease resides, as in Darier's disease, in defective desmosomal/tonofilament complexes. Since, additionally, the hereditary transmission is similar for both, this led to speculations that the former was just a variant of the latter. Microscopic examination dismissed that possibility, upon disclosing a distinctly different picture among these conditions, as can be realized by a microscopic comparison. Contrary to what happens in Darier's disease, in which suprabasal acantholysis is accompanied by all the elements of benign dyskeratosis (see Figs. 3.7 and 3.8), in

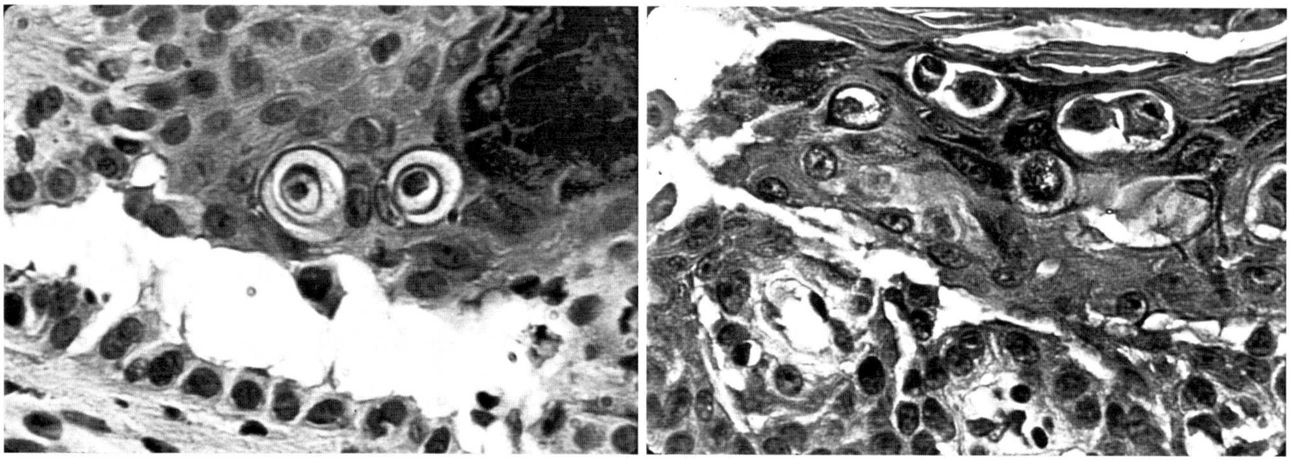

Fig. 3.8 Darier's disease. See details in the text. H&E ×400, o m

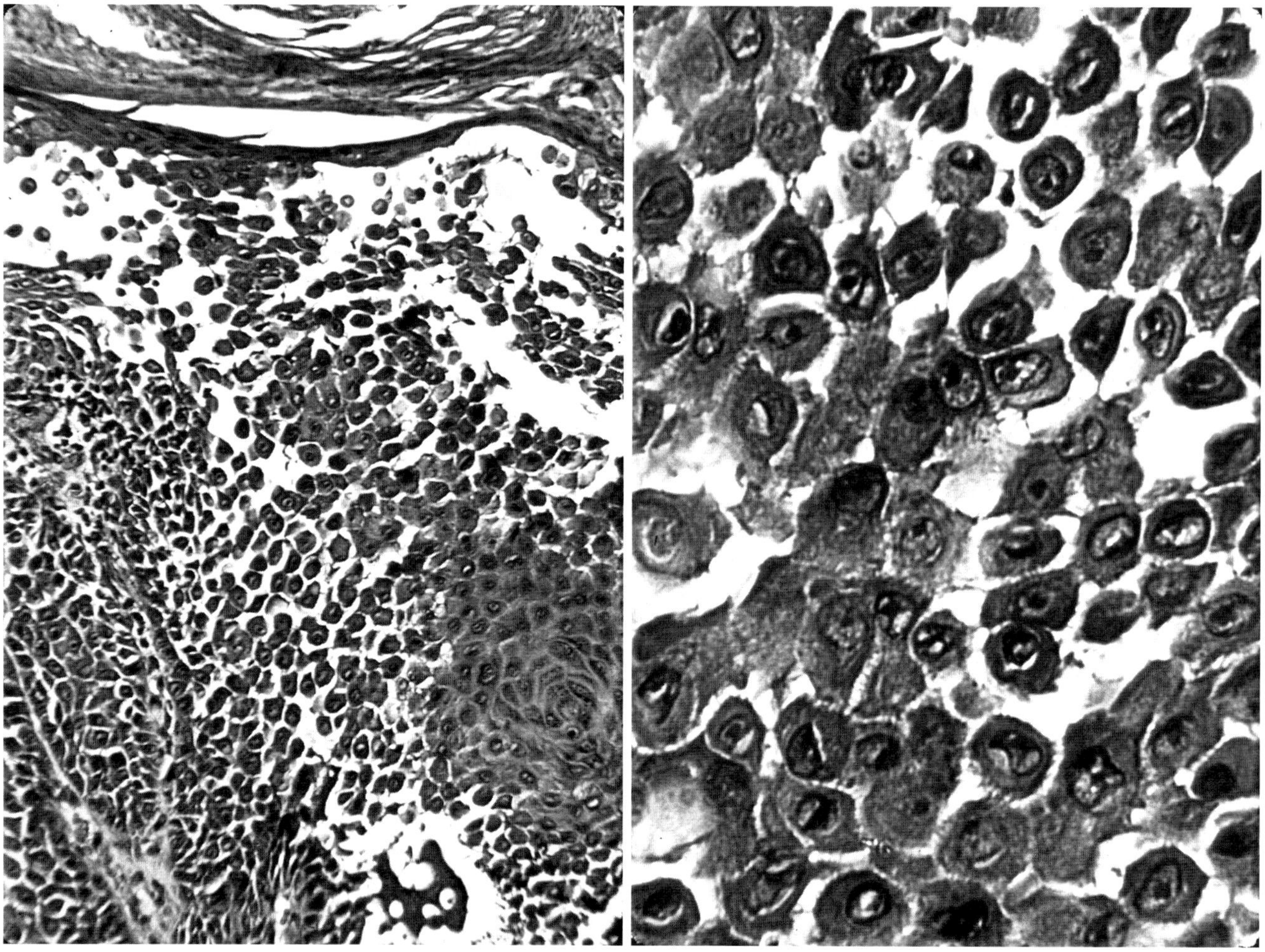

Fig. 3.9 Hailey-Hailey's disease. *Left*: The lesions show diffuse acantholysis with disintegration of the epidermis, but with no dyskeratosis. *Right*: The acantholytic keratinocytes which show little cellular distress are shown at higher magnification. H&E ×40; ×400, o m

Hailey-Hailey's disease, just a diffuse acantholysis occurs involving the entire thickness of the epidermis. It lacks parakeratosis and features a microscopic picture classically compared to "a dilapidated brick wall" (Fig. 3.9).

Lesions Associated to Genodermatoses of Low Epidermal Level of Expression

The lesions in the genodermatoses of low epidermal level of expression are conjointly denominated epidermolysis bullosa (EB). These are hereditary conditions caused by cutaneous defects revolving around the area of the dermoepidermal junction. The defects result in increased epidermal fragility, manifested by blistering after mild trauma, which under normal conditions would not have any adverse effect. Since these lesions are associated to trauma, they are frequently called "mecanobullae."

The technique of immunofluorescent mapping (see below) combined with EM inspection allows the determination of the level of dermoepidermal separation and the classification of the EB as being *above*, *through*, or *below the basement membrane*. This is also expressed as EB of epidermal, dermoepidermal, or dermal type. Some of the most classic examples of these entities are exposed in Table 3.4.

In the original direct technique of immunofluorescence (IF), fluorescent antibodies (Ab) (p. 193) corresponding to the antigens (Ags) (p. 193) under study are applied to fresh tissues. The labeled Abs are fixed specifically on the corresponding (Ags) if these happen to be present, forming deposits which upon UV irradiation under the microscope would emit fluorescent radiation allowing visual localization of the sought Ags.

The combined application of IF and EM in Fig. 3.10 shows highly schematically comparative details of the pathogenic mechanism leading to the formation of a bulla in an epidermal, a junctional, and a dermal type of EB.

Epidermolysis bullosa simplex: The defect responsible for development of the bulla in EB simplex is an intrinsic fragility of the basal keratinocytes. This anomaly is invisible to the analytic tools used in this study, and the area before trauma (left half of the left box) appears unremarkable. Therefore, incidentally, this left half box may be used as a normal reference for the situations that follow. After trauma, in EB simplex (right half of the left box), the basal keratinocytes undergoing necrosis break apart, and a separation of the epidermis from the BM ensues. The fact that the BM (LL+LD) remain unscathed in this process allows rapid epidermal regeneration, reason for which the prognosis of this condition is excellent.

Table 3.4 Epidermolysis bullosa congenital: examples, congenital defect, and hereditary transmission

Split level	Congenital defect	H.T.
Above the basement membrane		
Epidermolysis bullosa simplex	Fragility of keratinocytes	Aut.dom.
Epidermolysis of hand and foot	In the germinal layer	Aut.dom.
Within the basement membrane		
Epidermolysis bullosa letalis		Aut.rec.
Epidermolysis bullosa benign	Defective hemidesmosomes	Aut.rec.
Below the basement membrane		
Epidermolysis bullosa dystrophic, dominant	Diminution or absence of anchoring fibrils	Aut.dom.

Epidermolysis bullosa letalis: In EB letalis, EM inspection previous to the trauma (left half of the center box) already reveals sparse and faulty hemidesmosomes (compare with hemidesmosomes in the reference box). The failure of these structures to resist external trauma leads to a splitting through the LL with formation of a cavity: its roof, formed by the upper half of the LL, is attached to the cellular membrane of the keratinocyte above (M), whereas its base, formed by the lower half of the LL, remains attached to the LD (right half of the center box). Since the LD which is the most important structure concerning the favorable epidermal regeneration and the outcome of the lesion remains unaffected by the trauma, a satisfactory epidermal restoration could be expected. This would be the case, were it not for a grave circumstance: in EB letalis, not only the epidermis is affected but other epithelia as well, such as the urinary, the respiratory, and that of the GI tract, creating situations incompatible with life. There exists, however, an attenuated form of this condition EB generalisata atrophic benign, which allows the patient's survival despite the traumatic events.

Epidermolysis bullosa recessive: In the case of EB dystrophic recessive, EM examination before the trauma (left half of the right box) already reveals the absence of the anchoring fibrils from the sublamina densa space (compare with the features exposed in the reference box). In this case, the trauma will cause massive separation of the BL (LL+LD) from the superficial dermis, which will be found attached to the keratinocyte above (right half of the right box). Although the EB dystrophic recessive is not deadly in itself, the cutaneous disruption in this condition will prevent any sound epidermal repair, and after the trauma, only scars may be formed.

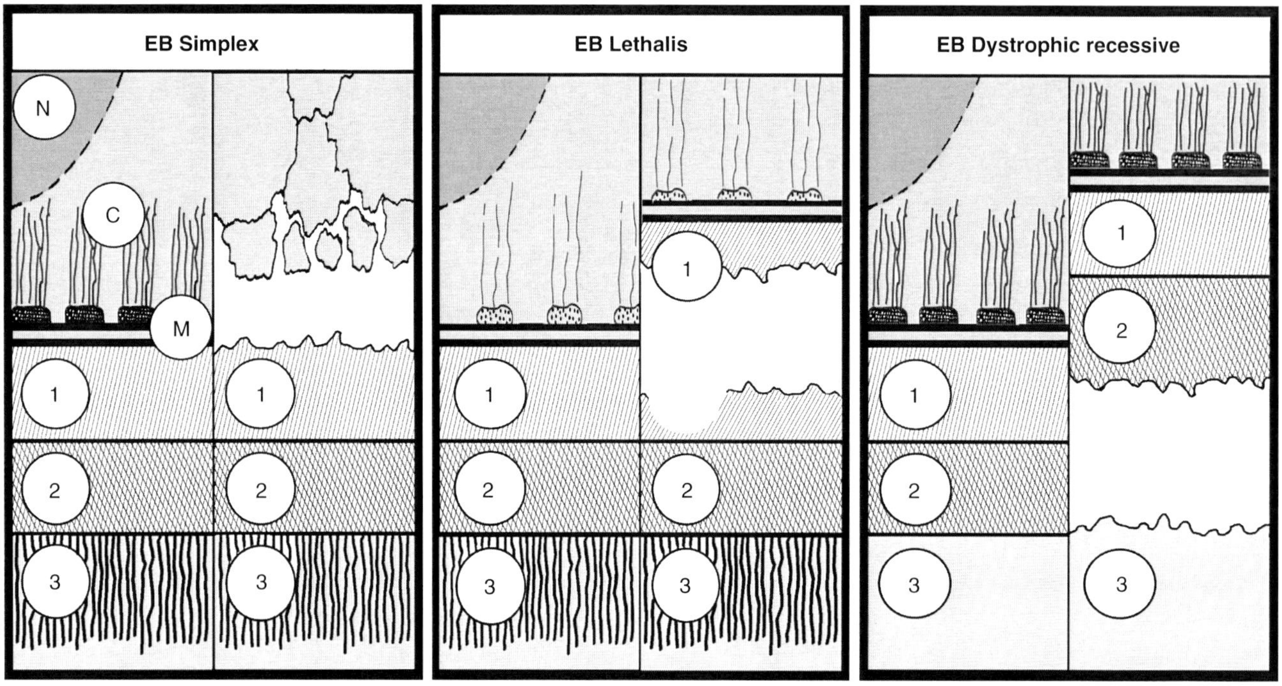

Fig. 3.10 Comparative IF/EM study of the pathogenesis of the bulla in the three types of EB. The entity under study is indicated above each of the three boxes: these are examples of epidermal, junctional, and dermal type of EB, respectively. In the left and right half of each box, details of a basal keratinocyte and the subjacent area before and after the triggering trauma are offered. *N* nucleus, *C* cytoplasm, *M* cellular membrane with desmosomes, *1* lamina lucida; *2* lamina densa, *3* anchoring fibrils in the sublamina densa space. 1, 2, and 3 are visualized by the use of labeled Abs against bullous pemphigoid Ag, collagen type IV, and collagen type VII, respectively. The empty space in the right half of each of the boxes indicates the place where the separation, that is, the bulla, occurs after trauma. The figure is not construed in scale and the proportions among the various elements are arbitrary

These do not offer any effective protection for the underlying osteotendinous structures, and after repeated traumatic events, the loss of digits and distal parts of the limbs ensues. As a consequence, these patients are transformed into invalids a few years after birth. As in the case of EB letalis, an attenuated form of EB dystrophic exists, known as EB dominant, in which the prognosis is not as grim as in the previous disorder.

It is important to realize that from a histopathologic viewpoint, the only form of EB actually deserving the title of "epidermolytic" is EB simplex: in this condition, a primary epidermal defect is responsible for the necrosis of the involved keratinocyte and the split formation. All other EB's are due to defects of mesenchymal structures which lead to the separation of cutaneous planes and, only secondarily, to the destruction of the epidermis [4].

At this point an incidental reference may be made to EB acquisita. This disorder (p. 84) must be clearly separated from the congenital EBs, since *it does not have a hereditary background*, being instead an autoimmune condition. In this condition, the destruction runs, *as in pemphigus vulgaris, within the epidermis instead of along the BMZ* [5] (p. 19).

Hereditary Polysystemic Disorders with Cutaneous Participation

The second group of entities mentioned in Table 3.1 is the hereditary polysystemic disorders with cutaneous participation (HPDwCP). Contrary to genodermatoses, which may be backtracked to faulty single genes, HPDwCP are polygenetic anomalies which affect the skin and extracutaneous organs. This is the reason for which they differ so widely in composition and clinical presentation from the genodermatoses.

As an introduction to this complex field, a representative gathering of HPDwCP was selected. According to their various forms of clinical presentation, they were tentatively separated into six groups as shown in Table 3.5. It must be realized that the terms "group" and "class" are hereby used as general descriptive terms, and not as "Group" and "Class" in a taxonomic sense, as would be in the classification of the cutaneous lesions. In its left column, the table states the various taxonomic criteria used for grouping the clinical entities. In the central column are clinical entities pertinent to each group, and in the right column, their hereditary transmission is shown.

Table 3.5 Hereditary polysystemic disorders with cutaneous participation grouped according to distinctive clinical features

	Clinic entity	HT
First group	LEOPARD syndrome	Aut.dom.
Distinctive feature	LAMB syndrome	Aut.dom.
Lentiginous component	Carney's syndrome	Aut.dom.
	Albright's syndrome	Dom.
Second group	Conradi's disease	X-1.dom.
Distinctive feature	Netherton's syndrome	Aut.rec.
Ichthyosiform rash	Refsum's syndrome	Aut.rec.
	Sjogren-Larsen's syndrome	Aut.rec.
Third group		
Distinctive feature	Gorlin's syndrome	Aut.dom.
Cutaneous malformations and neoplasias	Cowden's syndrome	Aut.dom.
	Muir-Torre's syndrome	Aut.dom.
Fourth group		
Distinctive feature		
Similar malformations as cutaneous and extra-cutaneous component	Buschke-Ollendorf's syndrome	Aut. dom.
	Rendu-Osler-Weber's syndrome	Aut.dom.
	Hemangiomatous blue nevus	
	syndrome	Aut. dom.
Fifth group		
Distinctive feature	Neurofibromatosis	Aut.dom.
Phakomas	Tuberous sclerosis	Aut.dom.
Sixth group		
Distinctive feature	Gardner's syndrome	Aut.dom.
Intestinal polyps	Peutz-Jeghers syndrome	Aut.dom.

The approach hereby used for the study of HPDwCPs is very simple and tentative. It must be considered as of a working character, susceptible of being modified by adding new entities to each group, by shifting the integrants of each group, or by creating new groups of entities, as needed.

The first group of HPDwCP in Table 3.5 is characterized by the presence of a lentiginous component. The group is headed by two clinical entities LEOPARD and LAMB syndromes. LEOPARD and LAMB syndrome are acrostics from their most significant manifestations, as shown below.

l entigines*	
e KG abnormalities	
o cular hypertelorism	*l* entigines
p ulmonary stenosis	*a* trial myxoma
a bnormalities of the genitalia	*m* yxomas cutaneous, papular
r etardation of growth	*b* lue nevi
d eafness (neural)	

The lentigines in these lesions are due to variable combinations of irregular melanocytes with large granules of this pigment, and their components do not totally respond to the definition of "*lentigo*" used in this chapter. For this reason, these lesions will be designated from here on in italics and quotation marks "*lentigo*" or "*lentigines*" (lentigines = plural of lentigo).

In addition to the "*lentigines*," LEOPARD syndrome is formed by a constellation of extracutaneous abnormalities among which the cardiovascular and neurologic are the most important ones. LAMB syndrome is clearly defined by its corresponding acrostic, formed by the initials of two cutaneous and two myxomatous components of the entity. Carney's syndrome is a related but more complex entity which comprises, in addition to the four elements of LAMB syndrome, adrenocortical, testicular, and pituitary tumors.

The existence of a Carney's or a LAMB syndrome in a patient is important for its caregiver to know, since these syndromes alert about the possible existence of atrial myxomas of potentially sudden and fatal outcome.

Albright's syndrome is another integrant of this group of conditions; this disorder, also called "hereditary dystrophy," is a complex entity, in which obvious skeletal anomalies are combined with endocrine disturbances and sexual precocity. The cutaneous component of this syndrome consists of pigmented spots, "lentigines," caused by the accumulation of abnormal melanocytes.

Following the group of HPDwCP with lentiginous component, the next group to be examined is characterized by an ichthyosiform component in addition to more specific features. Conradi's disease, which probably represents not one but a cluster of related entities, features epiphyseal and skeletal defects leading to dwarfism; Netherton's syndrome shows both an ichthyosiform rash and atopical dermatitis along with an anomaly of the hair known as "trichorrhexis invaginata," whereas Refsum's syndrome displays ataxia cerebelosa, polyneuritis, and retinitis pigmentosa. Sjogren-Larsen's syndrome, on the other hand, is characterized by spastic paralysis and mental retardation.

In the third group of HPDwCP in Table 3.5 are entities whose components present cutaneous malformations and neoplasias as distinctive features. Here, Gorlin's syndrome is placed first. This condition, also called "epithelioma basocellular nevoid syndrome," is manifested by the appearance of basal cell carcinomas in the second or third decade of life (instead of after 40 years of age as it usually happens). These are combined with palmar pits. The internal components of this syndrome include bone cysts in the jaws and ribs.

The detailed description of Gorlin's syndrome is necessary for its correct identification, since several entities have been described under this designation.

Cowden's syndrome exhibits multiple trichoepitheliomas (p. 56) as its cutaneous component. It is often associated with breast or thyroid carcinoma. Lastly, Muir-Torre's syndrome, exteriorized by sebaceous hamartomas and carcinoma, frequently presents colon adenocarcinoma as an internal component. For obvious reasons, these last two entities are regarded as cutaneous markers of internal malignancy.

Among the HPSwCP of the fourth Group, those characterized by similar mesenchymatous lesions as both external and internal component occupy the first place. Case in point is Buschke-Ollendorf's syndrome. These patients present mesenchymal hamartomas, exteriorized as firm cutaneous nodules and recognized internally by characteristic X-ray images called "osteopoikilosis" (osteo [L]+*poikilos* [G] uneven) in the long and pelvic bones, their usual location. Rendu-Osler-Weber's syndrome is caused by the presence of capillary hemangiomas. When these are attached to the skin, they are known as "nevi aracnei" and are just considered aesthetic defects. However, when localized on the respiratory or GI tract, inaccessible by appropriate instruments, they may cause serious problems if they happen to bleed. Hemangiomatous blue nevus syndrome is much more deforming than the previous lesion. This is due to the large caliber of the vessels from which it is formed. For similar reasons, its treatment is more difficult in a bleeding situation.

The fifth group of disorders in Table 3.5 are the phakomatoses. Phakomas are congenital retinal malformations visible by eye examination (*phakoma* [G] a malformation, a nevus) [6]. Some phakomatoses have cutaneous manifestations, reason for which these nosologic combinations are also called "neurocutaneous disorders." [7] Two of these are covered in this text, neurofibromatosis and tuberous sclerosis.

Neurofibromatosis (NF) was initially reported by F. D. v. Recklinghausen in 1882, based on the peripheral nerve tumors which these patients presented [8]. The pigmentary component in this disorder was reported by French authors, who popularized these under the name "*taches cafe* au *lait*" (cafe au lait spots).

Among the various forms of NF, the most important is the peripheric one (NF1) or v. Recklinghausen's disease (Fig. 3.11). NF1 represents 85 % of the total of these affections [9], followed by central neurofibromatosis (NF2), also called "acoustic neurofibromatosis" (Table 3.6).

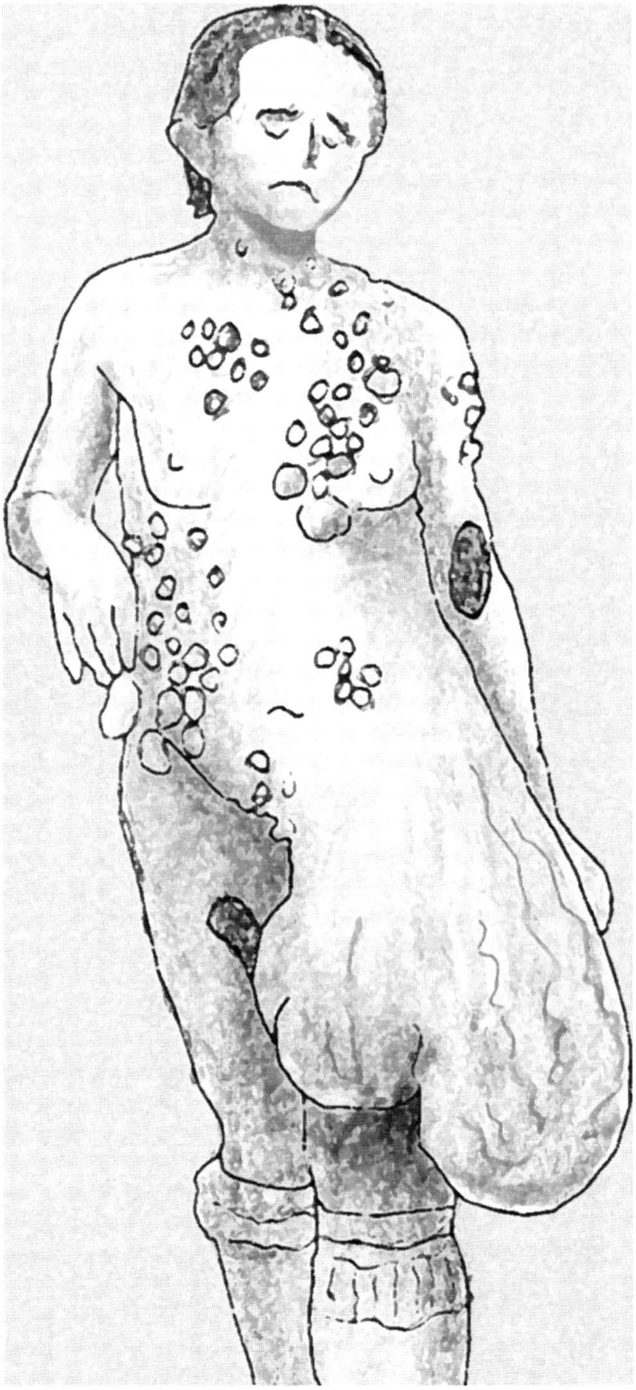

Fig. 3.11 v. Recklinghausen's disease. Picture copied from a R. Virchow publication in 1856, which shows a NF1 patient. The patient presents a pendulous plexiform neurofibroma as well as a large number of neurofibromas on the anterior and posterior part of the chest. Two pigmented spots ("*lentigines*"), one on the left arm and the other on the right thigh, are also visible

Once the medical community recognized the importance of the *cafe au lait spots* as signs of neurofibromatosis, the "incomplete" or "frustrated form" of this condition [10] – that is, the one that appears in the absence of neurologic manifestations – could be diagnosed whenever a patient features at least six of these spots with a greater dimension of 15 mm or more. Histologically, *cafe au lait spots* present large, irregular melanocytes, reason for which they fit under the definition of "*lentigines*."

Table 3.6 Manifestations of the peripheric (NF1) versus the central (NF2) forms of neurofibromatosis

Manifestation	NFl	NF2
Cafe au lait spots	4+	2+
Cutaneous neurofibromas	4+	1+
Plexiform neurofibromas	2+	0+
Malignant neurofibromas	1+	0+
Cutaneous schwannoma	0+	4+
Optic nerve astrocytoma	4+	1+
Bilateral acoustic schwannoma	0+	4+
Nisch's nodules	4+	0+
Skeletal malformations	3+	0+
Mental retardation	3+	0+

0+ = symptom absent
1+ = symptom present in up to 25 % of the cases
2+ = symptom present in up to 50 % of the cases
3+ = symptom present in up to 75 % of the cases
4+ = symptom present in over 75 % of the cases

The various nervous tumors which occur in connection with NF are dealt with in Chap. 6.

Tuberous sclerosis is also known as Bourneville's disease, in recognition of the individual who provided the most complete description of this disease. Tuberous sclerosis also goes by the name of "epiloia". This term, which is a combination of Greek and Latin words, brings up two of the most important manifestations of this condition, that is, epilepsy and mental deficiency. These, along with fibrovascular hamartomas and circumscribed areas of depigmentation commonly called "ash leaves," complete the symptomatic picture of this condition [11]. *Ash leaves* have a particular diagnostic implication: since they may be present at birth or shortly thereafter, they offer the earliest opportunity for diagnosing tuberous sclerosis. They may be found by naked eye or with help of Wood's light on the patient's skin.

The cutaneous hamartomas of tuberous sclerosis carry different names depending on their localization: the nasolabial ones, initially described by J. Pringle as "sebaceous adenomas" under the wrong impression that they were sebaceous *neoplasias*, are today called "Pringle's tumors." The sub- and periungual ones are nowadays designated as "Koenen's tumors," while the others, which appear as thickened areas of the skin, are known as "shagreen patches." The same type of mesenchymal hamartoma may be found in the kidney, the heart, and the meninges. From the latter derives the name "tuberous sclerosis" given to this condition by R. Virchow when he found them on the meninges of these patients. Phakomas, the distinctive feature of the phakomatosis, are in fact the same type of mesenchymal hamartomas, located on the retina.

The HPDwCP of the sixth and last group in Table 3.5 is distinguished by having an extracutaneous component in the form of intestinal polyps. Peutz-Jeghers syndrome is characterized by the combination of oral and perioral melanin pigmentations with hamartomatous jejunal polyps which are of benign nature but which may still be the cause of intestinal intrasusception.

Gardner's syndrome presents retention cysts (p. 40) as external components. These, in contrast to the common retention cysts, which are solitary (p. 186), are multiple in their appearance. The internal component of this condition are desmoid tumors (p. 159) of the abdominal wall. In Gardner's syndrome, the cysts and the desmoid tumors are combined with colonic polyps which in contrast to those in Peutz-Jeghers syndrome, are prone to undergo malignant degeneration.

Hereditary Metabolic Errors with Cutaneous Repercussion

These conditions (HMEwCR) are caused by inherited faulty enzymatic agents. These may affect the skin locally, through the accumulation of abnormal metabolic products or by triggering adverse reactions in this organ. Otherwise, they can affect the cutaneous metabolism, as a consequence of which abnormal skin would be synthesized.

Hereditary Metabolic Errors Associated to Cutaneous Lesions

Following his studies on alcaptonuria (from alcapton = homogenetic acid), A. Garrod advanced at the beginning of the twentieth century the idea that inherited defective material may be the cause of metabolic disorders, and based on the shortly before rediscovered Mendel's laws, he called these conditions "inborn errors of metabolism." [12]

Ochronosis (*ochron* + osis [G] yellow + condition), also called "alcaptonuria," a rare disorder of autosomal recessive transmission is due to the deficiency of a single enzyme, necessary for the oxidation of homogentisic acid into acetoacetic and fumaric acid. This leads to a urinary elimination of homogentisic acid and to its deposition on collagen and cartilage, with the consequent characteristic brown discoloration visible through the skin. The *exogenous* type of ochronosis, due to the topical application of hydroquinone, is considered in Chap. 7 (p. 183).

Phenylketonuria: Despite the fact that this condition only shows faint cutaneous manifestations, it is very instructive and of practical importance to compare it with ochronosis. Phenylketonuria is also an autosomal recessive condition caused by the lack of a single enzyme – in this case, active in the oxidation of phenylalanine into tyrosine. However, whereas the result of the deposition on the tissues of homogentisic acid in ochronosis causes only relatively minor problems to the patient, the presence of high levels of phenylanine in blood in phenylketonuria, if not corrected within the first months of life, leads to irreversible cerebral damage and mental deficiency in the patient, a condition called "phenylpyruvic oligophrenia."

The hyperlipoproteinemias and the porphyrias should be commented on next, since they are associated to conspicuous cutaneous repercussion.

Hyperlipoproteinemias are disorders in which the levels of circulating lipids and lipoproteins are altered and/or elevated. These disorders are divided into primary and secondary forms. Whereas secondary hyperlipoproteinemias are found as manifestations of diabetes or hypothyroidism, familial hyperlipoproteinemias are typically hereditary metabolic disorders caused by abnormalities in the synthesis, transport, and degradation of the plasma lipoproteins.

According to electrophoretic and ultracentrifugation studies, whose results overlap in general, five groups of familiar hyperlipoproteinemias were recognized. After further splitting group II, six groups, that is, types I, IIA, IIB, III, IV, and V, resulted [13].

The most common of these disorders are type IIA or familiar hypercholesterolemia, type IIB or combined hyperlipoproteinemia, and type IV or hyperprebeta lipoproteinemia. These are three disorders of autosomal dominant transmission. The three conditions, as well as the less frequent ones, are characterized by the formation of cutaneous xanthomas.

Xanthomas are deposits of lipid-laden histiocytes which may occur on the skin and extracutaneous locations. Xanthomas associated with the familiar hyperlipoproteinemias, that is, the metabolic or hyperlipidemic xanthomas, are of *reactive proliferative nature* and induced by high levels of lipids. In contrast, normolipidemic xanthomas represent neoplastic histiocytic proliferations to which diverse lipids are incorporated secondarily [14] (p. 127).

Upon external inspection, metabolic xanthomas offer a distinctive aspect which allow their differentiation: eruptive xanthomas, punctiform and multiple, are distributed on the gluteal regions and posterior surface of the thighs and show a clear tendency to regress upon improvement of the patients' condition; tuberous xanthomas, which may reach considerable volume, are found on osteotendinous planes such as the ones in elbows and knees; plane xanthomas are seen along palmar creases, whereas xanthelasmas show an elective palpebral localization. The microscopic images of these lesions are discussed in Chap. 6.

Porphyrias are disorders caused by alterations in the biosynthesis of heme, the prosthetic nucleus of hemoglobin and other metalloproteins. Due to the deficiency or absence of certain enzymes, the biosynthetic chain of heme may be interrupted at different levels. The various intermediate metabolites, which cannot be processed beyond the blockage point, are eliminated, totally or in part via feces or urine, to which they impart a brown-reddish discoloration. This gave rise to the general nomenclature of these disorders as "*porphyrias*," which derives from *porphyreos* ([G] purpura). Otherwise, these metabolites are fixed on the tissue.

These disorders may occur as isolated, extemporary episodes following accidental events (alcohol ingestion and other forms of intoxications) being then called "secondary porphyrias." Otherwise, they may display a familiar pattern of transmission. These are the inborn or familiar porphyrias, from which eight principal forms are recognized (Table 3.8).

Since heme biosynthesis occurs mainly in the liver, bone marrow, or in both organs simultaneously, porphyrias may be classified as of hepatic, erythropoietic, or hepatoerythropoietic types [15].

Clinical manifestations of the porphyrias – in addition to the red discoloration of feces and urine – are classified as *cutaneous* and *neuropsychiatric*. The cutaneous manifestations of the porphyrias, considered generally as "cutaneous photosensitivity," amount, in the acute phase, to pruritus with blister formation following UV radiation. In the long term, the skin becomes scarred, mutilated, and pigmented, exhibiting hirsutism.

The primary damaging mechanism of cutaneous photosensitivity is related to "phototoxic metabolites" generated by the faulty metabolic cycles. These are fixed on the superficial dermis, very close to the epidermis and within reach of UV radiation [16]. The metabolites are excited by UV radiation from the sun or other sources and upon returning to their basal state they emit longer wave radiations which damage tissues by a mechanism akin to the one of thermal burns.

The neuropsychiatric manifestations of the porphyrias consists of abdominal colics and vomiting, with burning feeling and lacinant pain along the limbs, and of a complex of neuropsychiatric manifestations, which range from a bizarre behavior to transient episodes of dementia as those suffered by George III of England from whom it was said that he carried so much blue blood in his veins that some used to spill into his urine... The pathogenesis of these symptoms, in contrast to those of cutaneous photosensitivity, has not been clarified to date.

The symptomatic spectrum of the hepatic porphyrias exposed in Table 3.8 ranges from exclusively cutaneous as in porphyria cutanea tarda to mixed in porphyria variegata and coproporphyria hereditaria, ending with the purely neuropsychiatric form of porphyria, the porphyria intermittent acuta or Swedish porphyria.

The clinical manifestations in the erythropoietic and hepatoerythropoietic porphyrias reside exclusively at the cutaneous level.

Porphyria cutanea tarda (PCT) is the paradigm of the cutaneous porphyrias. The lesions associated with it may be backtracked to the deposition close to the BM of phototoxic metabolites. Their UV activation results into the destruction of the BM, which leads to dermoepidermal separation with formation of a space, that is, a *subepidermal bulla* [17] (p. 87).

Erythropoietic porphyria, or Gunther's disease, deserves a short comment. This condition, the first porphyria to be described, belongs to the group of the erythropoietic ones and contrasting with most of the other porphyrias, is of autosomal recessive transmission; it causes severe destruction and mutilation, with scarring, digit synechiae, and hirsutism. Indeed, patients of Gunther's disease were eventually associated, due to their external aspect, to the saga of *werewolves*.

Fabry's disease, located below the porphyrias in Table 3.7, belongs to the group of the sphingolipidosis. All these conditions are disorders related to the malfunction of enzymes involved in the metabolism of diverse sphingolipids. Since these cannot be processed, they accumulate in the body causing severe problems. Nieman-Pick's and Gaucher's disease are among the best known of these inborn metabolic errors, but since they have little or no cutaneous repercussion, these are only mentioned in this chapter. Fabry's disease, to the contrary, has a peculiar cutaneous localization and deserves a short comment. Fabry's disease, a condition of X-recessive transmission, is due to the deficiency of the enzyme necessary for the splitting of a determined sphingolipid. As a consequence, it accumulate in endothelial cells and pericytes. This causes irregular dilation of the involved vessels. In the skin, this leads to reactive hyperkeratosis, also called "angiokeratoma corporis diffusum."

Among hereditary metabolic errors, a separate mention should be made of the inherited form of gout. This, contrary to the secondary form of this condition, is a disorder ultimately related to hereditary deficiency of enzymes involved in purine metabolism, which leads to hyperuricemia and to the deposition of urates in soft tissue and joints. The name of the condition "gout" derives from the form of pain the patient suffers during the attacks, with an imperturbable rhythm comparable to that of "water dripping in a cavern." The presence of urate crystals in the tissues (Fig. 3.12) causes strong but localized foreign body granulomas, the "*tophi*" (*tophus* [L] calcareous deposit), whose characteristics are described in Chap. 7.

The hereditary form of hemochromatosis is of autosomal recessive transmission. It is a condition associated with a cutaneous pigmentation caused by the presence of iron in the body. This is actually a disorder of the intestinal mucosa which causes an increased uptake of this element, followed by its deposition in the liver, pancreas, and on the skin. The slate gray discoloration it produces on the skin, along with *liver cirrhosis* and *diabetes mellitus*, gives rise to the symptomatic combination known as "bronze diabetes [18]."

Table 3.7 Inborn metabolic errors

With cutaneous lesions
Ochronosis
Phenylketonuria
Hyperlipoproteinemias
Porphyrias
Fabry's disease
Gout
Hemochromatosis
With defective skin
Ehlers-Danlos' syndromes
Cutis laxa

Table 3.8 Familiar porphyrias: division, clinical manifestations, and hereditary transmission

Division and clinic examples	C	N	HT
Hepatic			
Porphyria cutanea tarda	3+	0+	Aut.dom.
Porphyria variegata	2+	2+	Aut.dom.
Coproporphyria hereditaria	2+	3+	Aut.dom.
Acute intermittent porphyria	0+	3+	Aut.dom.
Erythropoietic			
Erythropoietic porphyria	3+	0+	Aut.rec.
Erythropoietic protoporphyria	3+	0+	Aut.dom.
Erythropoietic coproporphyria	3+	0+	
Hepatoerythropoietic			
Hepatoerythropoietic porphyria	3+	0+	Aut.

The frequency of a symptom goes from 0+ to a maximum of 3+
C cutaneous, *N* neuropsychiatric, *HT* hereditary transmission

Hereditary Metabolic Errors Associated with Defective Skin

As previously mentioned, this second group of hereditary metabolic errors with cutaneous repercussion is not characterized by discrete cutaneous lesions, but by a generalized defective skin caused by a faulty biosynthetic pathway which affects the production of structural proteins, namely, collagen and elastic fibers.

Ehlers-Danlos syndromes (EDS) are examples of disorders caused by defects in the synthesis of the various types of collagen. All these characteristically feature *skin overextension*. The first three forms of EDS are autosomal dominant; types IV and VII are dominant/recessive, while type VI is recessive and type IX is X-linked.

Cutis laxa is a heterogeneous group of conditions characterized by coarse folds of lax skin derived from the faulty production of elastic fibers.

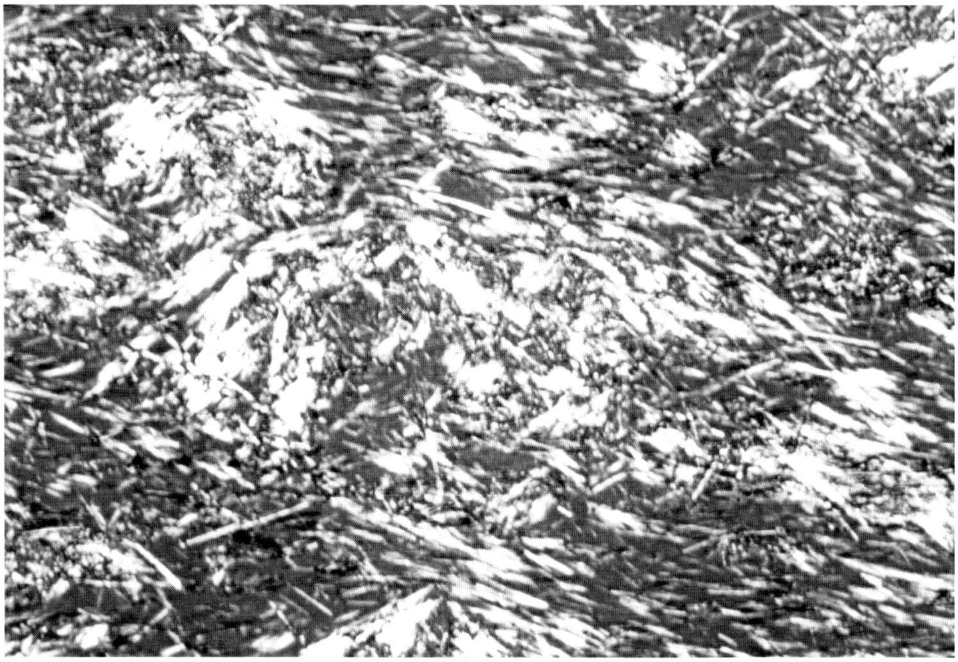

Fig. 3.12 Uric acid crystals in synovial fluid. Polarized light ×400, o m

Cutaneous Lesions Resulting from Hereditary Impaired Control and Defense Mechanism

As an example of a failure in homeostasis control, mention may be made of hereditary angioedema. This disorder results from the hereditary lack of the inhibitor of the activated C1 fraction of complement. If unchecked, to the activation of C1, the triggering of the whole cascade may follow, with diffuse edema of the subcutaneous tissue as a first consequence.

Lesions due to the Failure in Repair of the Organism

Xeroderma pigmentosum is an example of this situation, insofar as the congenital lack of DNA-repair enzyme allows the irrestricted proliferation of mutant clones in these patients. This gives rise to basal and squamous cell carcinoma as well as melanoma, not different from those described in Chap. 6.

References

1. Pinkus H, Mehregan AH. A guide to dermatohistopathology. New York: Appleton-Century-Crofts; 1973. p. 407.
2. DiGiovanna JJ. In: Freedberg IM, et al., editors. Fitzpatrik dermatologia en medicina general, 5th ed. Buenos Aires: Editorial Medica Panamericana; 2001. p. 616–24.
3. Mehregan AH, Hashimoto K, editors. Pinkus' guide to dermatohistopathology. 5th ed. Norwalk: Appleton & Lange; 1991. p. 403–9.
4. Mehregan AH, Hashimoto K, editors. Pinkus' guide to dermatohistopathology. 5th ed. Norwalk: Appleton & Lange; 1991. p. 168.
5. Lever WF, Schaumburg-Lever G. Histopathology of the skin. 7th ed. Philadelphia: J.B. Lipppincott; 1990. p. 79.
6. Braun-Falco O, Plewig G, Wolff WW, Burgdorf WHC, editors. Dermatology. 2nd ed. Berlin: Springer; 2000. p. 840.
7. Barkowich AJ, Kutzniewsky RI. In: Goldman L, Ausiello D, editors. Cecil textbook of medicine, 22nd ed. Philadelphia: Saunders; 2004. p. 2361–3.
8. Enzinger F, Weiss SW. Soft tissue tumors. 3rd ed. St. Louis: Mosby; 1995. p. 851–63.
9. James WD, Berger TG, Elston DM, editors. Andrews' diseases of the skin. 10th ed. Philadelphia: W.B. Saunders; 2006. p. 552–4.
10. Darier J. Precis de dermatologie. 4th ed. Paris: Masson et Cie, Editeurs; 1928. p. 455.
11. Goldsmith LA. In: Freedberg IM, et al., editors. Fitzpatrik dermatologia en medicina general, 5th ed. Buenos Aires: Editorial Medica Panamericana; 2001. p. 2275–8.
12. Elsas II LJ, In: Goldman L, Ausiello D, editors. Cecil textbook of medicine, 22nd ed. Philadelphia: Saunders; 2004. p. 185–91.
13. James WB, Berger TG, Elston DM, editors. Andrews' diseases of the skin. 10th ed. Philadelphia: W.B. Saunders; 2006. p. 533–4.
14. Braverman IM. Skin signs of systemic diseases. 3rd ed. Philadelphia: W.B. Saunders Co.; 1998. p. 467–74.
15. Harber LC, Bickers DR. In: Thiers BH, Dobson RL, editors. Pathogenesis of skin diseases. New York: Churchill Livingstone; 1986, p. 341–57.
16. Lever WF, Schaumburg-Lever G. Histopathology of the skin. 7th ed. Philadelphia: J.B. Lipppincott; 1990. p. 462–5.
17. Lever WF, Schaumburg-Lever G. Histopathology of the skin. 7th ed. Philadelphia: J.B. Lipppincott; 1990. p. 464.
18. Braun-Falco O, Plewig G, Wolff HH, Burgdorf WHC, editors. Dermatology. 2nd ed. Berlin: Springer; 2000. p. 1335–6.

Malformative Lesions

4

The individual members of this division of cutaneous lesions are called "malformations." Malformations occur during ontogenesis and are therefore *congenital*; they may or may not be hereditary. According to the time at which they occur, cutaneous malformations may be subdivided as early or late malformations (Fig. 4.1).

Early Malformations

Early malformations are the result of dynamic problems such as interruption of migratory processes, misdirected or incomplete shifts, and defective fusions or obliterations of embryonal parts. They frequently reflect the pernicious effects of environmental factors (radiation and other forms of contamination) on embryonic structures. They can also reflect iatrogenic, hormonal, or carential factors as well as the effects of infectious agents on the embryo. These lesions may be classified as melanocytic, fusion line cysts, and vestigial structures.

Table 4.1 offers examples of early malformations. In the designation of some of the lesions, the term "*nevus*" is applied. This term is used here in a general, traditional context, as already explained in p. 5.

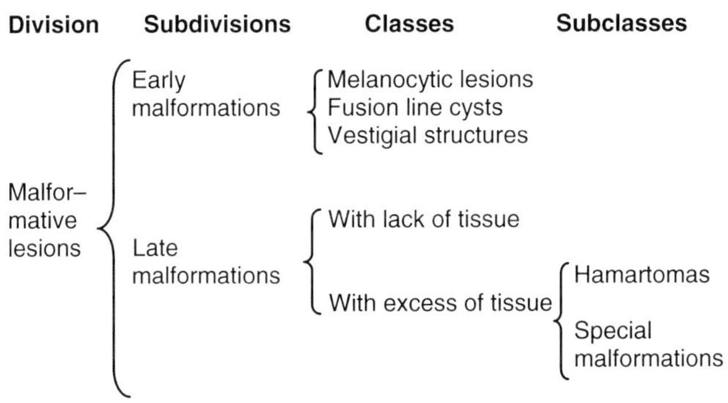

Fig. 4.1 Malformative lesions: Subdivisions, Classes, and Subclasses

Melanocytic Lesions

Melanocytic lesions, the first Class of early malformations, are the result of disturbances which prevent melanocytes to complete their migration from the neural crest to the epidermis, forcing these to remain within the dermis or even at lower planes. The presence of melanocytes is recognized in the five mentioned examples listed in Table 4.1 by a slate gray discoloration of the overlying skin.

Blue nevus receives that particular name from the bluish discoloration of its external surface. The lesion is formed by bundles of elongated melanin-loaded melanocytes, frequently located around pilosebaceous complexes and sometimes reaching the subcutaneous fat or even deeper planes (Fig. 4.2).

Combined nevus is a lesion which should be mentioned in connection with blue nevus: it is formed by the combination of a blue nevus with an overlying lentigo [1]. The three lesions, Mongolian spot, nevus Ota, and nevus Ito, offer a similar microscopic picture, characterized by scattered

Table 4.1 Early malformative lesions: classes and examples

Melanocytic lesions
Blue nevus
Combined nevus
Mongolian spot
Nevus Ota
Nevus Ito
Fusion line cysts
Pilonidal cyst
Dermal cyst
Branchial cyst
Cyst of the penile raphe
Vestigial embryonal structures
Mesonephric remnants
Papilliferous cyst of the vulva
Omphalomesenteric cyst
Thyroglossal duct cyst
Syringocystadenoma papilliferum
Warty dyskeratoma

E. Zappi, E.A. Zappi, *Dermatopathology*,
DOI 10.1007/978-1-4471-2894-6_4, © Springer-Verlag London 2013

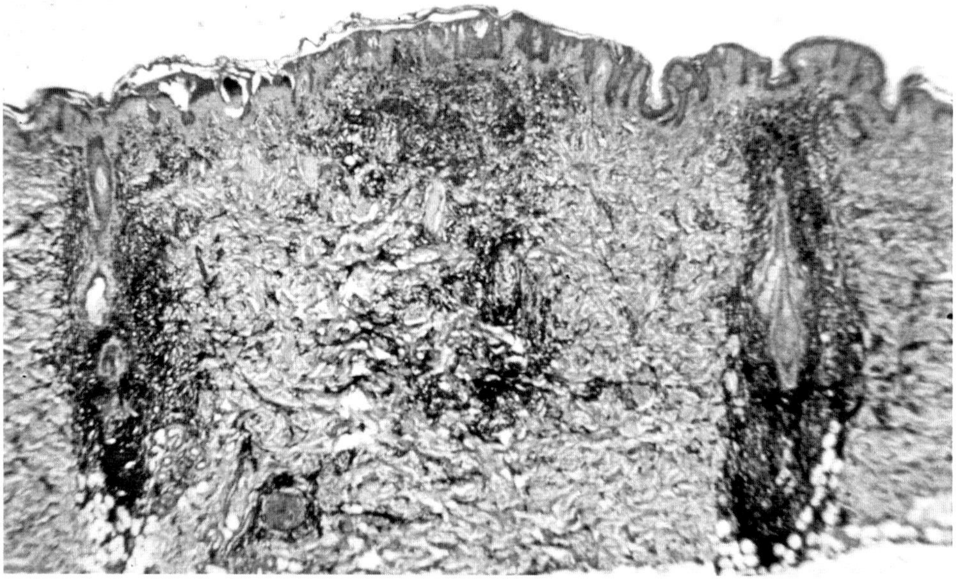

Fig. 4.2 Blue nevus. Two separate blue nevi are noted, formed by packed melanocytes located around hair complexes. MP×100, o m

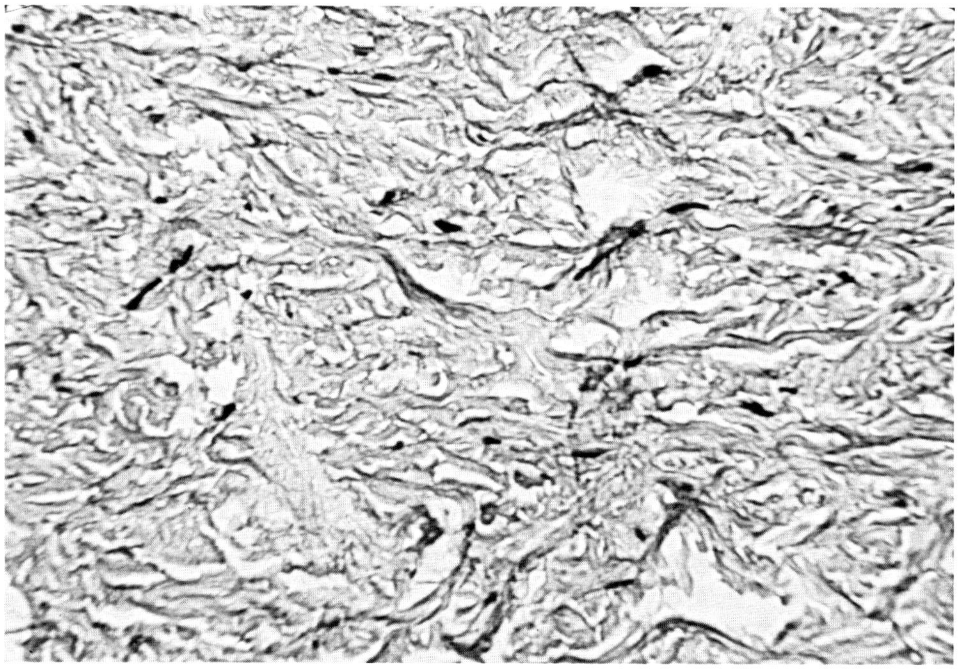

Fig. 4.3 Mongolian spot. Scant melanocytes are noted scattered in the dermis of the specimen. This nonspecific picture does not allow the identification of any of the three entities mentioned above. MP×1,000, o m

melanocytes dispersed in the dermis. This nonspecific histologic appearance does not allow the microscopic identification of these lesions. This can easily be accomplished otherwise, considering their anatomic localization: Mongolian spot appears on the sacral region, while nevus Ota and nevus Ito are found on the face and shoulder, respectively, following a trigeminal and brachial plexus distribution (Fig. 4.3).

Fusion Line Cysts

A cyst (kystis [G] a sac or a bladder) is a cavity surrounded by its own capsule and lined in the inside by its own tissue. Its lumen may be secondarily filled by debris or other material shed into the cavity, but a cyst is, primarily, a *hollow*, not a *solid* structure.

The cysts that the dermatologists are concerned with may be formed in embryonal or extrauterine life. According to their pathogenesis, the former is called here "*fusion line cysts*" and the latter "*retention cysts*." Fusion line cysts are discussed in the next paragraphs, whereas the study of the retention cysts shall be postponed to Chap. 6. The entity studied in gynecology under the name "*dermoid cyst*" is not a cyst but a "teratoma" [2], representing one of the most frequent ovarian tumors totally unrelated to dermatopathology.

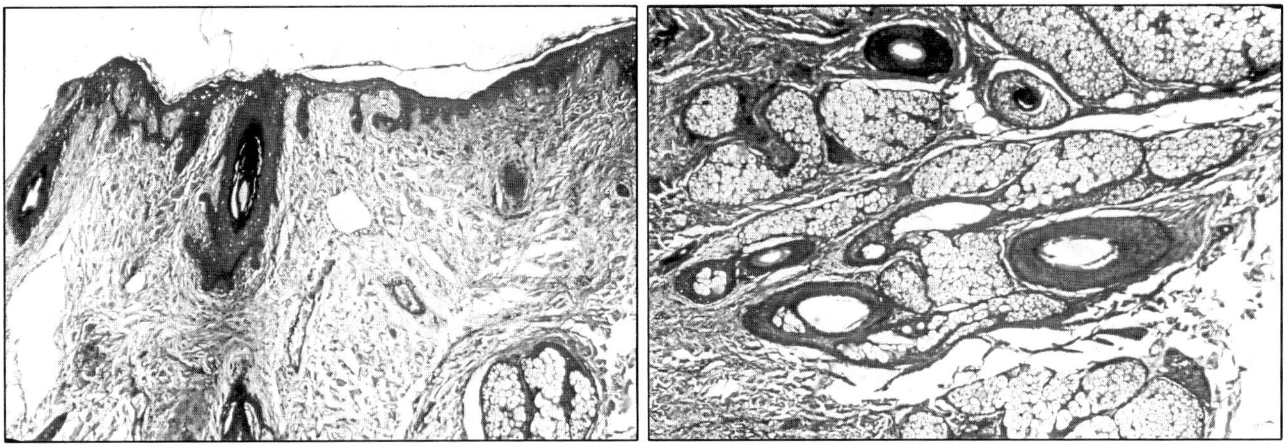

Fig. 4.4 Pilonidal cyst. Note the abundant pilosebaceous complexes included in the wall of the cyst. H&E; ×100, o m

Fig. 4.5 Branchial cyst. Note the subtle brush on the external surface of the pseudostratified epithelium lining the cystic space. H&E ×400, o m

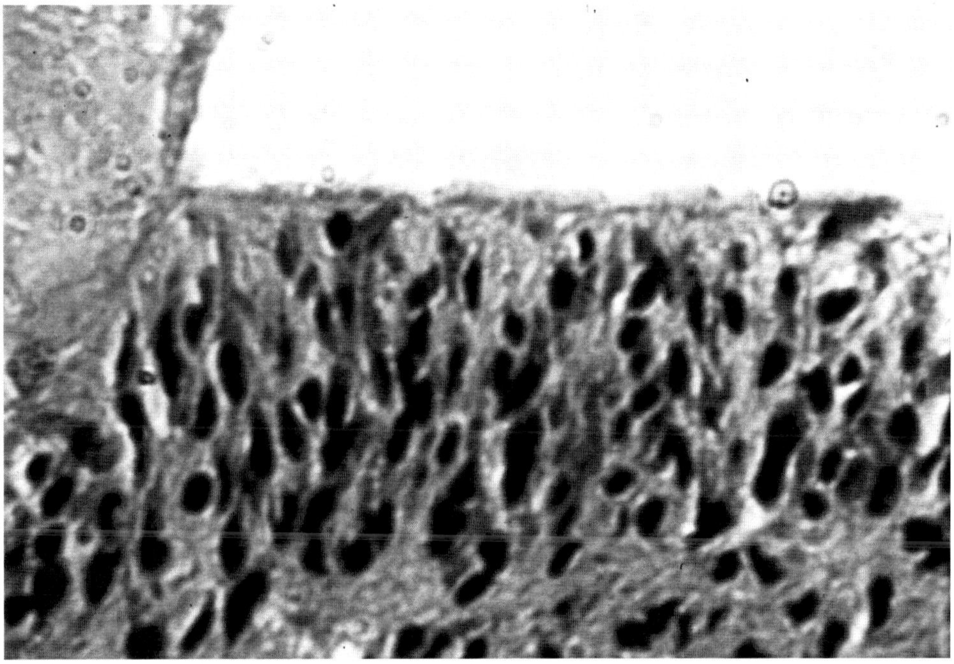

Fusion line cysts originate during early ontogenesis from fragments of tissue interposed and trapped in the line of fusion of developing embryonal parts. The sequestered tissue, if viable, may spread out, to line the wall of the cleft left by the faulty apposition, forming a cystic cavity.

The prototypic and not infrequent fusion line cyst is the pilonidal cyst, located on the sacrococcygeal region. It is formed during closure of the neural tube and features in its wall a large number of pilosebaceous complexes disposed in disarray (Fig. 4.4). Pilonidal cysts may be secondarily infected, developing into painful abscesses.

Another not uncommon fusion line cyst is that known currently as "dermal cyst." It sits on the temporal region and derives from defects in the embryonal development of the face.

Branchial cyst – or fistula, if it happens to open to the exterior – falls also under the class of embryonal cysts. The formation of this lesion derives from the maldevelopment of the neck. This lesion is lined by the ciliated, pseudostratified epithelium found in that area (Fig. 4.5).

Cyst of the raphe of the penis is another example of embryonal cyst. It is formed upon the closure of the male urogenital groove, featuring the transitional epithelium of the urethra as its inner lining (Fig. 4.6).

Vestigial Embryonic Structures

The third class of early malformations (Table 4.1) is formed by remnants of embryonic structures which did not entirely

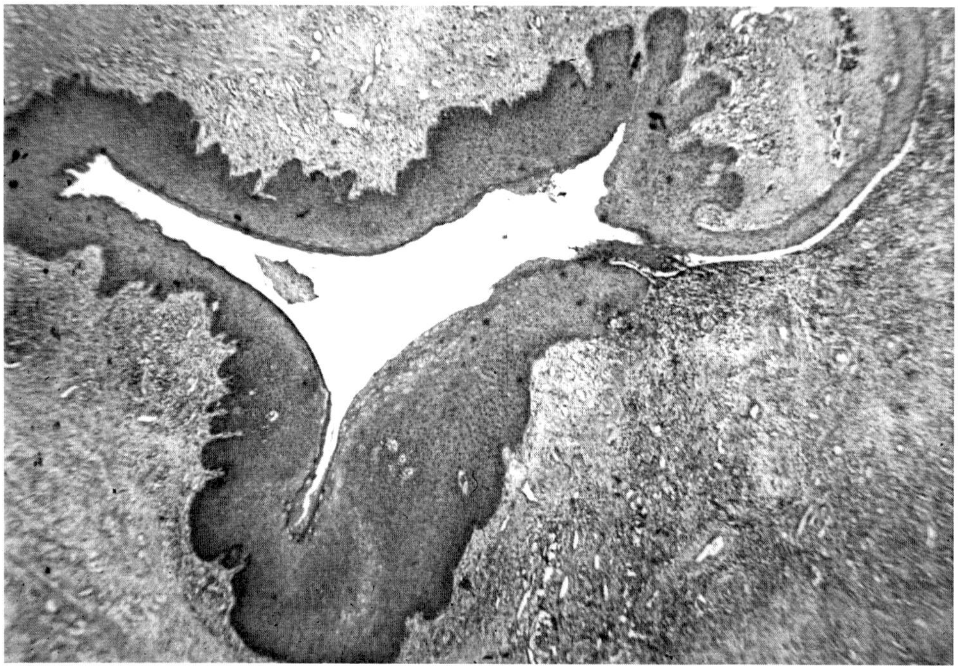

Fig. 4.6 Cyst of the raphe of the penis. Note the triangular-shaped cavity and the thick layer of transitional epithelium lining it. Observe the fistulous tract arising from the right upper corner of the cavity. H&E ×20, o m

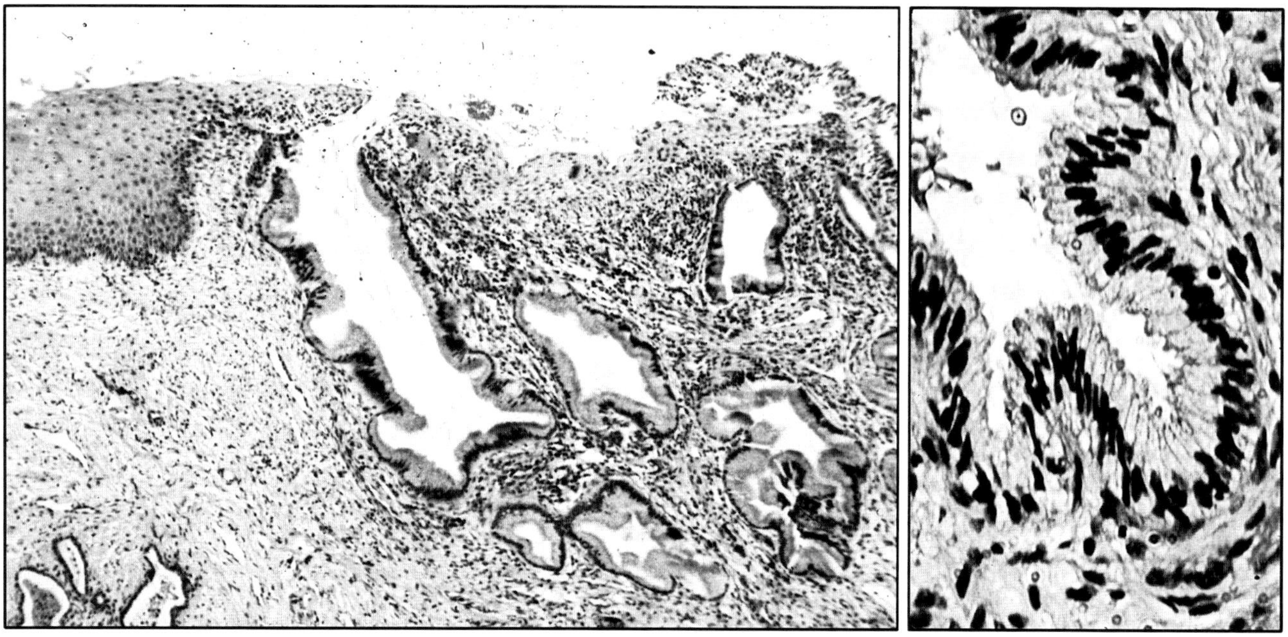

Fig. 4.7 Mesonephric ductules (*left*). This lesion, found in a female perineum, is formed by a group of disconnected ductules located in a fibrous stroma (*right*). The lining epithelium, devoid of malignant features, is formed by tall cylindrical cells with basal nuclei. H&E ×40; ×400, o m

follow their programmed involution during the ontogenesis: several of these are associated to the development of the female urogenital system. This is the case of the mesonephric ductules which may eventually be found in adult women in the broad ligament and the perineum (Fig. 4.7).

A second of these vestigial structures, eventually a remnant of the Mullerian tube, is shown in Fig. 4.8.

Papilliferum cyst of the vulva is a third vestigial structure associated to the development of the female urogenital system. This lesion (Fig. 4.9) shows a high level of organization, faithfully repeated from one specimen to another. It lacks aggressivity, which belies the neoplastic connotation given to it by the original name "hidradenoma papilliferum of the vulva."

Two other vestigial structures whose origin is obvious are omphalomesenteric remnants and thyroglossal duct. Omphalomesenteric remnants may appear as periumbilical oozing nodules on lactating or young babies. They are formed

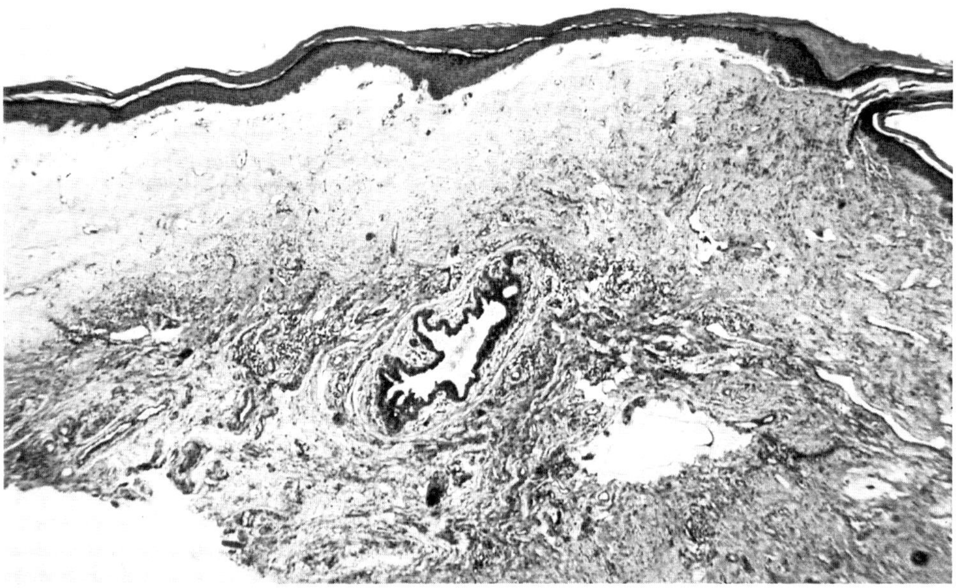

Fig. 4.8 Remnants of a Mullerian tube. Sectioned tubes are found, in this particular case, in the vulva of a patient affected by *kraurosis vulva*. Note the highly edematous dermis, surrounding the ducts and separated from the atrophic epidermis by a cleft. H&E ×40, o m

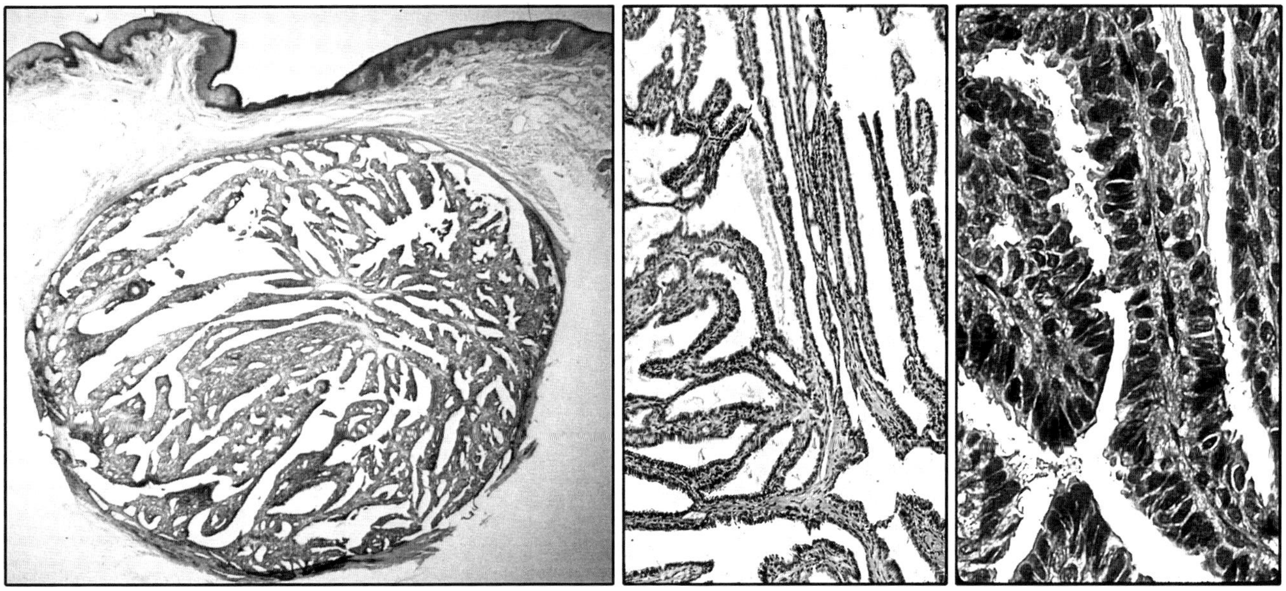

Fig. 4.9 Papilliferum cyst of the vulva (*left*). The lesion appears surrounded by a fibrous capsule and is clearly separated from the surrounding stroma. It is lined by a cylindric epithelium devoid of malignant changes or mitotic activity, thrown as long folds into the center of the cavity. Higher magnification images (*center and right*) show details of the lesion. H&E ×4; ×100; ×400, o m

by remnants of the omphalomesenteric duct, which normally involutes and disappears by the second month of embryonal life. Upon microscopic examination, they appear as fibrous nodules covered on the top by primitive intestinal epithelium, in direct continuation with the epidermis (Fig. 4.10).

The existence of thyroglossal duct remnants is usually denoted by the appearance of one or several nodules in a linear disposition along the midline above the sternal notch. They correspond to localized dilatations of the thyroglossal duct, and under the microscope, they show a cavity lined by the cuboidal single-layered thyroid epithelium. The cavity may eventually contain colloid in the lumen.

In order to complete the discussion of the early malformations, syringocystadenoma papilliferum and warty dyskeratoma should now be considered. Both of these are generally solitary nodules on the head and nape of neck, frequently reaching the size of a pea. The complex and organized structures of these two lesions are closely reproduced in separate cases. Their indolent character – which leads them to remain unchanged for years after reaching their maximal size – indicates that they are not actively proliferating structures. The taxonomic problem faced upon trying to classify them is that there are no embryonal structures to which they may be homologized. For this reason, their putative vestigial

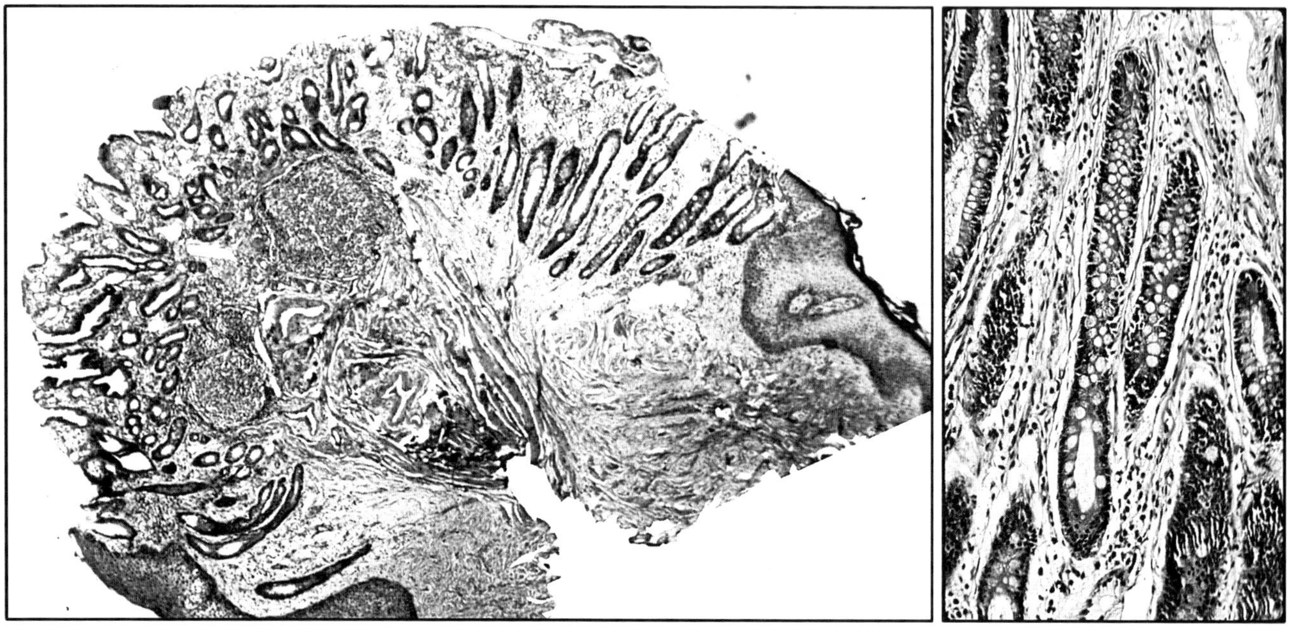

Fig. 4.10 Omphalomesenteric duct remnants (*left*). The lesion is formed by a vascularized fibrotic nodule showing a couple of germinal centers. It is overlaid by primitive intestinal epithelium prolonged on both slopes by normal squamous epidermis (*right*). Details of the intestinal glands are given. H&E ×40; ×100, o m

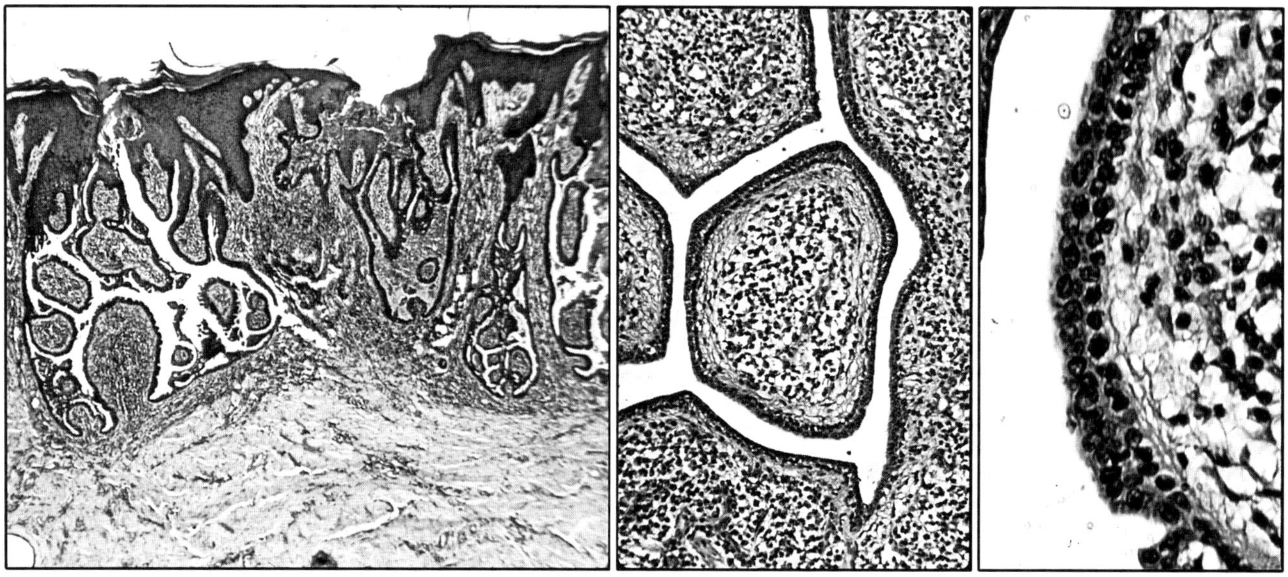

Fig. 4.11 Syringocystadenoma papilliferum (*left*). The lesion, encased in the skin and surrounded by a dense cellular infiltrate is formed by thick, irregular cords. Higher magnification shows its double-layered epithelium (*center*) and its plasmacytic infiltrate (*right*). H&E ×40; ×100; ×400, o m

nature cannot be further supported. These two lesions could be alternatively placed with the "special malformations" (Table 4.4), but, at any rate, the important thing is to lay them in Chap. 4, in order to emphasize their *malformative* rather than *neoplastic* character, as is frequently claimed.

Syringocystadenoma papilliferum appears upon microscopic examination as a rather circumscribed and organized structure set deeply in the skin. It is formed by broad tissue projections originating from the bottom and reaching the external surface of the skin. Under cross-section examination, the projections feature a polygonal contour, being delimited by a characteristic double-layered epithelium formed by a lower layer of cuboidal elements, overlaid by a second one of short cylindrical ones. In the stroma of the projections, there is an almost pure collection of plasma cells (Fig. 4.11).

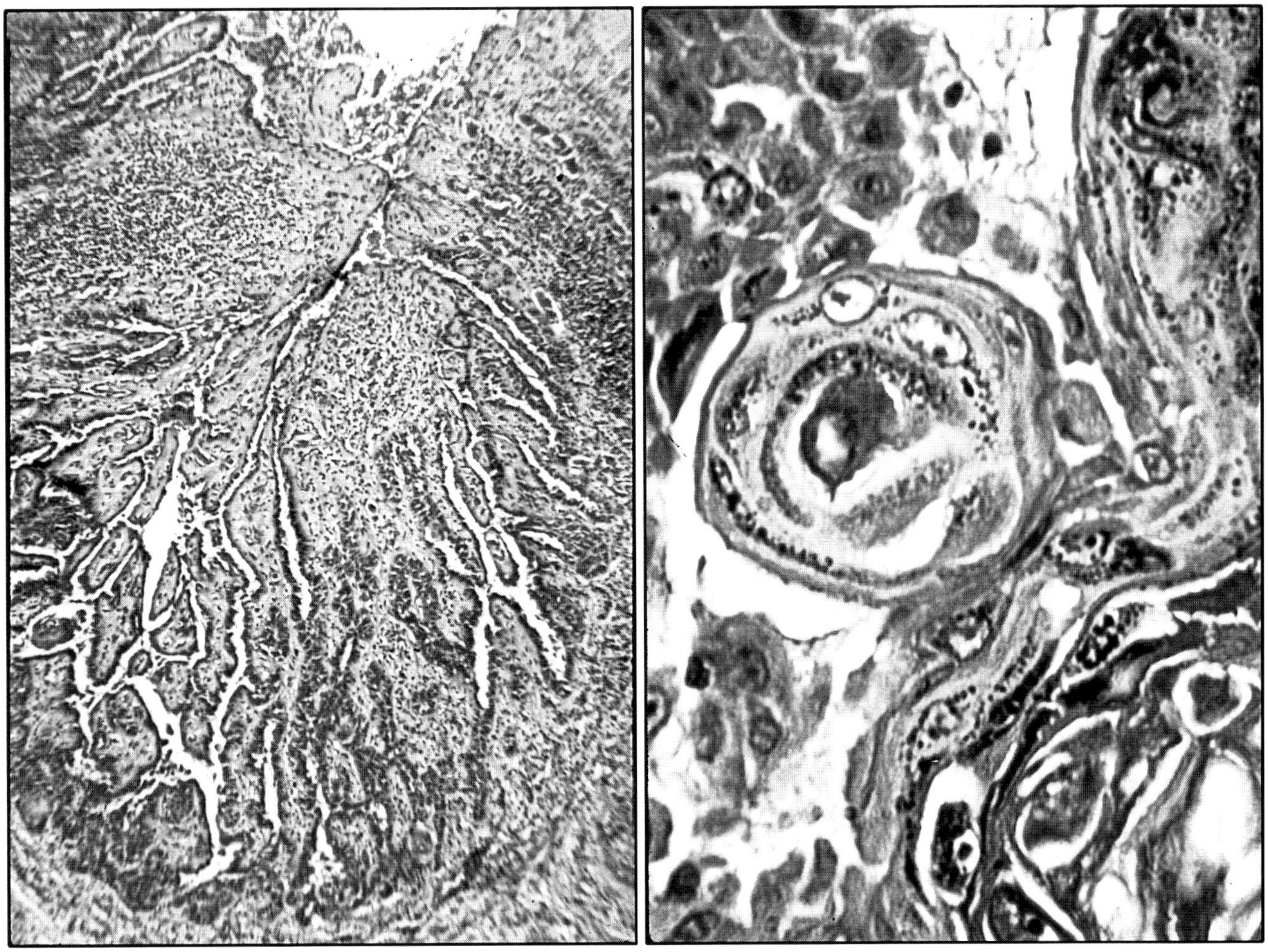

Fig. 4.12 Warty dyskeratoma. Note the crusted external surface of the lesion. Observe the irregular clefts and the suprabasal acantholysis within the high cellular lesion (*left*) and the dyskeratotic elements (corps ronds and grains) similar to the ones in Darier's lesion (*right*). H&E ×40; ×400, o m

Warty dyskeratoma exhibits a crateriform structure encased in the skin, often with a fistulous tract connecting it to the outside. The lesion is lined by squamous stratified epithelium featuring suprabasal acantholysis and benign dyskeratosis. These two features make this lesion microscopically comparable to that associated with Darier's disease (p. 28) (Fig. 4.12).

Late Malformations

Late malformations are hereby simply called "malformations" so as to differentiate them from "early malformations." Malformations do not have the dynamic implication nor the depth of the latter. They are generally of a superficial and circumscribed character and may occur either in a sporadic, isolated fashion or associated to hereditary disorders, as discussed in Chap. 3. They may be hypothetically considered products of fortuitous "aberrant embryonal centers," as proposed by P.G. Unna many years ago [3].

In the Subdivision of late malformations, two Classes may be recognized. These are the ones which lack of, or have an excess of, normal components of the skin. They are therefore known as *minus* and *plus malformations*, respectively (Fig. 4.1).

Minus Malformations

Minus malformations are characterized by the absence in circumscribed areas of the skin of some or all of the normal cutaneous components. Table 4.2 presents examples of these entities: because of their obvious character, they do not deserve detailed microscopic descriptions.

Plus Malformations

In the Class of plus malformations, two Subclasses must be distinguished: hamartomas and special malformations (Fig. 4.1).

Table 4.2 Malformation with missing tissues

Lesion	Missing element
Nevus alopecicus	Pilosebaceous complex
Nevus anemicus	Blood vessels
Nevus atrophicus	Collagen tissue
Depigmented nevus	Melanocytes
Aplasia cutis congenita	Entire skin

Table 4.3 Cutaneous hamartomas: groups and examples

Dermoepidermal
Nevus verrucosus
Linear epidermal nevus
Adnexal
Nevus sudoriparus
Nevus pilosus
Nevus sebaceous
Mesenchymatous
Nevus araneus*
Hemangioma, capillary
Hemangioma, cavernous*
Port wine spot
Cirsoid aneurism
Angiokeratoma Mibelli's
Arteriovenous fistula
Pringle's tumor*
Koenen tumor*
Ash leaves*
Nevus elasticus
Combined
Nevus sebaceous Jadassohn

Note: *Denotes an eventual dysgenetic background in the lesion

Hamartomas

Hamartomas are common occurrences in the dermatologic practice. Their distinctive microscopic character is the *disorder* in which their components are disposed (*hamartia* [G] an error). Hamartomas (a) are circumscribed masses of tissue; (b) are of benign nature and (c) have autolimited growth; (d) are formed by components indigenous to the organ where they occur; and (e) appear in disarray and (f) without reproducing the structure of any organ.

According to their predominantly histologic composition, hamartomas may be grouped as: dermoepidermal, adnexal, mesenchymatous, mixed, and combined (Table 4.3). The nomenclature of hamartomas is heterogeneous and varied: it includes, along with eponymic names, other names simply descriptive of their gross features or histologic composition. Hamartomas may appear in an extemporary fashion or related to hereditary conditions. The latter possibility is indicated in Table 4.3 by the asterisk attached to the name of each item.

Dermoepidermal Hamartomas

The prototypical dermoepidermal hamartoma is nevus verrucosus, a lesion generated by focal, disorganized, and synergic dermoepidermal proliferation. LM examination of the lesion reveals a combination of hyperkeratosis, acanthosis, and papillomatosis (Fig. 4.13), featuring an image almost indistinguishable without clinical help, from that of seborrheic keratosis.

On occasion, the papillomatosis in nevus verrucosus leads to the formation of recesses which, even if lacking a significant microscopic expression, may change the external image of the lesion, which appears dotted by black spots. This may lead to its descriptive, although incorrect,

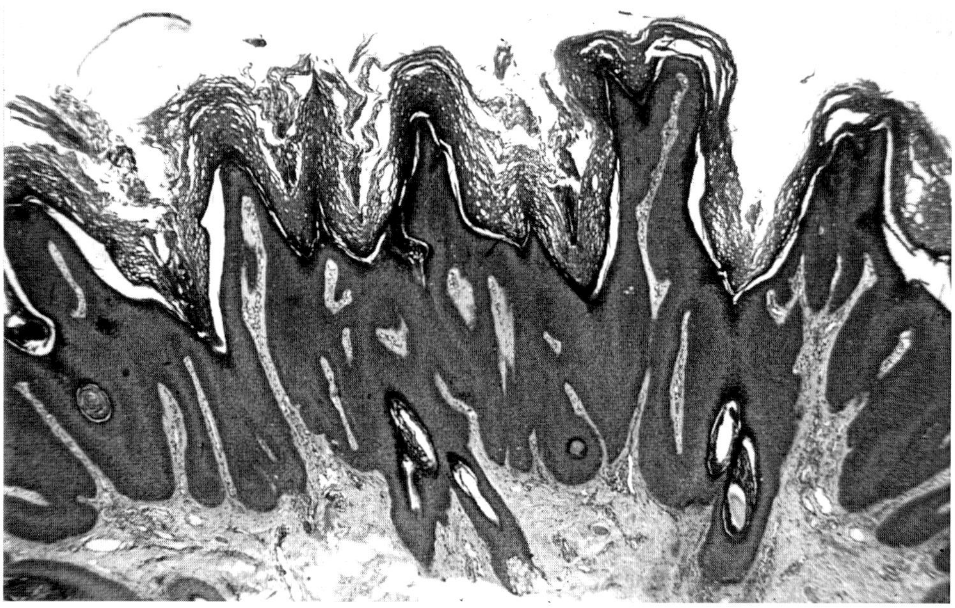

Fig. 4.13 Nevus verrucosus. See details in the text. H&E ×40, o m

diagnosis as "nevus comedonicus" (see p. 186 for the definition of comedo).

Instead of its usual focal character, nevus verrucosus may present a linear appearance known clinically as "linear epidermal nevus." If a mononuclear cell infiltration is found under microscopic inspection, the lesion may be called "inflammatory linear verrucous epidermal nevus," abbreviated as "ILVEN," although the mononuclear infiltrate probably does not respond to an inflammatory reaction, being a malformative component of the lesion instead. ILVEN may even be associated to warty dyskeratoma or present epidermolytic hyperkeratosis.

Adnexal Hamartomas

The histologic composition of the adnexal hamartomas is clearly defined by their names, nevus pilosus, nevus sebaceous, nevus sudoriparous, etc., as demonstrated in Fig. 4.14, which also shows the characteristically disorganized structure of these lesions.

Mesenchymal Hamartomas

The simplest of the mesenchymal hamartomas is capillary hemangioma, a particular example of which is rubi spot, frequently seen on the abdomen of aged people. It consists of a tuft of dilated capillaries (Fig. 4.15, left). Spider angioma made up of dilated vessels exiting from a central point on the skin is also a capillary hemangioma. It may appear disconnected from any ongoing condition in the patient, or forming part of a hereditary syndrome, as previously explained (p. 34).

Nevus Flammeus: This lesion is a capillary hemangioma as well but whose elements appear as a thick, diffuse matt. It is most frequently found on the posterior neck and head: whereas the one on the neck is in general devoid of further significance, the one on the lateral face may represent a port-wine stain, that is, a component of Sturge-Weber-Dimitri syndrome. The internal counterpart of this syndrome are ipsilateral, diffuse vascular malformations involving the meninges and cerebral cortex. Since these malformations may extend to the retina, featuring *phakomas* (p. 34), Sturge-Weber-Dimitri syndrome is sometimes considered a phakomatosis. This assumption is incorrect since this condition is not transmitted (as phakomatoses should) via Mendelian patterns.

Cavernous hemangiomas are vascular hamartomas formed by blood vessels of large caliber (Fig. 4.15, right). They appear on the skin surface or internal organs, most frequently as isolated, sporadic lesions. They may also be seen in the congenital – though not hereditary – Maffucci syndrome, associated to dyschondroplasia, or otherwise, forming part of some of the HPDwCPs mentioned before.

As an unexpected complication in patients bearing cavernous hemangiomas, mention must be made of the purpuric syndrome of Kasabach-Merritt, of fearful consequences. It is triggered by the sequestration and destruction of blood platelets within a cavernous hemangioma which may lead to uncontrollable hemorrhages and the demise of the patient.

Cirsoid aneurysm and arteriovenous fistula are related vascular hamartomas, hereby worthy of mention. Cirsoid aneurysm (*kyros* [G] varix) is a special type of cavernous hemangioma formed by a pack of vascular elements of thick and irregular walls (Fig. 4.16, left). This lesion may only be recognized through LM, since it does not present any external feature which may allow its clinical diagnosis. According to some authors, this lesion constitutes a real aneurysm originated in a defective vessel [4]. Arteriovenous fistulas consist of conglomerates of irregular blood vessels with thickened walls and variable caliber (Fig. 4.16). Since these lesions are associated to an excessive blood flow, they may lead to cardiac hypertrophy and insufficiency. In the congenital Klippel-Trenaunay syndrome, whose most significant components are arteriovenous fistulas, these lead to localized gigantism of the patient's limbs affected by the increased blood flow.

In the review of cavernous hemangiomas, angiokeratomas must be included. Angiokeratoma was originally described by V. Mibelli as multiple papules sitting on the dorsum of fingers and toes. Its LM examination shows dilated blood vessels fully occupying dermal papillae and in direct contact with the epidermis which outline these. Fordyce's angiokeratoma, found on the scrotum or vulva, shows essentially the same composition (Fig. 4.17, left and right).

At the end of the review of vascular hamartomas, lymphangiomas should now be briefly discussed. The bulkiest one of these is the cavernous, also known by the name of cystic hygroma (Fig. 4.18). This is a structure formed by dilated vessels in intimate contact with the epidermis. In contrast to arterial or venous malformations – and for obvious reasons – this lesion appears devoid of erythrocytes.

In the discussion of mesenchymal hamartomas, the three types associated with tuberous sclerosis (p. 35) should be included. These are Pringle's tumor, Koenen tumor, and ash leaf. These three have a similar fibrovascular composition and can only be distinguished by their anatomic location. Because of their similarity, the description shall be limited to Koenen tumor: its microscopic examination shows a fibrovascular nucleus of tissue overlaid by a hyperkeratotic epidermis (Fig. 4.19).

Lastly, in this discussion of mesenchymal hamartomas, mention should be made of mastocytoma. This lesion, appearing as multiple papules in cases of infantile urticaria pigmentosa, usually regresses without leaving major problems. Since mast cells are mesenchymal elements and appear in disarray, it seems justified to classify an infantile mastocytoma – formed by a cluster of mast cells – as a *mesenchymal malformation* (Fig. 4.20).

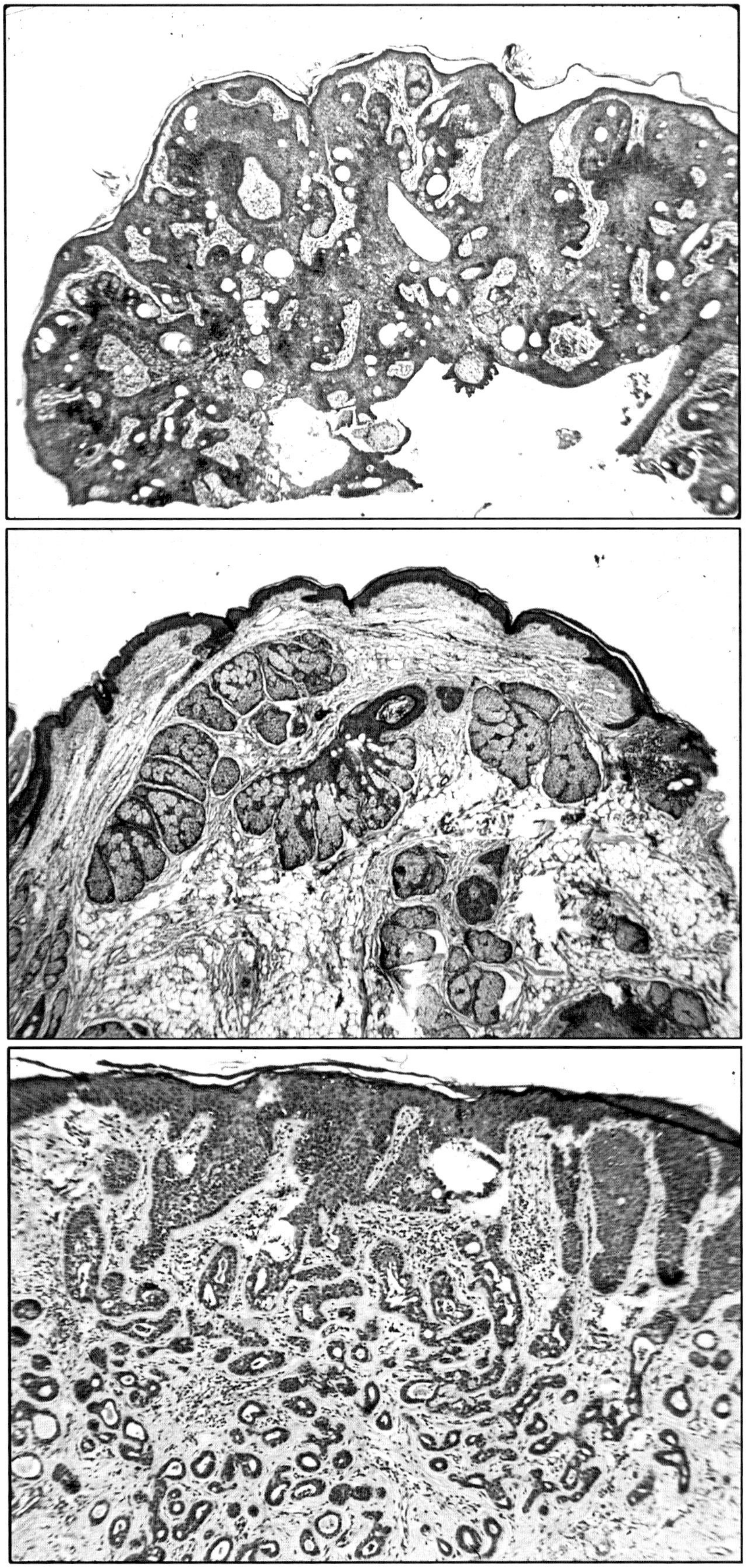

Fig. 4.14 Nevus pilosus, nevus sebaceous, and nevus sudoriparus (*upper*, *mid*, and *low*). Note the predominant histologic component of the three lesions: rudimentary pilar follicles, irregular clusters of sebaceous glands, and eccrine excretory ducts, respectively, in a characteristically disarrayed fashion. H&E ×40, o m

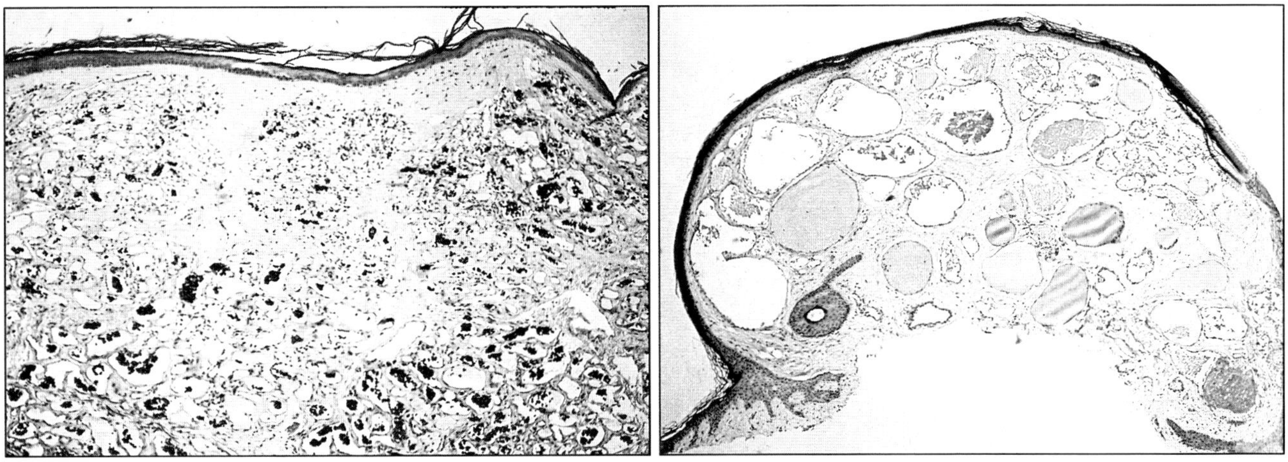

Fig. 4.15 Rubi spot and cavernous hemangioma. The rubi spot (*left*) is formed by multitude of capillaries diffusely occupying the dermis, which appears covered by a flat, uninvolved epidermis. Contrast the caliber of the vessels in this lesion with that of the cavernous hemangioma (*right*). H&E ×40, o m

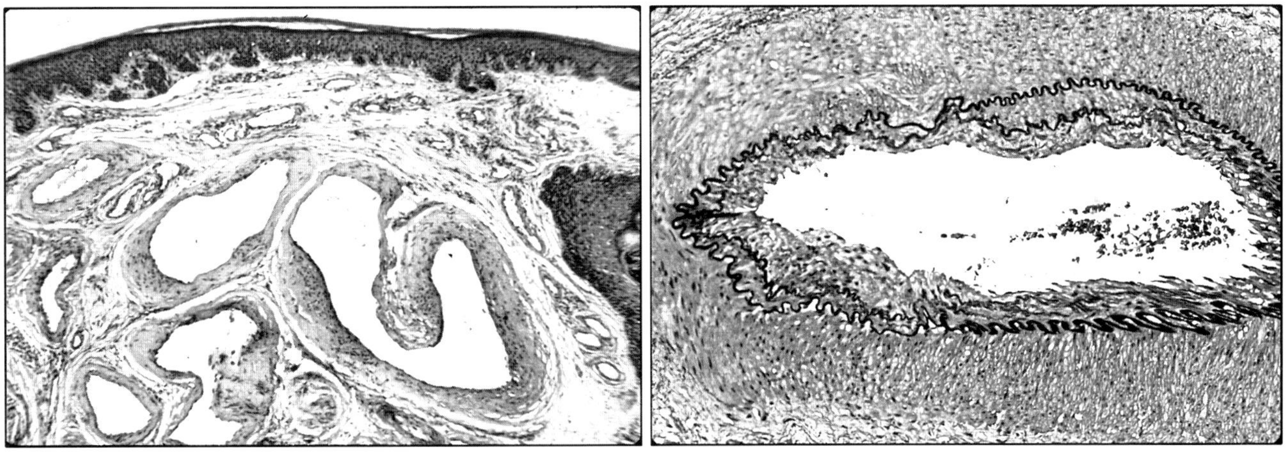

Fig. 4.16 Cirsoid aneurysm and arteriovenous fistula. Cirsoid aneurysm (*left*) shows an agglomeration of convoluted blood vessels of thickened walls and variable caliber. The isolated blood vessel (*right*) is part of an extensive arteriovenous fistula not shown in the picture. Its wall shows an irregular thickening of the muscular layer and a duplication of the elastic coat. H&E ×40; EvG ×100, o m

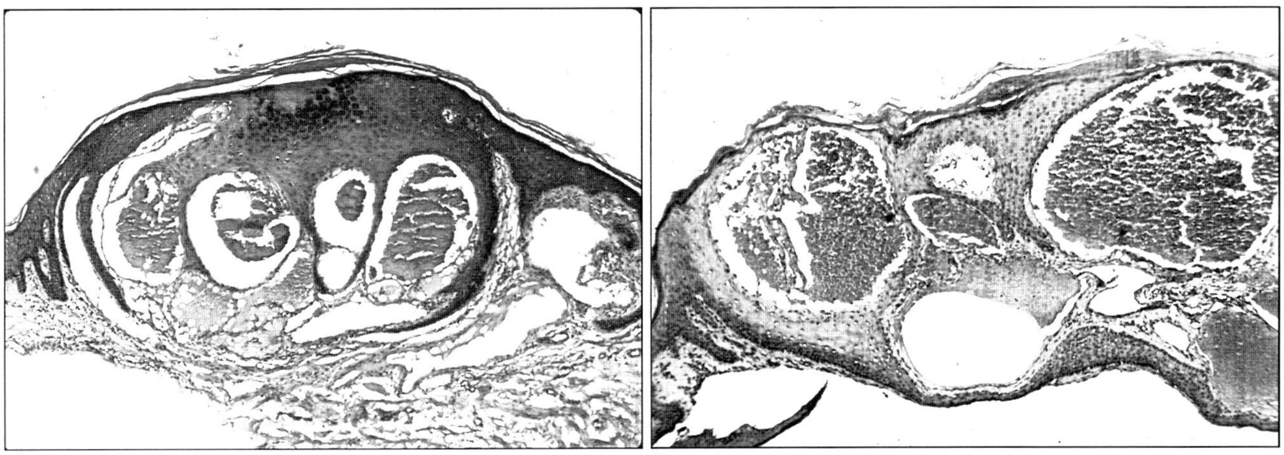

Fig. 4.17 Angiokeratoma Mibelli and Fordyce. Both lesions (*left and right*, respectively) show an essentially similar picture, characterized by large blood vessels totally occupying dermal papillae and in direct contact with the overlying epidermis. This one appears hyperkeratotic, partially outlining the vessels. H&E ×40, o m

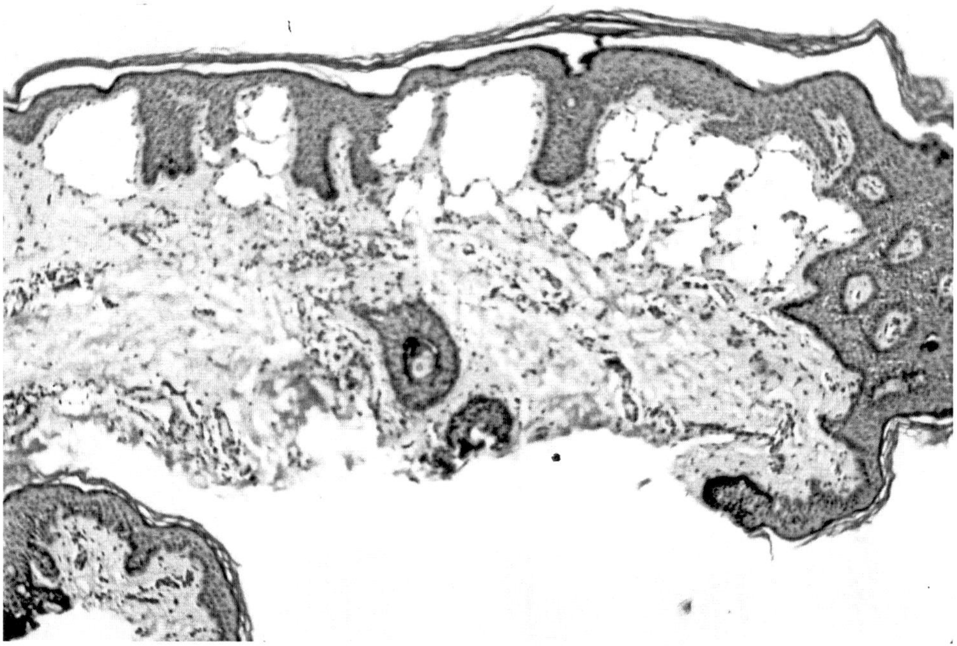

Fig. 4.18 Cystic hygroma. See details in the text. H&E ×40, o m

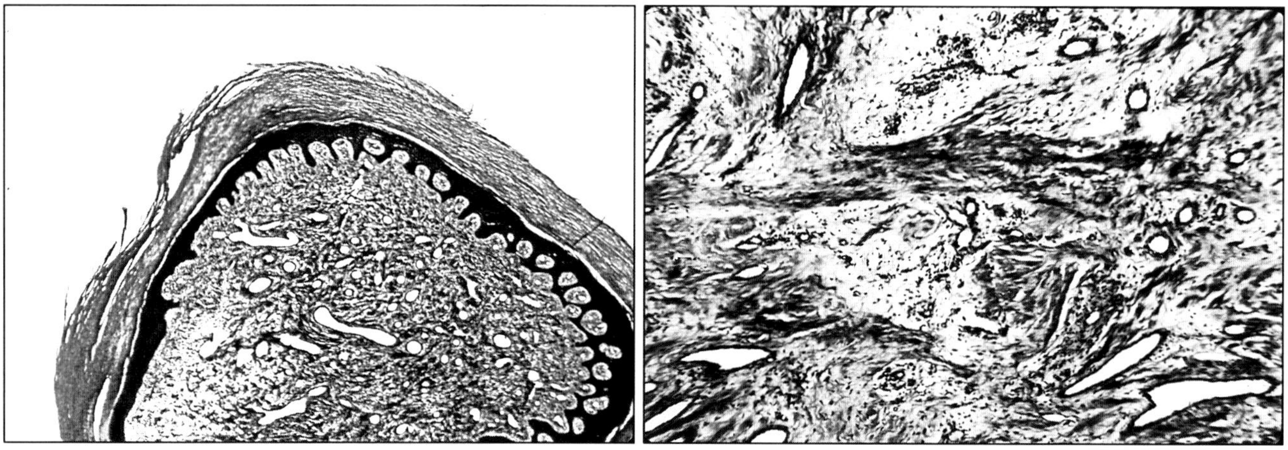

Fig. 4.19 Koenen tumor. A low and a high magnification picture of the lesion (*left and right*) reveals its fibrovascular composition. Note the regular stunt epidermal ridges (*left*), characteristic of the epidermis of the finger tips, from where the biopsy was taken. H&E ×40; Tri ×400, o m

Combined Hamartomas

In this group, only one lesion is included, known as nevus sebaceous of Jadassohn. This lesion is different from all the previously discussed hamartomas, in that it develops in three phases. In the initial one, seen in young patients, it is only a papillomatous growth sitting on the scalp. In the second phase, when the patient reaches puberty, a sebaceous component is added. Lastly, the third phase is manifested during young adulthood. At this stage, a basal cell carcinoma develops, which imparts a pathognomonic character to this lesion. Since the lesion features a double components, that is, a malformative and a neoplastic one, the qualification of "combined hamartoma" was devised for its designation (Fig. 4.21).

Special Malformations

Plus malformations which do not fulfill all the requisites set in the definition of "hamartomas" (p. 46) should be considered as belonging to the Subclass of special malformations. To the four groups of special malformations listed in Table 4.4, a fifth one was added for reasons which shall be explained below.

Malformations with Extracutaneous Components

The first group of special malformations (Table 4.4) is that of the nevocytic nevi. As explained in the previous chapter, nevocytes, or nevus cells, *are not normal components of the skin* (p. 8), and that is the reason for considering them "malformations with an extracutaneous component" rather than hamartomas.

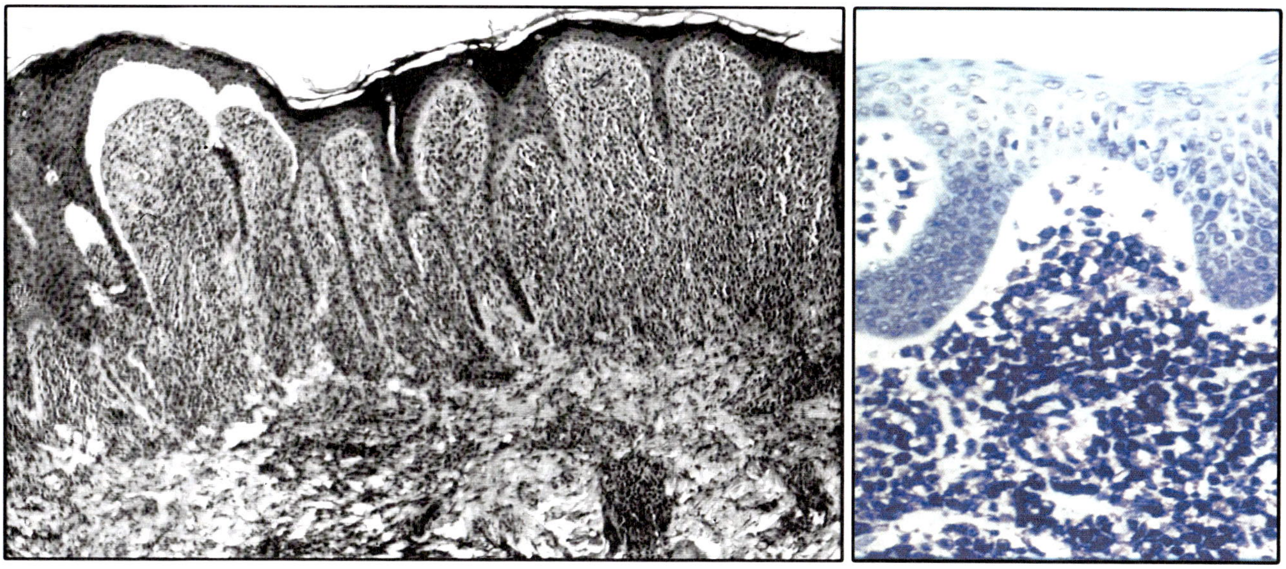

Fig. 4.20 Mastocytoma. The microscopic examination (*left*) reveals a fragment of skin with elongated dermal papillae fully occupied by mononuclear elements. These, upon staining with toluidine blue (*right*), yield a strong purple metachromasia, identifying them with mast cells. H&E ×40; TB ×100, o m

Fig. 4.21 Nevus sebaceous Jadassohn. The lesion, in the third stage of development, shows a central basal cell carcinoma. H&E ×100, o m

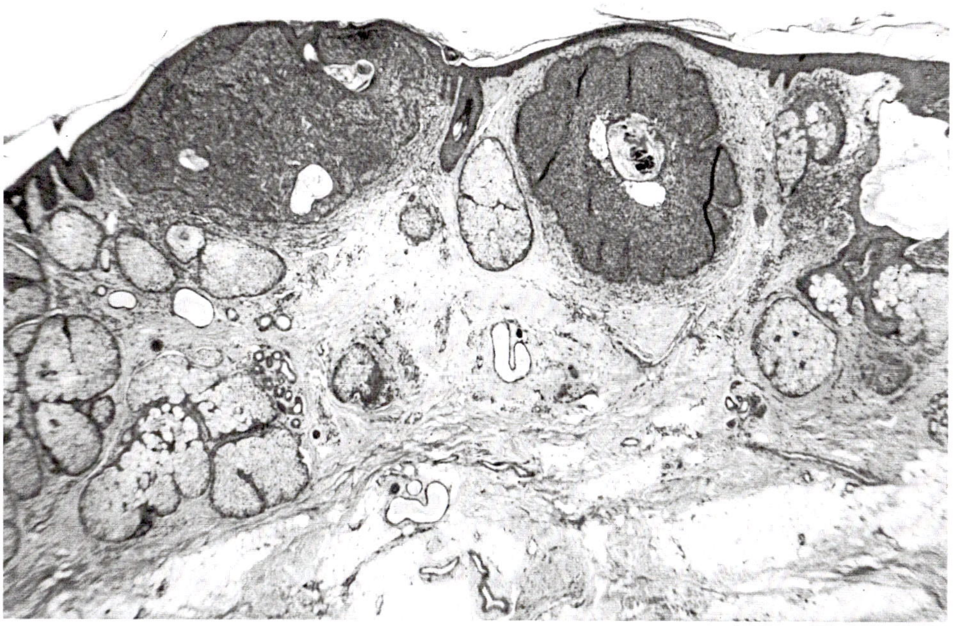

P.G. Unna placed within the "soft nevi" of his classification a group of lesion formed by the "nevocytes," which he had previously described (p. 51). In his interpretation, nevocytes were *epithelial cells* which, after proliferating in their initial position at the dermoepidermal level, expanded toward the upper level of the epidermis and, in a third step, "squeezed" or "dropped down" in the opposite direction in order to find their final position in the dermis. The resulting lesions were then successively called "junctional," "compound," and "intradermal nevi." It must be pointed out that "*compound nevus*" is not equivalent to "*combined nevus*": as formerly discussed, the latter results from the combination of a blue nevus with an overlying heavily pigmented lentigo (p. 39).

Unna's conception, fanciful although acceptable by the public at the time in which it was postulated, was presented under the name of "Abtropfen Theorie" ("dropping down theory") [5]. It was accepted enthusiastically and without reservations by the dermatologic community. Dermatologists consider that postulate still valid [6, 7], one hundred years later(!), in spite of the words of Claude Bernard, "the father of the experimental medicine," who several decades prior to Unna wrote: "Upon formulating a theory in our sciences, the

Table 4.4 Special malformations: groups and examples

With extracutaneous elements
Nevocytic nevus
Neuronevus
Nevocytic nevus, congenital
Spitz nevus
Choristoma
With high level of organization
Trichofolliculoma
Trichoepithelioma
With defective production of epidermal elements
Solitary acantholytic acanthoma
Solitary acanthoma with benign dyskeratosis
Solitary acanthoma hyperkeratotic with epidermolysis
Ephelides
With reproduction of anatomic structures
Supernumerary breast
Supernumerary nipple
Supernumerary digit
Supernumerary tragus
With tendency to spontaneous resolution
Berry angioma
Juvenile xanthogranuloma

only thing we may be sure of, is that the particular theory, in absolute terms, will turn out to be wrong" [8]. C. Bernard continued his dissertation by saying that theories are only working tools which reflect our knowledge on a certain topic at the moment when they are postulated and that they should be discarded when they prove to be inaccurate. Indeed, the *neural* origin of these cells, already suggested by Soldan in 1899, was firmly established by P. Masson in 1926 [9].

It is interesting to present the anecdotal aspect of the problem, as explained in the words of P. Masson himself [10]. He stated: "At the beginning of my career (...) I had plainly and completely adopted Unna's classic theory: 'nevus cells are nothing but proliferated epithelial cells that migrated to the dermis by a sort of 'dropping down' (*Abtropfung*). In those days I was invited to present a paper regarding nevocytes and malignant melanomas (...) but while preparing it, I felt it was necessary for me to study nevi more attentively and, more importantly, with different staining techniques." This became for him, in his own words, sort of "a trip to Damascus" in reference to the biblical episode of Paul who, falling from his horse on his way to that town, had a sudden revelation about the truth of Christianity, to which he was suddenly converted, and for which he turned into a passionate apostle.

Mason's ideas triggered a lively controversy among his followers. This was centered not so much on the *neural* origin of nevocyte but rather on the details related to their identity. In fact, some hold the viewpoint that nevocytes were Schwann cells, whereas others contended that they were immature melanocytes or nevocytes (melanoblasts or nevoblasts, respectively). This diverted the authors' attention from an important practical conclusion: if nevocytes are *of nervous and not epithelial origin, the lesions they form could not be built up by their dropping from an epidermal position in which they are actually not present but rather by their upward migration from the neural crest*, just like melanocytes, in order to reach the skin during embryonic development.

Meanwhile, the nervous origin of nevocytes has been definitively accepted, categorically invalidating the "dropping down theory." Therefore, Unna's original conception about the nature and building up of nevocytic nevi, as well as its related nomenclature, should have been declared obsolete many years ago, although this has still not occurred.

Nevocytic Nevus: In spite of this lesion being the most frequent malformation in the human species, its exact nature and origin are still unsettled and it is still being speculated whether they are aberrant neural or sensorial structures, remnants of some embryonal organ, or otherwise... Moreover, the variegated structure of these lesions, along with their highly variable histologic picture, makes one wonder if nevocytic nevi actually represent one sort or more than one – of vestigial – entities.

Nevocytic nevi may in some cases appear as exophytic or pedunculated fleshy masses, whereas in other cases they show up as sessile or flattened plaques. Their external pigmentation, ranging from pale pink to blackish brown, simply reflects their erratic melanogenic capacity, without constituting an index of their malignancy. It may be incidentally said that the jet black lesions sent to the laboratory under the presumptive diagnosis of "junction nevi" (a remnant of Unna's classification) are most frequently *not nevocytic nevi* – since they are not formed by nevocytes – but rather lentigines, which are benign proliferations of melanocytes, as already explained on p. 134.

Halo nevus, also called "leukodermia centrifuga acquisita" or "Sutton nevus," falls under that category of lesions that can be diagnosed by their external features, without resorting to microscopic examination. This lesion starts as a pigmented mole which develops a halo of depigmentation around it. In a matter of weeks, the depigmentation spreads to the center, causing the nodule to disappear, leaving a depigmented spot in its place. The pathogenesis underlying halo nevus is presumed to be an autoimmune cellular reaction triggered against a nevocytic nevus. LM examination lends support to this assumption by revealing a lymphohistiocytic infiltration in the affected area, with remnants of nevus cells and melanin granules.

A nevocytic nevus is occasionally presented as a pigmented mole with a hairy component, reason for which it may be called "hairy nevus" or "nevus hirsutus." This qualification helps to distinguish it from "*nevus pilosus*," a

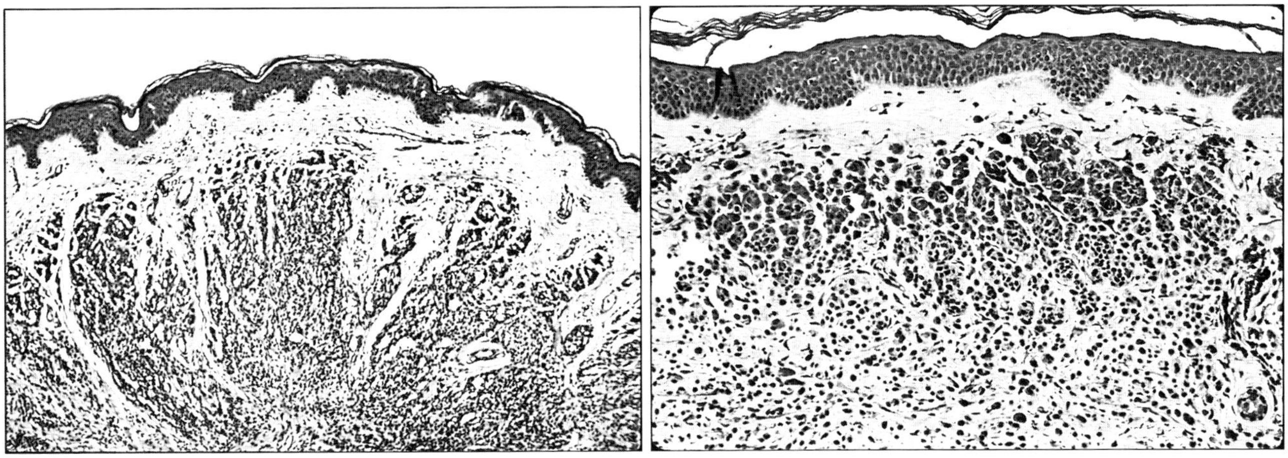

Fig. 4.22 Nevocytic nevus (*left and right*). See details in the text. H&E ×40, o m

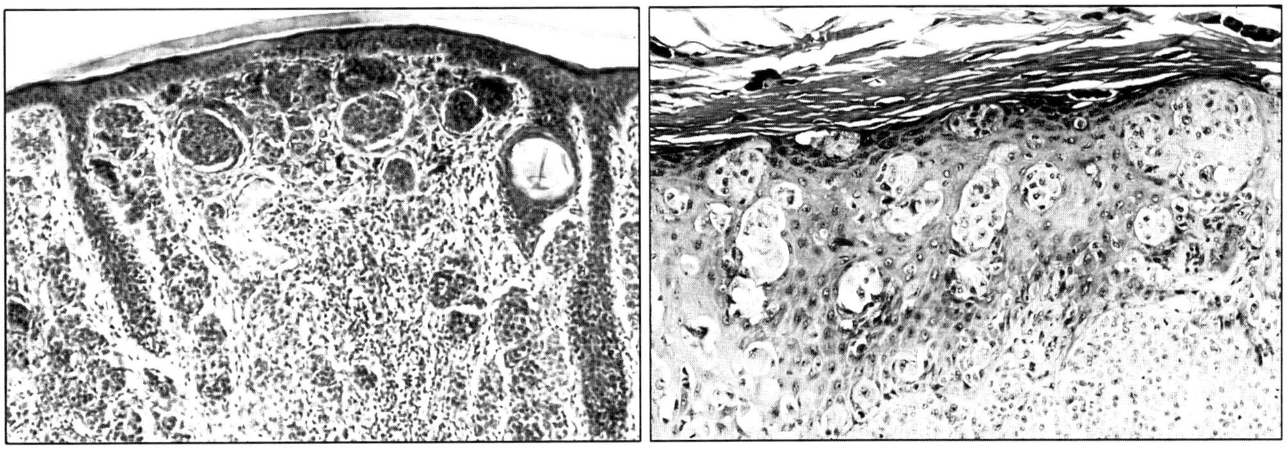

Fig. 4.23 Nevocytic nevus, epidermotrophic, and superficially spreading malignant melanoma. Whereas in the first case (*left*), nevocytes press the BM without penetrating it, in the second case (*right*), the malignant cells have destroyed that structure and are freely invading the epidermis. H&E ×40, o m

hamartoma with a prominent pilar component but devoid of nevocytes (p. 52). In this regard, Becker's nevus *is a hairy nevus* of elective localization around the shoulder. It is formed by a flat, pigmented nevocytic nevus, with a pilar component.

Nevocytic nevi show a highly variable microscopic picture. The two featured in Fig. 4.22 seem to be *ascending from the depth*: the one to the left in an expanding arborescent fashion and the one to the right in a broad advancing front loaded with melanin granules. Both are separated from the overlying epidermis by an acellular band. This last detail fully supports Masson's concept about the *extraepidermal origin* of these lesions.

In daily practice, however, it is not uncommon to find nevocytic nevi in close vicinity to the epidermis: these are the "epidermotrophic" nevocytic nevi (Fig. 4.23, left). That position may blur the dermoepidermal limits, inducing the observer to believe that these lesions are actually "*compound* nevi" – in Unna's terminology – present simultaneously in the dermis and epidermis of the specimen. In order to illustrate the differences between an epidermotropic nevocytic nevus sitting in the superficial dermis but not invading the epidermis and a superficially spreading malignant melanoma in which the epidermis has been actually invaded (xxx), two of these lesions are comparatively presented in Fig. 4.23.

A distinctive microscopic pattern of nevocytic nevus is the "pseudoalveolar" one. In it, cords of nevus cells are seen, loosely arranged, and featuring irregular confluent spaces of a vague vascular or pseudoalveolar aspect (Fig. 4.24).

Another frequent microscopic pattern adopted by nevocytes is the "neuroid" one, characterized by delicate membranes concentrically located and reminiscent of Vater-Pacini's corpuscles (Fig. 4.25).

Neuronevus: This distinctive pattern of nevocytic nevi is characterized by a loose stroma, frequently enclosing adipose lobes and showing, as a pathognomonic feature, "neuroid bodies." These are rounded multinucleated structures with a neural appearance (Fig. 4.26). Neuronevi should not

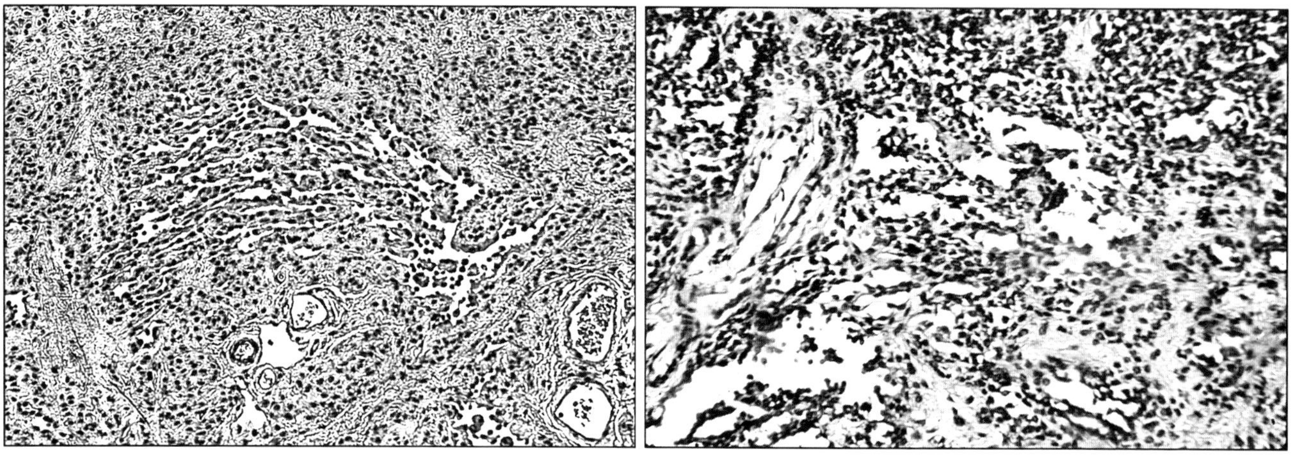

Fig. 4.24 Nevocytic nevus, pseudoalveolar. The lesion is formed by a collection of small, pyknotic nevocytes (*left*). In the center of the lesion, cellular cords are noted in a loose arrangement, featuring irregular spaces, shown at higher magnification to the *right*. H&E ×40; ×100, o m

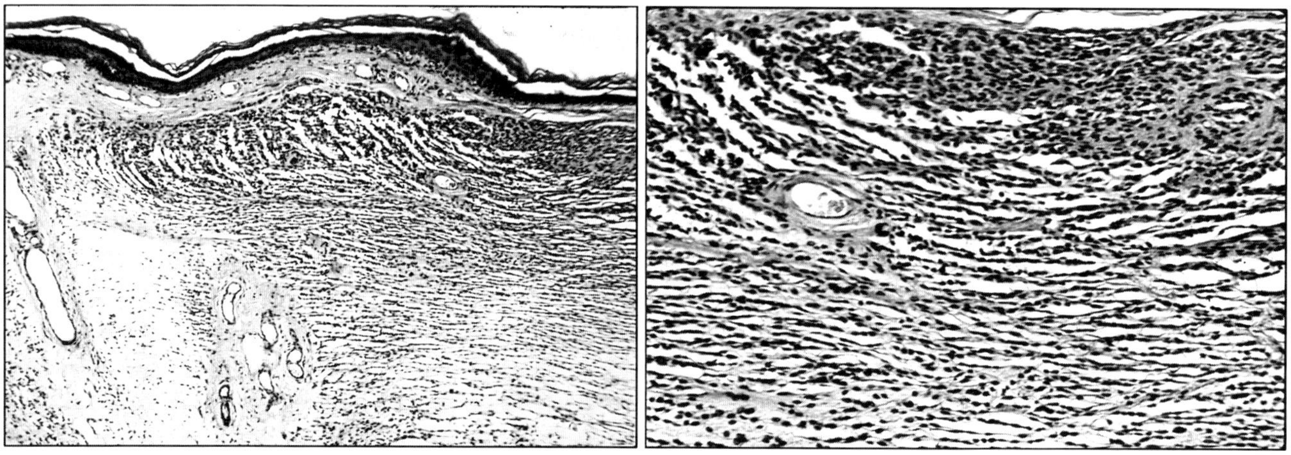

Fig. 4.25 Nevocytic nevus, neuroid type (*left and right*). See details in the text. H&E ×40; × 100, o m

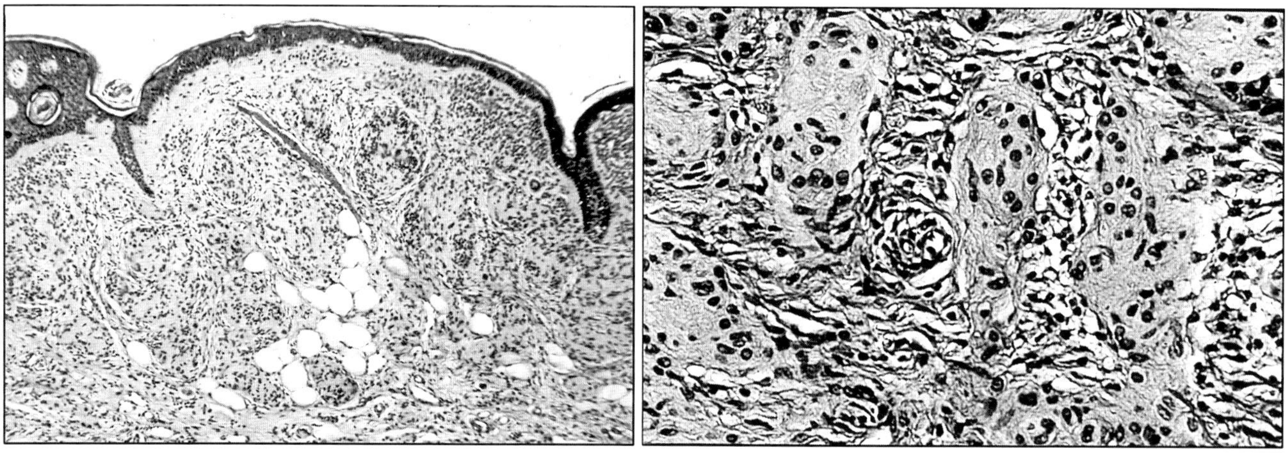

Fig. 4.26 Neuronevus. Note the presence of fatty tissue in the lesion (*left*) and of rounded polynuclear, pathognomonic structures, the "neuroid bodies" seen at higher magnification at the *right*. H&E ×40; ×100, o m

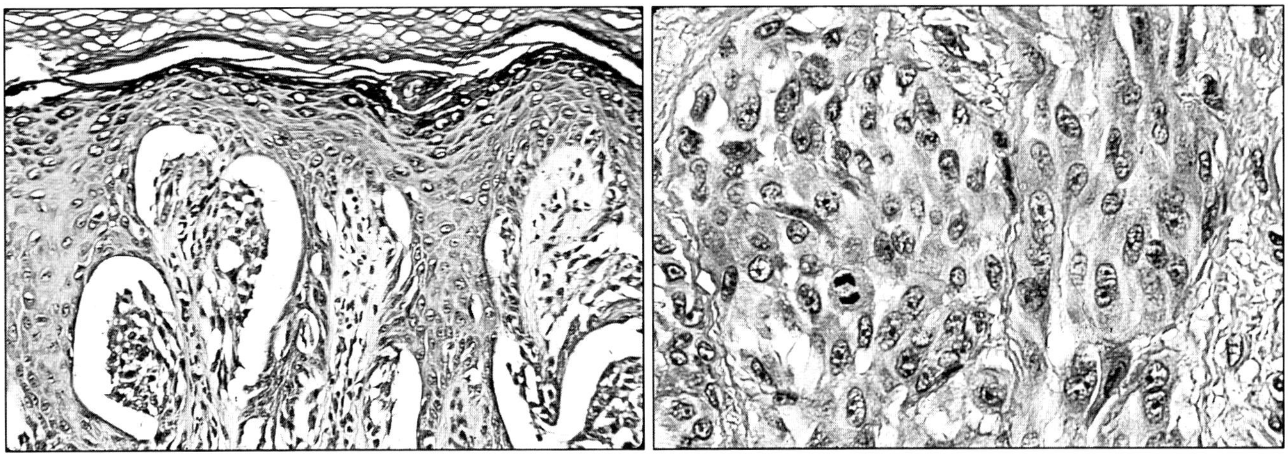

Fig. 4.27 Spitz nevus (*left*). The most characteristic feature of the lesions is the cellular loops occupying the dermal papillae but leaving narrow clefts that separate them from the surrounding stroma (*right*). This picture illustrates the typical spindle-shaped/epithelioid composition of the lesion and also its active mitotic rate. H&E ×100; ×400, o m

be mistaken for the above-mentioned "*neuroid type*" of nevocytic nevi.

Spitz nevus [11] deserves a mention among the lesions dealt with in this section. This is a frequently encountered lesion, particularly in the young population. Due to the presence of melanosomes in their bizarre-looking cells, and their active mitotic rate, these lesions were considered to be malignant melanomas. However, the fact that they prove to have an overwhelming benign outcome was a reason to change the initial opinion regarding their malignancy and instead call them "benign juvenile melanomas." This designation was later modified, also in tribute to its initial reporter, S. Spitz, to the eponymic name "Spitz nevus" (Fig. 4.27).

The peculiar composition of the lesion justifies its alternate name of "epithelioid and spindle-shaped nevus." Indeed, based on this histopathologic detail, this lesion has been alternatively considered to be a benign tumor of peripheral nerve, a "*neurotekheoma*" [12] (p. 170).

Congenital nevocytic nevi are characterized in the author's opinion not so much for being present at birth but for having an associated hamartomatous component of mesenchymatous and adnexal elements, which appear in profound disarray. The previously mentioned Becker nevus may be regarded as minimal forms of congenital nevocytic nevi.

Congenital nevocytic nevi may reach monstrous proportions, totally covering the back or trunk of the patients, from which the terms "bathing trunk nevus" and "giant nevocytic nevus" derive. These lesions appear as coarse and redundant skin folds, often with a pilar component that along with the pigmentation ranging from light brown to blackish brown – caused by a heavy load of melanin – imparts in the patient's skin the appearance of an *animal hide*. Upon microscopic examination, gross alterations are noted in the lesion. These include, along mesenchymatous malformations of every possible sort, an irregular epidermis with an excess of adnexal abnormalities, including large pilosebaceous and eccrine elements. The lesions usually display, along with a disproportionately high amount of nevocytes and melanocytes of large and irregular contour, extremely heavy loads of melanin. In addition to the serious social problems that these lesions burden the patients with, there is the frequent malignant degeneration of these lesions into malignant melanomas.

Choristomas: Among the special malformations with foreign elements, choristomas should also be mentioned. These are masses of tissue normally absent from the organ where they occur (*chorystos+oma* [G] separated+tumor). Due to their extremely low incidence, these lesions hereby only deserve mention.

Malformations with High Level of Organization

The second group of special malformations (Table 4.4) includes those with a high level of organization. The group is headed by trichofolliculoma.

Trichofolliculomas are malformations of a clear pilosebaceous progeny located most frequently on the face and particularly on the tip of nose. They appear as solitary nodules from which a bunch of thin hairs emerge. The microscopic examination of a meridian section of one of these lesions (Fig. 4.28) reveals a central cavity surrounded by a crown of miniature hair follicles. This is an appearance closely repeated in unrelated lesions. This *constant reproduction* of the same microscopic structure to the last detail greatly favors the *malformative* versus the *neoplastic* character of the lesion – a rule of thumb for the microscopist while dealing with proliferative lesions.

Trichoepithelioma is the second component of this group of lesion. This lesion (Fig. 4.29, left) may appear as a solitary extemporary nodule, or as an array of these, in which case it may represent the cutaneous component of Cowden syndrome. The lesion is formed by central keratinous nuclei

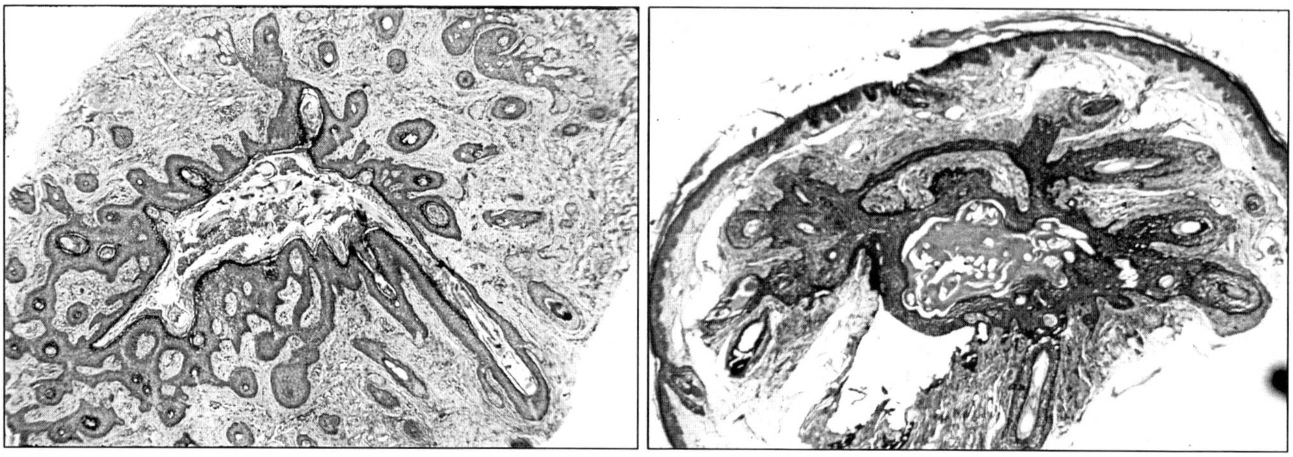

Fig. 4.28 Trichofolliculoma. The microscopic examination of the lesion to the *left* reveals a central cavity surrounded by miniature hair follicles which present, except for their size, the structural details of normal hair follicles. This picture is reproduced with amazing fidelity in the unrelated specimen to the *right*. H&E ×40, o m

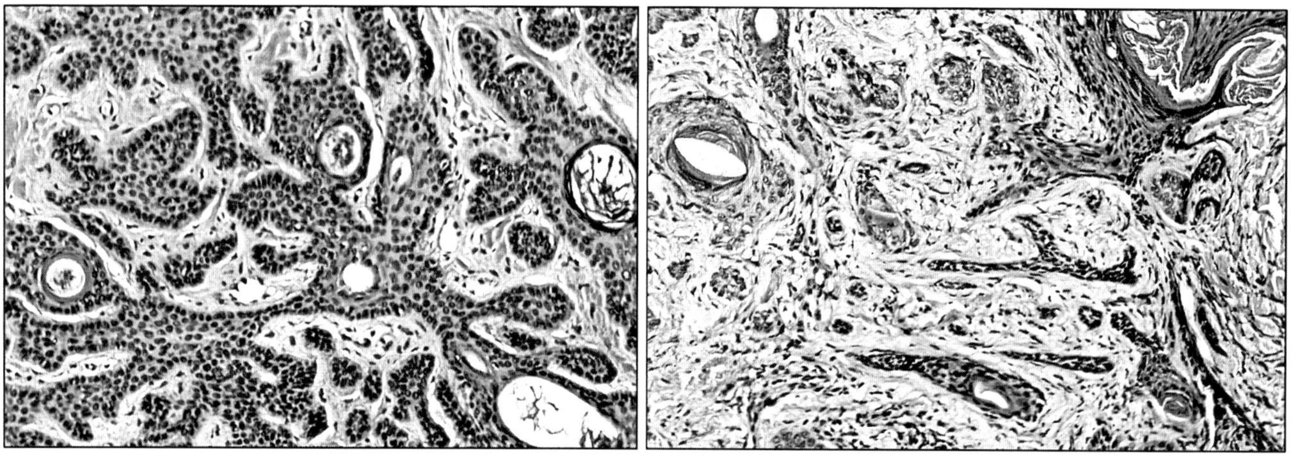

Fig. 4.29 Trichoepithelioma (*left*). Note the network of cellular cords and the keratinous cysts (*right*). A "tadpole figure" is seen at the bottom of the figure, toward the center. For more details see the text. H&E ×40; ×100, o m

surrounded by mantles of basophilic cells devoid of keratohyalin granules, connected by cellular cords to similar surrounding structures, and forming continuous networks. Trichoepithelioma may present an exaggerated component of fibrous stroma compressing its components and turning them into filiform cords, giving rise to the entity known as desmoplastic trichoepithelioma (Fig. 4.29, right). Desmoplastic trichoepitheliomas constitute an important differential possibility in cases of "morphea type of basal cell carcinoma" (p. 147).

Malformations with Defective Production of Epidermal Elements

Whereas the lesions in the two previous Subgroups in Table 4.4 have a static, structural quality, the lesions in this third Subgroup have a dynamic character since they are the result of a constant, faulty production of an epidermal element, mainly keratinocytes. These lesions are exteriorized as solitary, inconspicuous papules which under the microscopic examination turn to be acanthomas of any of the three types featured in Table 4.5. This table exposes the lesions just discussed, including their relevant histopathologic feature and the lesions that may be included as differential diagnostic possibilities in each of the cases.

In the absence of any supportive clinical information, the diagnosis of any of the three solitary acanthomas in Table 4.5 remains questionable. Based on LM study (Fig. 4.30) and supported by clinical information, the final diagnosis of these papules should be those stated on the central column of Table 4.5.

As far as ephelides are concerned, these lesions, as Pinkus indicated, result from a transient increase in the production of melanin by hyperactive melanocytes excited by UV radiation [13]. They may be regarded as dynamic anomalies, reason for which they may be incorporated into the group of lesions featured in Table 4.5.

Table 4.5 Special malformations due to defective organogenesis

Entity	Relevant histopathologic feature	Conditions of comparable histopathologic features
Solitary acantholytic acanthoma	Acantholysis	Hailey-Hailey disease and pemphigus vulgaris
Solitary benign dyskeratotic acanthoma	Acantholysis and benign dyskeratosis	Warty dyskeratoma, Darier's disease, Grover's disease
Solitary hyperkeratotic and epidermolytic acanthoma	Epidermolytic hyperkeratosis	Bullous congenital ichtyosiform Erythroderma ichthyosis hystrix
Ephelides	Melanocyte proliferation	Lentigo simplex Lentigo maligna

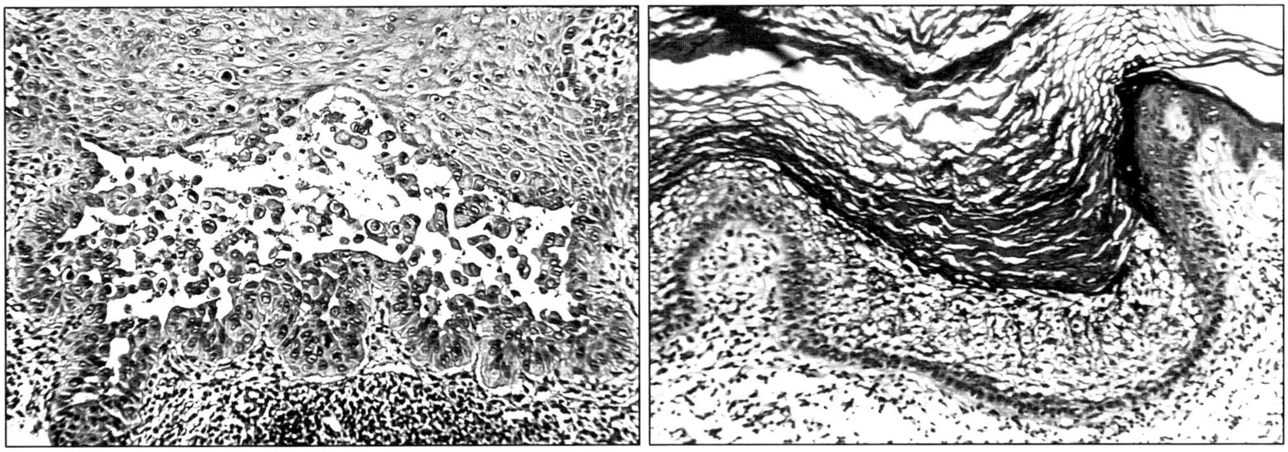

Fig. 4.30 Solitary acantholytic acanthoma (*left*) and solitary hyperkeratotic epidermolytic acanthoma (*right*). H&E ×40, o m

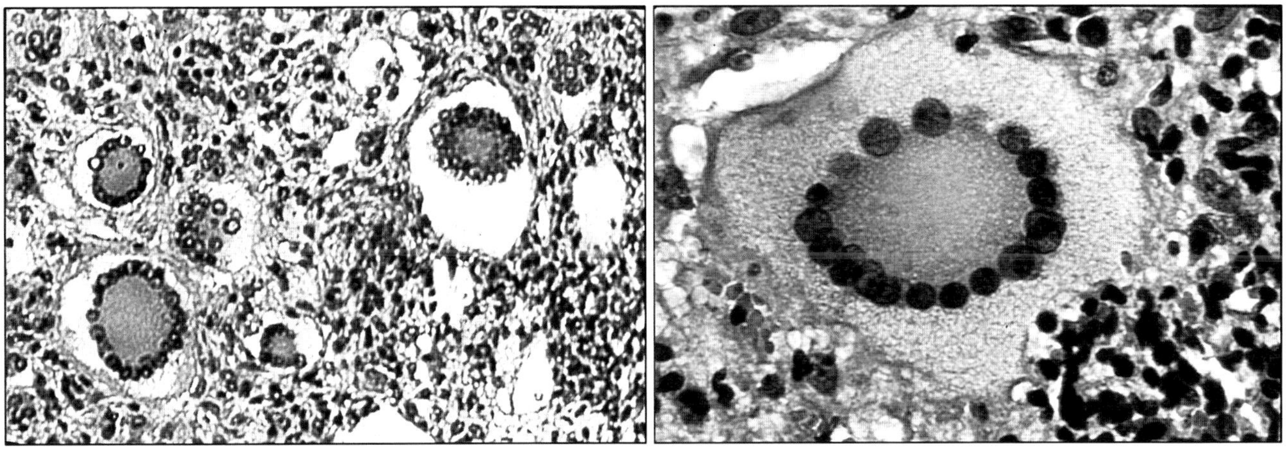

Fig. 4.31 Touton's giant cells (*left and right*). See details in the text. H&E ×40; ×400, o m

Malformations Reproducing Organs

The integrants of this group of special malformations (Table 4.4) are distinguished from hamartomas because, contrary to those, they faithfully reproduce anatomic structures, such as breast, nipple, digits, or tragus, whose descriptions are hereby not necessary.

Malformations with Tendency Toward Spontaneous Resolution

This fifth group of special malformations (Table 4.4) includes two lesions. These are juvenile xanthogranuloma and strawberry angioma. These two lesions are benign, sporadic, and congenital or perinatal in their form of appearance. They present a histiocytic/vascular structure. In this context, it should be mentioned that juvenile xanthogranuloma presents a distinctive microscopic feature, that is, Touton's giant cells (Fig. 4.31), which will be further discussed.

The purpose of including these two lesions *in* a special *group* of malformations is to highlight their tendency to spontaneous resolution. This designation should indicate to the practitioner the advisability of waiting until the lesion has reached its maximal expected regression, before undertaking any therapeutic measure.

References

1. Lever WF, Schaumburg-Lever G. Histopathology of the skin. 7th ed. Philadelphia: J.B. Lipppincott; 1990. p. 778.
2. Rosai J. Rosai and Ackerman surgical pathology. 9th ed. Edinburgh: Mosby; 2004. p. 1687.
3. Unna PG. Histopathologie der Hautkrankheiten. Berlin: Hirschwald Verlag; 1894. p. 1145.
4. Pinkus H. In: Mehregan AH, Hashimoto K, editors. Pinkus' guide to dermatohistopathology, 5th ed. Norwalk: Appleton & Lange; 1991. p. 646.
5. Unna PG. Histopathologie der Hautkrankheiten. Berlin: Hirschwald Verlag; 1894. p. 1148.
6. McCarty A. Histopathology of skin diseases. St. Louis: C.V. Mosby; 1931. p. 408–9.
7. Allen AC. The skin. St. Louis: C.V. Mosby; 1954. p. 838.
8. Bernard C. Introduction a l'etude de la medicine experimentale. Paris: J.B. Bailliere et fils; 1865. p. 63–5.
9. Masson P. Les naevi pigmentaires, tumeurs nerveuses. Ann Anat Pathol. 1926;5:417–53.
10. Masson P. My conception of cellular nevi. Cancer. 1951;4:9–38.
11. Lever WF, Schaumburg-Lever G. Histopathology of the skin. 7th ed. Philadelphia: J.B. Lipppincott; 1990. p. 766–8.
12. Scheithauer BW, Woodruff JM, Erlandson RA. In: Rosai J, editor. Atlas of tumor pathology, 3rd series, fascicle 24. Washington, D.C.: Armed Forces Institute of Pathology; 1999. p. 236–48.
13. Pinkus H. In: Mehregan AH, Hashimoto K, editors. Pinkus' guide to dermatohistopathology, 5th ed. Norwalk: Appleton & Lange; 1991, p. 392.

5 Inflammatory Cutaneous Lesions

The inflammatory lesions of the skin may be solitary and constitute by themselves the whole diagnostic problem faced by the microscopist. On the contrary, they may be multiple, representing part of a cutaneous disease or of a systemic condition involving several organs, including the skin.

At the time inflammatory lesions of the skin are removed for microscopic examination, they may be in an evolutive phase or otherwise, after having ended that stage without complete reestablishment of the affected area, they may be in a postevolutive, inactive phase. Still some other lesions, at the time of their removal, may be in a transitional phase at the end of which, if they had not been previously removed, they may have had eventually emerge as overt malignancies. Accordingly, three Subdivisions of inflammatory lesions are recognized in this classification. These are referred to as evolutive, postevolutive, and transitional.

In order to establish a first separation among the evolutive inflammatory lesions, a topographic criterion was adopted. In this way, five Classes of them may be recognized, which are the ones with epidermal, junctional, dermal, subcutaneous, or adnexal localization. Evolutive lesions, however, are localized only with rare exceptions. Instead, they affect surrounding areas of the skin with variable intensity. For this reason, to each of the postulated five Classes, resulting from a rather rigid approach, the prefix "*predominant*" must be attached to adapt the classification to reality.

In the case of the postevolutive lesions, the alterations suffered by the tissues during the active inflammatory process along with vascular proliferation, collagen deposition, and other reparative changes deeply distort the affected site, erasing the microscopic hallmarks on which the previous taxonomic scheme was based and making necessary another approach for their classification. In this way, dystrophic, atrophic, and cicatricial lesions are recognized (Fig. 5.1). Insofar as the transitional lesions, they are arranged at the end of this chapter in three separate Groups of histiocytic, Langerhans, and T cell lesions.

Concerning the pathogenesis of the inflammatory cutaneous lesions, either isolated or as part of more complex nosologic processes, several factors may be responsible. Among them should be mentioned physicochemical agents such as UV radiations, heath and cold, acid and basic solutions, and traumas of every sort which the skin, due to its exposed situation, may ineludibly confront. Following physicochemical agents, viruses must be considered. Figure 5.2 presents the group of viruses of major importance regarding dermatopathology.

After viruses, the next agents to be mentioned in cutaneous pathology are bacteria, arthropods and other ectoparasites, and, finally, adverse immune reactions. These deserve a special comment.

Although the immune system is primordial for the defense of the body, in some cases such as hypersensitivity and autoimmune reactions, its activity may result into severe damage and even in the death of the affected person [1].

Hypersensitivity may be defined as an exaggerated or inappropriate immune response which would rather harm than protect the host. Hypersensitivity reactions were categorized by Coombs and Gell as of types I, II, III, and IV [2]. A fifth type of immunogenic reaction was later added, the "stimulating hypersensitivity reaction," which is however of minor importance in dermatology and hereby needs no further comment. Hypersensitivity reactions do not always occur as isolated events but may befall in combination, difficulting the interpretation of the ongoing events.

In hypersensitivity reactions, an *afferent phase* and an *efferent phase* are distinguished. The afferent phase covers

Subdivisions	Classes
Evolutive	Predominantly epidermal Predominantly junctional Predominantly dermal Predominantly subcutaneous Predominantly adnexal
Post-evolutive	Dystrophic Atrophic Scars
Transitional	

Fig. 5.1 Inflammatory cutaneous lesions: subdivisions and classes

E. Zappi, E.A. Zappi, *Dermatopathology*,
DOI 10.1007/978-1-4471-2894-6_5, © Springer-Verlag London 2013

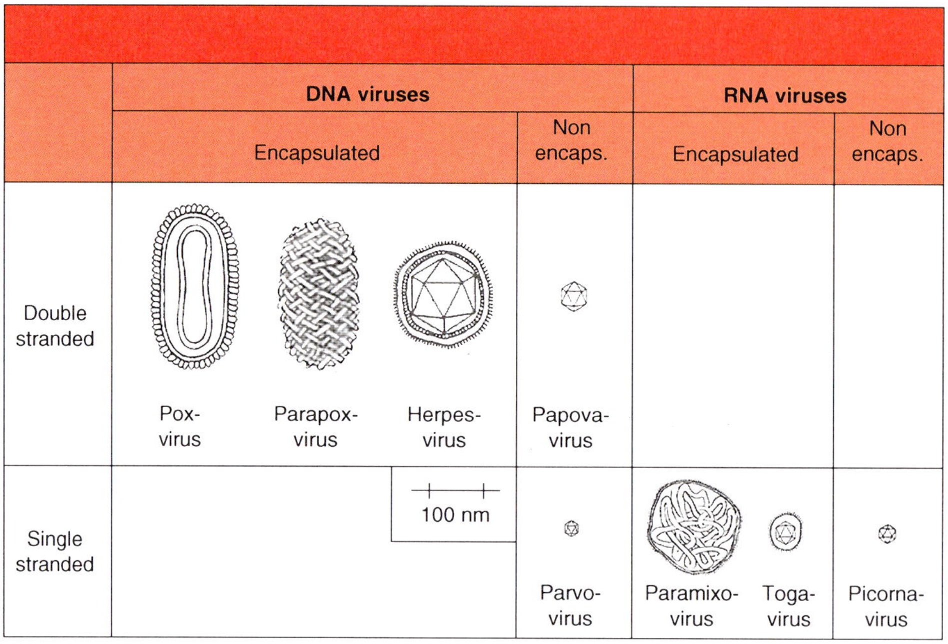

Viral agent	Clinical manifestation
Poxvirus	Smallpox vaccinia
Parapoxvirus:	moluscum contagiosum ectima contagiosa milker's nodule
Herpesvirus:	herpes simplex varicella/zoster sixth disease

Viral agent	Clinical manifestation
Papovavirus	Verruca condiloma acuminatum epidermodispl. verrucif.
Parvovirus	Fifth disease
Paramixovirus	Measles German measles
Picornavirus	Foot, hand and mouth disease Gianotti-Crosti syndrome

Fig. 5.2 Representative group of epidermotrophic viruses. Encapsulated viruses are shown in sagittal sections in order to expose their interior. In the case of parapox virus, its external surface is shown to illustrate its characteristic woven exterior

all the preparatory changes determined by the initial, primary contact of an immunogenic agent, that is, the antigen (Ag) (p. 193) with an immunocompetent organism. The efferent phase, that is, the immune response, is triggered by a reiterated contact of the Ag with the meanwhile sensitized host.

In hypersensitivity types I to III, the interval between the secondary contact and the immunoresponse is brief, occurring in terms of minutes or hours. In type IV, to the contrary, the interval between the secondary contact and the immunoresponse takes days, weeks, or even longer to occur. For that reason, it is considered that reactions I to III cause "immediate hypersensitivity" reactions, while type IV produces "delayed hypersensitivity." The pathogenic mechanisms of immediate hypersensitivity reactions are antibody (Ab)-mediated, while those of delayed hypersensitivity are cell mediated. Indeed, experimentally, whereas immediate hypersensitivity may be transferred from a sensitized to an unsensitized animal by injection of serum of the first into the second, delayed hypersensitivity of a sensitized animal may be passed down to an unsensitized one by transfer of lymphocytes from the first to the second. (For the record, it may be stated that the converse experimental maneuvers do not succeed in the transfer of hypersensitivity).

Type I is the allergic type of hypersensitivity. Its afferent phase starts with the introduction of an Ag usually through the respiratory mucosa of a *predisposed* person. With the help of antigen-presenting cells (APC) and helper T cells (T_H cells), B cells are induced to the production of IgE, which is liberated into the circulation. The IgE molecules are fixed by their C fraction (p. 194) to special receptors on the surface of tissue-fixed mast cells and their circulating equivalents, basophilic polynuclears. If the pertinent Ag is reintroduced into the circulation, it will be specifically bound by the Ab fraction of the previously fixed IgE, bridging neighbor Ab molecules and providing a signal for the mast cells to degranulate, causing the liberation of histamine, serotonin, and other vasoactive amines. The signal also causes the activation

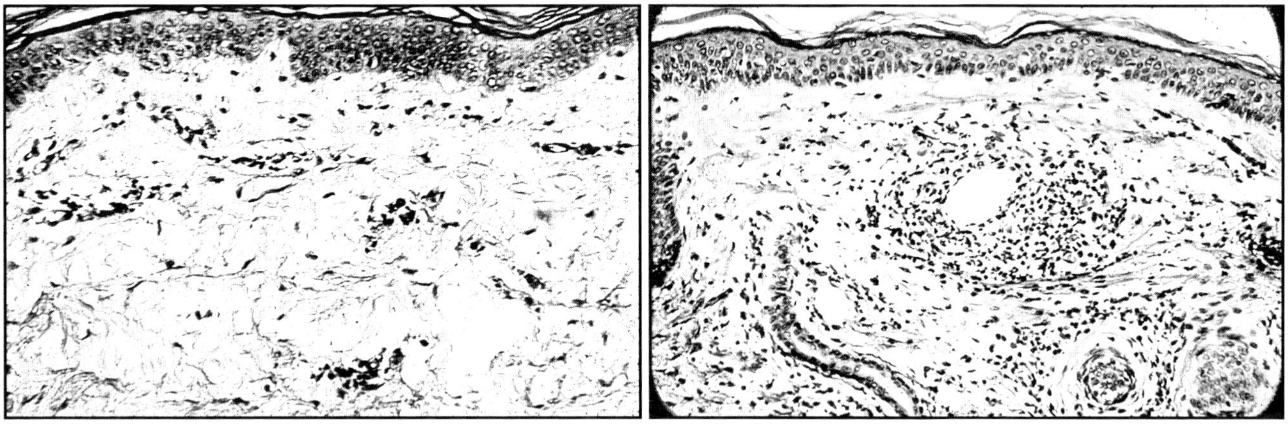

Fig. 5.3 Urticarial papule and vasculitis. The urticarial papule (*left*) corresponds to type I allergic hypersensitivity due in this particular case to food intolerance. The picture shows a section of skin with a faintly eosinophilic dermis and dilated lymphatics. Note that in spite of its intensity, edema remains within the dermis, without transgressing the BM to invade the epidermis, which in fact appears undisturbed. For comparative purposes, a case of vasculitis corresponding to a type III hypersensitivity is shown (*right*). It is caused by circulating immunocomplexes within the framework of secondary syphilis. In this case, besides the usual changes for vasculitis, that is, the damaged venule surrounded by abundant acute inflammatory elements and nuclear dust, the lesion also shows strong edema. This, again, remains restricted to the dermis, as in the case of the urticarial papule (*left*). H&E × 40 o m

of the arachidonic acid pathway, with production of prostaglandins, etc., which cause vasodilatation, bronchiolar constriction, and other alterations which constitute the base of the clinical manifestations of allergies (Fig. 5.3).

Type II hypersensitivity, the "cytotoxic" type, occurs upon the fixation of circulating Ab, usually of the IgM or IgG class onto tissue-fixed Ags. In human pathology, the simplest example of this reaction occurs when an individual receives a transfusion of mismatched blood. Under this condition, the afferent phase of the reaction is reduced to the fixation of the Abs of the recipient blood groups – which are already circulating – onto the surface Ags of the mismatched red blood cells. At that point, activation of the complement system (C) occurs, with agglutination and hemolysis. The destruction of the donor's erythrocytes is fulfilled during the later sequence of C activation, to which opsonization (p. 194) and related events contribute.

An example of a cytotoxic reaction much more pertinent to dermatopathology is the one that occurs in pemphigus vulgaris. This is an autoimmune disorder in which Abs are raised against the patient's own glycocalyx. The circulating Abs are fixed in the interstitial spaces of the target epidermis, with the ultimate result of its destruction (p. 79).

Type III hypersensitivity, the immunocomplex-mediated hypersensitivity, is associated to disorders which evolve with production of circulating immunocomplexes (p. 194). Under normal conditions, immunocomplexes are rapidly cleared from circulation by the reticuloendothelial system. If for any reason this does not occur, these complexes can be deposited onto inappropriate structures and in the particular case of the skin, on the endothelium of the smallest venules coming immediately after the capillary bed. The frequently used term "postcapillary venules" is redundant and incorrectly applied in this particular case as explained elsewhere. The deposition of immunocomplexes leads to local C activation, with production of anaphylotoxins and attraction of neutrophils and eosinophils to the area, as in the course of the process classically known in immunopathology as "*vasculitis*" (p. 88) (Fig. 5.3, right). Inflammatory elements liberated during the course of the reaction lead to irreversible endothelial damage, with thrombosis and neutrophil destruction resulting in "nuclear dust" – an important element of the histopathologic picture of this lesion. Vasculitis is a frequent finding under conditions in which circulating immunocomplexes are known to occur, such as rheumatoid arthritis, syphilis, and allergic granulomatosis.

As regards type IV hypersensitivity, the delayed type, several subtypes have been found after this reaction was initially reported. The best characterized are the tuberculoid and the granulomatous one, as well as contact dermatitis. An experimental type IV hypersensitivity reaction has also been described, the Jones-Motte reaction whose discussion shall not be pursued further in this text.

In the afferent phase of a type IV reaction, a particular Ag is captioned by antigen-presenting cells (APCs) and presented, combined with products of the major histocompatibility complex (MHC) (p. 194) to T_MCells. These process the Ag further, and as a result, memory T cells (T_MCells) against that Ag are raised. If the pertinent Ag happens to make contact again with the T_M cells, these will respond by proliferating into a clone, initiating the effector phase of the reaction. *Interleukins* of various types and other factors will be generated. These attract to the area macrophages and other cellular effectors, which will try to eliminate the intruder.

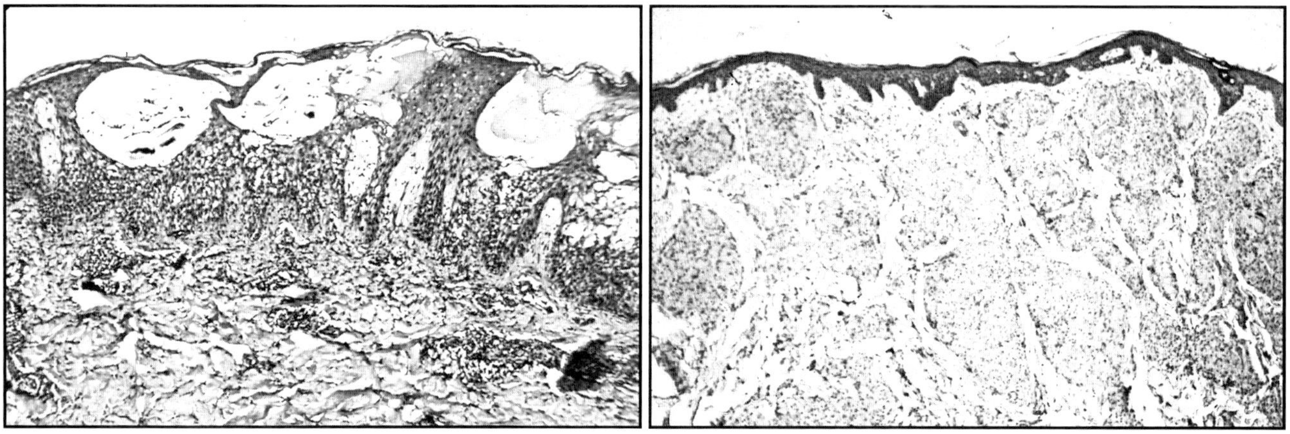

Fig. 5.4 Contact dermatitis and sarcoidosis. In contact dermatitis (*left*), a typical instance of type IV hypersensitivity, the lesion – which is localized in the epidermis – is characterized by extreme spongiosis. In sarcoidosis (*right*), another typical instance of type IV hypersensitivity, the lesion, which is localized in the dermis, is formed by tightly apposed "sarcoidal granulomas", leaving the overlying epidermis almost undisturbed. H&E ×40 o m

Even if the lesions in all subtypes of the type IV hypersensitivity have the same underlying pathogenic mechanism, their microscopic appearance differs widely from case to case, depending on the terrain in which the response develops and on the influence of several additional agents involved (Fig. 5.4).

A miniform of tuberculoid reaction is provoked in sensitized individuals injected for diagnostic purposes with tuberculin. The microscopic appearance of this lesion, which only shows the active mobilization of macrophages, barely matches that which occurs in real life – in tuberculoid granuloma – frequently caused by infections with TB or comparable bacilli. The tuberculoid granuloma is characterized by a core of epithelioid histiocytes eventually displaying central necrosis, surrounded by a heavy rim of mononuclear cells.

Concerning the before-mentioned autoimmune reactions, it is important to keep in mind that the hypersensitivity reactions, in addition to being caused by external factors, may be also triggered by components of an individual. This occurs if a "self" component is altered for some reason and is recognized by its own immunogenic system as "*nonself*": in that case, the organism may develop hypersensitivity reactions similar to the ones discussed above. Moreover, *normal* components may be recognized as "*nonself*" by a defective immunogenic system and subjected to a destructive process. All these alterations and aberrations are the basis of the autoimmune diseases encountered in dermatology as in other branches of medicine.

Evolutive Inflammatory Lesions

Upon analyzing the inflammatory cutaneous lesions, the epidermis is distinguished from the other layers of the skin in the variety of responses that it may generate against diverse aggressions. This is explained by the fact that the epidermis is the most complex and specialized component of the skin. The responses it may yield, however, can only occur if its reactive capacity has not been abrogated by the intensity of the aggression, in which case the destruction of the epidermis will ensue.

In contrast to the epidermis, the basement membrane (BM) is an acellular, defenseless structure, unable to react against any aggression. It may be destroyed along with other tissues in inflammatory processes in that area. In other cases, the BM may be the specific target of an immunoaggression, which will cause its selective destruction, leading to detachment of the epidermis from the dermis and to the formation of a space between them, known in this text as a *subepidermal bulla*.

The dermis, in turn, being a mesenchymatous structure endowed with abundant vascular and inflammatory elements both fixed and motile, has a great potential of reaction, being able to render intense, although nonspecific inflammatory responses. The subcutaneous panniculus, despite its mesenchymal constitution, is a labile structure, unable to react to any aggression, which leads to its diffuse, nonspecific necrosis, modified by the eventual presence of inflammatory infiltrates.

The different structure of the cutaneous adnexae accounts for the bountiful array of microscopic pictures that can be observed following their aggression by different noxious agents.

Lesions of Predominant Epidermal Localization

The lesions of this complex Class are divided into five Subclasses: *exfoliating*, *spongiotic*, *necrotizing*, *with inflammatory infiltration*, and *epidermolytic*, according to their

Subclasses	Groups	Subgroups
Exfoliating	Exogenous	
	Endogenous	
Spongiotic	Exogenous	
	Endogenous	
	Miscellaneous	
Necrotizing	Exogenous	
	Endogenous	Superficial
		Massive
With acute inflammatory infiltrate	Infectious	
	Non infectious	
Epidermolytic	Infectious	
	Non infectious	

Fig. 5.5 Class of inflammatory lesions of predominant epidermal localization: Subclasses, Groups, and Subgroups

histopathologic characteristics. The lesions in the first two Subclasses reflect active responses of the epidermis to aggressions of low intensity. These responses usually subside after short periods of time, without leaving drastic changes, and with the complete restoration of the original conditions in the affected area. The last three Subclasses of lesions attest to the incapacity of the epidermis to withstand the assault, resulting in significant epidermal alterations and destruction.

Further taxonomic classification of the lesions in the five Subclasses follows variable criteria. The exfoliating lesions may be grouped as responsible insult. The spongiotic lesions are separated into three groups: exogenous, endogenous, and miscellaneous. Necrotizing lesions may again be conveniently grouped as externally or internally mediated, with the latter group even subgrouped as having superficial or massive necrosis. The lesions with inflammatory infiltration, as well as the epidermolytic types, may be more conveniently grouped as infectious and noninfectious (Fig. 5.5).

Exfoliating Lesions

The qualifying term "exfoliating" used in this text to describe the lesions in this first Subclass has a clinical rather than a pathologic character. It was chosen because of the impossibility in finding a suitable pathologic term that fully and concisely summarizes the histopathologic changes which characterize this type of lesion. These alterations, that is, thickening of the epidermis with increased mitotic rate and concomitant thinning of the granular layer with hyperkeratosis and scaling, reflect a transient activation of the keratinocyte's vital cycle, due to

Table 5.1 Pathogenic agents of exfoliating and spongiotic lesions

Exogens
Physicochemical
UV radiation, mild
Acid and basic solutions, weak
Infectious
Dermatophytes
Endogens
Infectious
Viral
Noninfectious
Allergens

a mild, tolerable stimulation. In these lesions, the dermis simply shows an increased irrigation and a mild, diffuse infiltration by mononuclear cells.

Mononuclear cells is an objective and uncommitted term which refers to the components of cellular infiltrates, whose only common feature, as they appear under LM examination of standard-stained tissue sections, is the possession of only one nucleus. Covered by the term "mononuclear" are – with the exception of plasma cells and mast cells, which may be identified by LM inspection – lymphocytes of any progeny, macrophages, histiocytes, etc., whose actual nature can only be ascertained with the help of analytic techniques of no current use in the histopathology diagnostic laboratory.

Regarding "polynuclear cells," these are hereby designated in shorthand as "neutrophils," "eosinophils," and "basophils" based on the reaction of their specific cytoplasmatic granules.

Exfoliating and spongiotic lesions are associated to mild pathogenic agents, some of which are mentioned in Table 5.1.

Exfoliating Lesions, Exogenous

The microscopic image of lesions resulting from brief solar exposure, clinically designated as "solar erythema," "first degree burn," etc., fully correspond to the above-depicted histopathologic changes in exfoliation.

Dermatophytic infections lead, in the simplest cases, to exfoliation of the epidermis. It must hereby be pointed out that "dermatophytosis" is the general term assigned to *superficial fungal infections*. These are frequently produced by *Trichophyton* and *Pityrosporum* species. These thrive among keratin scales, without penetrating into the dermis. The term "dermatomycosis" on the other hand refers to *deep fungal infections* caused by organisms able to grow deep in the tissues [3]. In dermatophytosis (Fig. 5.6), the most striking details of the images are at the level of the horny layer, which at low magnification shows a loose appearance, the so-called *basket weave pattern*. In cases favorable to the observer, the examination of simple H&E-stained sections is enough to disclose the presence of fungal elements, allowing an unequivocal diagnosis of "dermatophytosis." Otherwise,

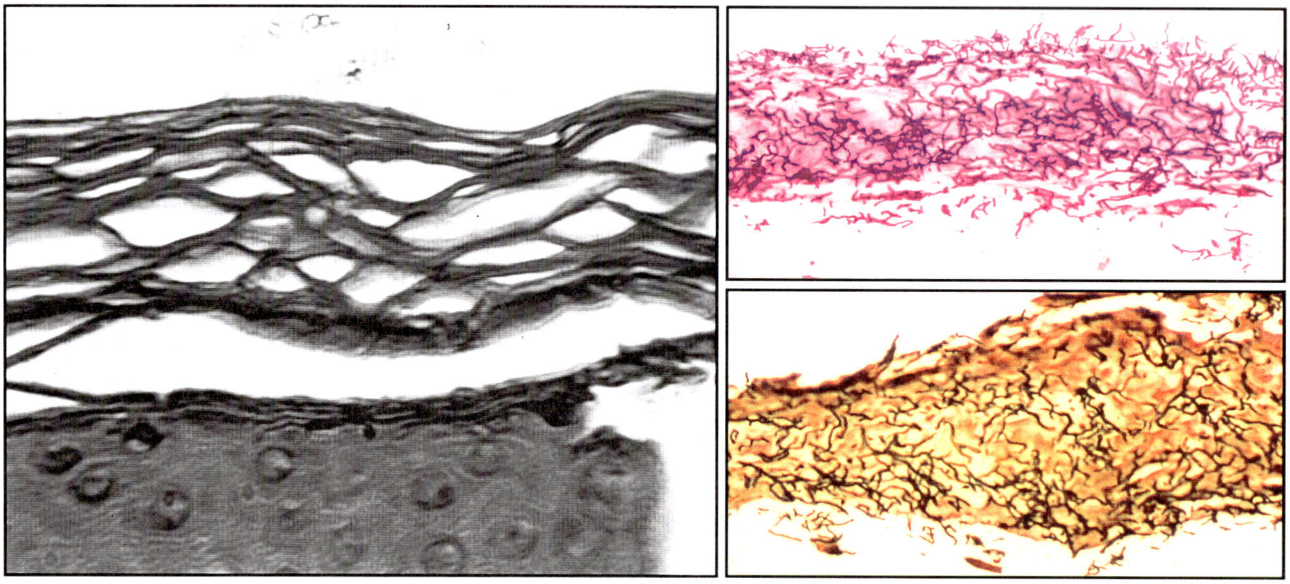

Fig. 5.6 Dermatophytosis. (*Left*) H&E-stained specimens at low magnification reveal looseness and irregular thickening of the horny layer, configurating a "basket weave" pattern. (*Right*) Horny layer pervaded by dermatophytes, stained with PAS (*top*) and GMS (*bottom*) ×40; ×100; 100 o m

PAS staining or GMS staining techniques are of great help to the microscopist in substantiating the diagnosis (Fig. 5.6).

In spite of primary confinement in the horny layer, dermatophytoses are able to cause allergic reactions of variable intensity in deeper-seated tissues via sensitization.

Exfoliating Lesions, Endogenous

At the beginning of the nineteenth century, A.J.I. Brocq designated the integrants of a group of disorders which did not convincingly look like psoriasis or lichen planus, "parapsoriasis" [4]. A condition was retrieved later on from the large Group of the parapsoriasis and called "pityriasis lichenoides" [4] based on the external aspect of its lesions (*pityriasis* [G] brann or dandruff + *lichenoides* [L] alike lichen). According to its evolution, this condition was split into pityriasis lichenoides acuta and pityriasis lichenoides chronica. Pityriasis lichenoides chronic (PLC) or "Juliusberg disease" shows a nonspecific microscopic picture characterized by acanthosis with parakeratin crusts, focal spongiosis, exocytosis, and perivascular cuffs of mononuclear cells (Fig. 5.7, left). Pityriasis lichenoides acuta, to the contrary, features an acute picture with epidermal necrosis, reason for which it shall be discussed along with other necrotizing dermatitides.

Parapsoriasis en plaque was derived too from the previously mentioned conglomerate of papulosquamous disorders. Based on subtle differences not easily perceptible by the dermatology layman, several "*parapsoriases*" were described. For the sake of simplification, this condition tends to be divided into two main entities: *small-plaque parapsoriasis* of benign character and *large-plaque parapsoriasis* [5], which may eventually undergo transformation into *mycosis fungoides*. Small-plaque parapsoriasis is characterized histologically by "exocytosis," that is, infiltration of the epidermis by mononuclear elements, combined with spongiosis, acanthosis, parakeratosis, and crusting, resulting in a microscopic picture which does not allow its separation from the above-mentioned PLC (Fig. 5.7, right). Large-plaque parapsoriasis will be discussed further in this chapter (p. 73).

Spongiosis may be defined as *the changes in the epidermis brought about by the interstitial accumulation of fluid*. In this regard, the term "*edema*," frequently used in the discussion of spongiotic lesions, should be reviewed. Edema, as laid down by E. H. Starling at the turn of the century, is the accumulation of fluid in the extravascular space as a consequence of an imbalance between hydrostatic and osmotic pressure across a semipermeable membrane, that is, the endothelium [6]. Being a purely vascular phenomenon, edema cannot be envisaged as developing in the epidermis, which is an eminently avascular layer. For this reason, the simplistic habit of interpreting spongiosis as if it were a form of edema, as in the terms "intracellular edema" or "extracellular edema," frequently used in discussing the pathogenesis of spongiotic lesions, is totally wrong. Even if the term "edema" itself only means "a swelling" (*oidema* [G] a swelling), it is convenient to use it strictly in the original sense proposed by its author. In fact, in light of our present knowledge regarding the role of the epidermis as an immunogenic organ, the striking cellular changes observed in spongiosis should be interpreted as consistent with those recalled in keratinocytes by a type IV immunoresponse (Fig. 5.8).

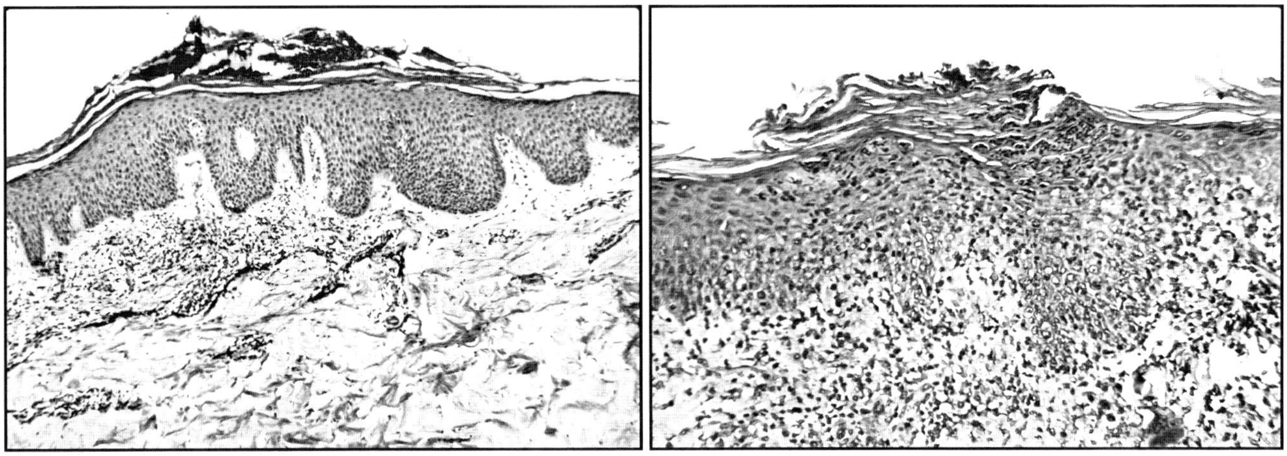

Fig. 5.7 Pityriasis lichenoides chronica and small-plaque parapsoriasis. In the first lesion (*left*), there is acanthosis with crusting and mild perivascular cuffs of mononuclear elements. In the second (*right*), the mentioned features are more accentuated but not enough for determining a picture consistently different from the previous one, H&E ×40; ×100 o m

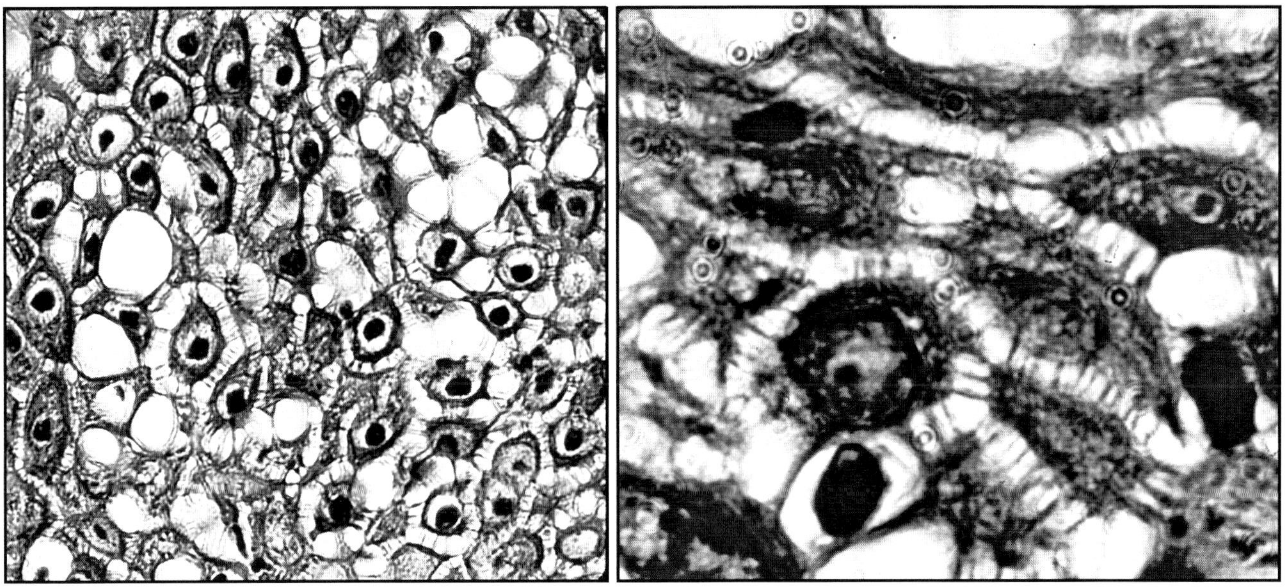

Fig. 5.8 Spongiotic reaction, early phase. (*Left*) Observe the pyknotic nuclei of the affected keratinocytes, surrounded by rings of clear cytoplasm. Note also the wide interstitial spaces in the lesion, dilated by the presence of fluid and crossed by spanned intercellular bridges. (*Right*) A higher magnification offers details of the lesion. Note the presence of three mononuclear elements, intimately contacting keratinocytes. H&E ×100; ×400 o m

The changes noted in Fig. 5.8 are of an irreversible character and lead to the destruction of the epidermis, with formation and elimination of necrotic epidermal straps, featuring the picture known as "reticular degeneration" shown in Fig. 5.9.

Spongiotic Dermatitides: Itchy conditions with vesiculation used to be designated in the clinic as "eczema." This term, however, after being arbitrarily applied to an extensive range of different conditions, ended up losing any coherent and specific meaning [7]. Nowadays, it tends to be replaced by the name "dermatitis." In order to emphasize the microscopic character of the dermatitides, the prefix "spongiotic" is frequently attached to that name.

For practical purposes and without following any specialized scheme, spongiotic dermatitides are hereby divided according to their origin, as either *exogenous* or *endogenous*, as shown in Table 5.2. The *miscellaneous* spongiotic dermatitides also included in the table will be dealt with at the end of this section.

Exogenous spongiotic dermatitides are the "contact dermatitides." These may be the direct effect of an irritating agent on the skin, being then called "primary contact dermatitis," in order to differentiate these from those resulting from a previous sensitization process. The latter type is called "allergic contact dermatitis." Endogenous spongiotic

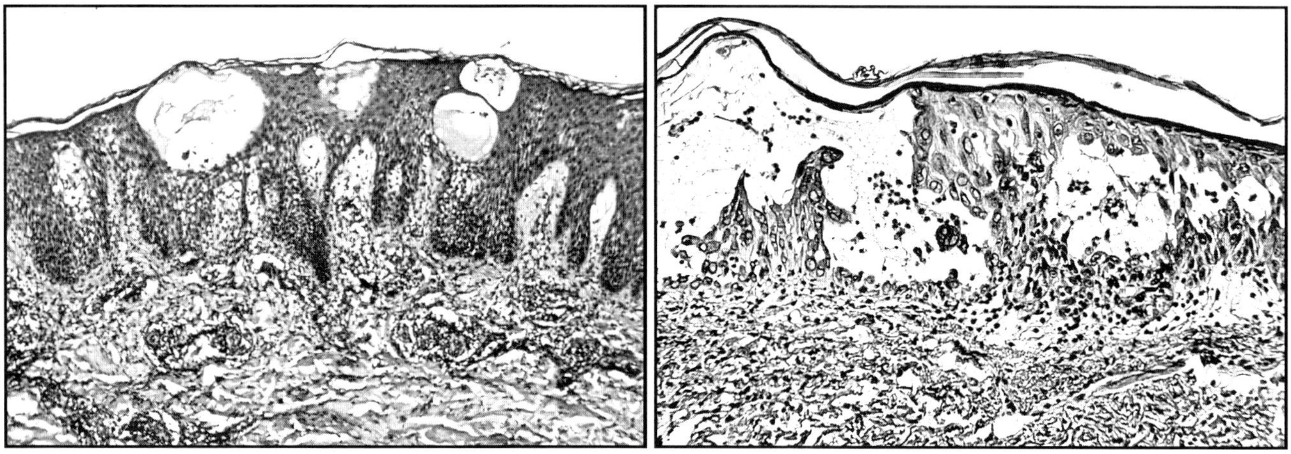

Fig. 5.9 Epidermis in an advanced stage of spongiosis. (*Left*) The coarse vesiculation of the epidermis is the actual feature on which the term *spongiosis* is based. (*Right*) The destructive process is completed by the elimination of necrotic epidermal straps building in the image of reticular degeneration. H&E ×40 o m

Table 5.2 Spongiotic dermatitides

Exogenous
Primary contact dermatitis
Allergic contact dermatitis
Photocontact dermatitis
Endogenous
Allergic dermatitis
Photodermatitis
Miscellaneous

dermatitides are considered here to be of allergic nature and called in consequence "allergic dermatitis." When allergic dermatitides occur in response to solar radiation, they are known in this classification as "photocontact dermatitis" and "photodermatitis," respectively.

Spongiotic Lesions

The lesions in the purported Groups of spongiotic dermatitis (Table 5.2) do not show significant histologic difference among each other, requiring help from the clinic in order to reach meaningful diagnoses.

Spongiotic Lesions, Exogenous

In lesions associated with primary contact dermatitis, devitalization and necrosis may take preeminence over all other changes mentioned. This is exemplified by the lesion featured in Fig. 5.10, left, of a primary irritant contact dermatitis, in a case of scabies infection. The necrosis and heavy inflammatory infiltration below the mite conceal the spongiosis of the lesion, more visible at the periphery. The picture in Fig. 5.10, right, presents a lesion in a classic case of allergic contact dermatitis, following external sensitization to the nickel-plated back of a wrist watch. Note the thickened epidermal ridges featuring mild spongiosis and exocytosis. A significant component of this lesion is crusting, which results from serous oozing.

The lesion in Fig. 5.11, left, features the image of another classic instance, this time of photocontact dermatitis. This is a case of "beach party dermatitis," after sun exposure of an individual, previously sensitized to lime juice, who attended a beach party. An explosive combination occurred, as may be appraised! The cellular infiltration of the deep dermis is always tantamount of the intervention of solar radiation in the pathogenesis of the lesion. The lesion to the right shows the spongiotic lesion pertaining to an endogenous allergic dermatitis related in this case to food intolerance.

Spongiotic Lesions, Endogenous

Food and drugs administered via enteral and parenteral pathways to sensitized patients most frequently results in endogenous dermatitis. Spongiosis may take a prominent role in the histopathologic picture, as seen in the lesion in Fig. 5.11, right, corresponding to a case of food intolerance. The lesion also shows a dense inflammatory infiltrate with abundant eosinophils, a finding always supportive of the allergic nature of a lesion.

Spongiotic Lesions, Miscellaneous

In this third Group of miscellaneous dermatitides (Table 5.2), chronic dermatitis should be considered first. As acute dermatitis does not subside and is prolonged into chronicity, the histopathology of its lesions changes accordingly. Spongiosis tends to diminish, almost disappearing from the microscopic picture, whereas hyperkeratosis, acanthosis, and increase in thickness of the granular layer occur simultaneously. There is elongation and bifurcation of the epidermal ridges, which appear surrounded by a fibrotic dermis featuring a diffuse inflammatory infiltrate. This description

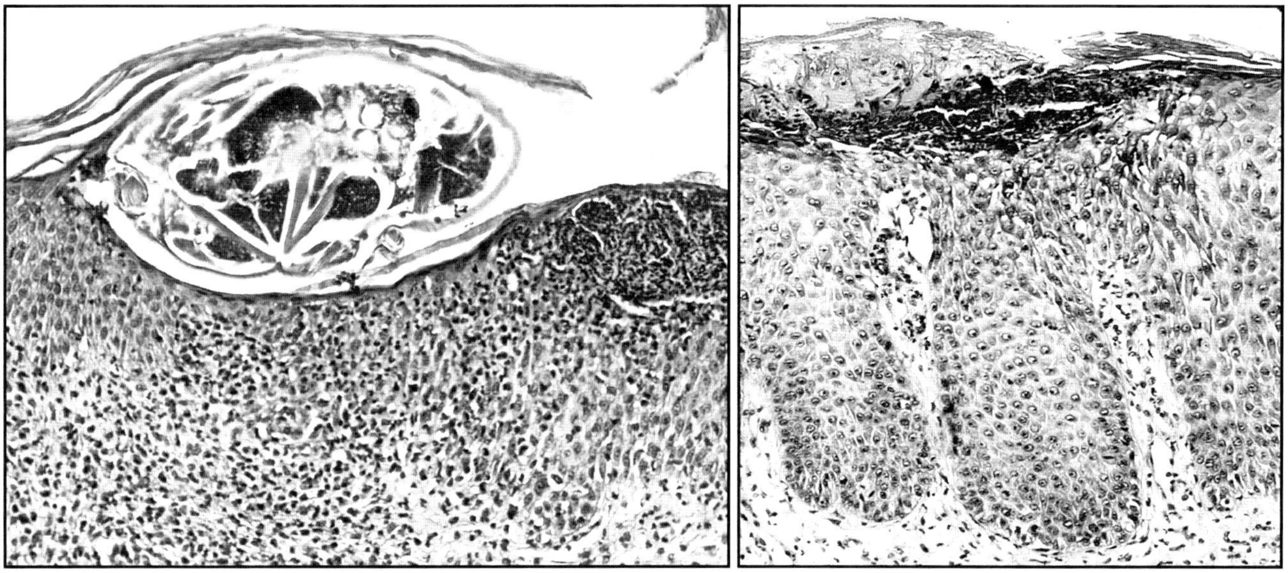

Fig. 5.10 Primary irritant and allergic contact dermatitis. (*Left*) Note the scanty keratin scales covering the sarcoptes mite, which, otherwise, does not penetrate into the skin. (*Right*) Observe the spongiosis, exocytosis, and crusting of the lesion. H&E; ×100

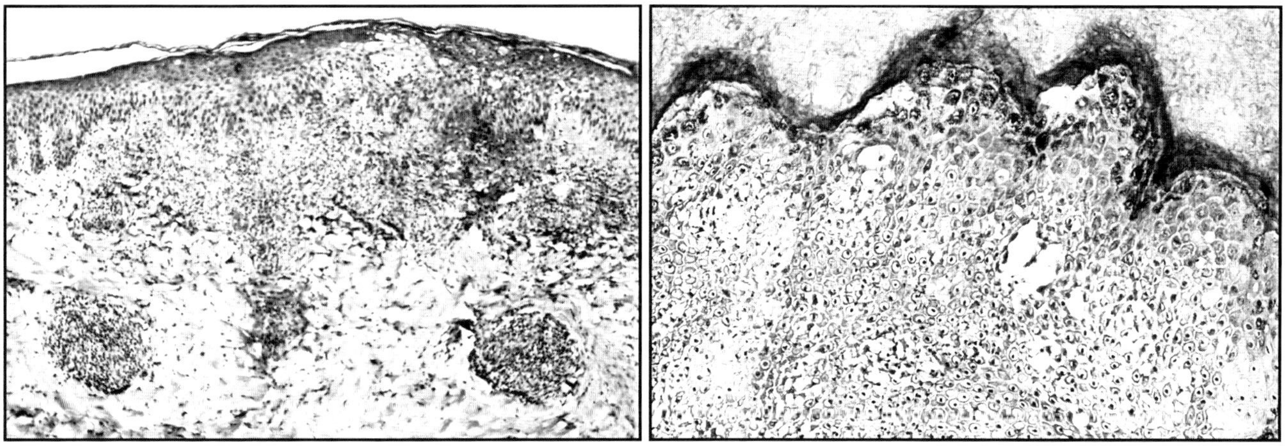

Fig. 5.11 Photocontact and allergic dermatitis. The first lesion (*left*) shows combined spongiosis and necrosis of the epidermis along with strong edema and mononuclear cell infiltration of the superficial and deep dermis. The second lesion (*right*) shows spongiosis with vesiculation of the epidermis, which appears crusted and invaded by a dense infiltrate spreading out from the dermis. H&E; ×100 o m

of chronic dermatitis fully matches the lesions of nummular eczema and picker's nodule (Fig. 5.12).

After chronic dermatitis, a series of conditions of diverse nature should be considered, all of whose lesions feature spongiosis as a constant microscopic detail. In all of these cases, clinical information is essential in order to arrive at a correct final diagnosis of the lesion under study.

Id-lesions: The term "*id*" derives from "*eczematid*," a name given by the French school to entities whose lesions resemble eczema, although without being totally identifiable with it [8]. Id-lesions are probably distant, secondary localizations to a primary focus of sensitization located elsewhere on the body. Although LM images of id-lesions show spongiosis as an indispensable requisite, the absence of the sensitizing agent is **sine qua non** for the diagnosis. For instance, a lesion considered to be in the "id"-category would lose its denomination in favor of "dermatophytosis" if fungi happens to be discovered in it.

Fixed drug eruption is a condition characterized by a recurrent lesion on the exact same anatomic site, following the administration of some medication, phenolphthalein being the prototypic example. The reason for the bizarre behavior of these lesions has not been clarified to date, except for considering them instances of "somatization." The usual chronic look of the lesion under LM may become more acute in case of its exacerbation.

Seborrheic dermatitis is also included in this group because of the spongiotic character of its lesions. This disorder is eventually due to a low-grade cutaneous infection in a *predisposed* individual. The combination of elongated rete

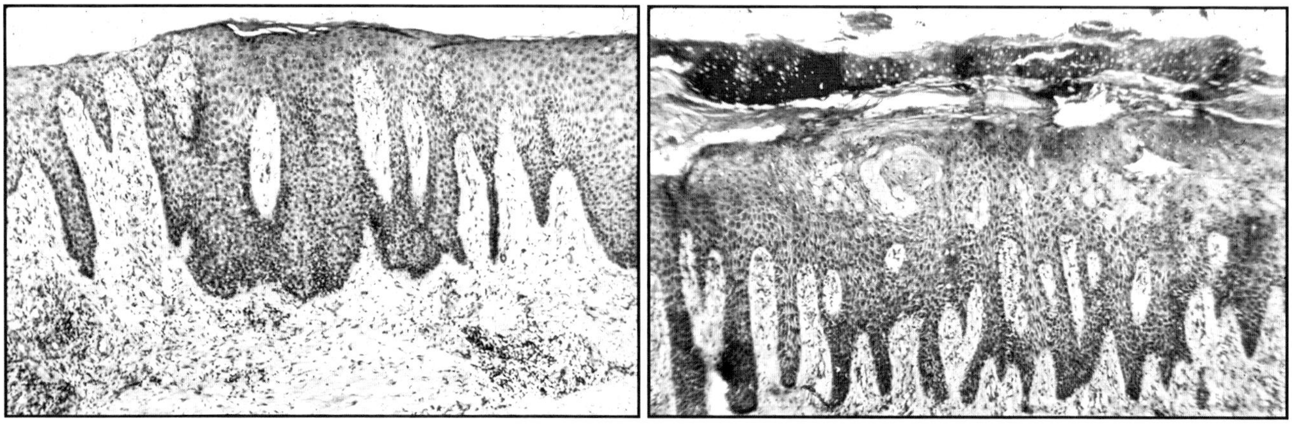

Fig. 5.12 Nummular eczema and picker's nodule. Nummular eczema (*left*) is shown in an exacerbation phase. To the acanthosis, rete ridge elongation, and chronic inflammatory infiltrate customarily seen in this lesion, moderate spongiosis and crusting are added here as an expression of the reactivation of the lesion. Picker's nodule (*right*) shows a picture essentially comparable to the one to the left, except for the considerable crusting, related to the self-inflicted damage of the patient. Note in both lesions the deep alteration with bifurcation of the epidermal ridges, a sign indicative of the tendency to chronicity of the lesion. H&E ×40 o m

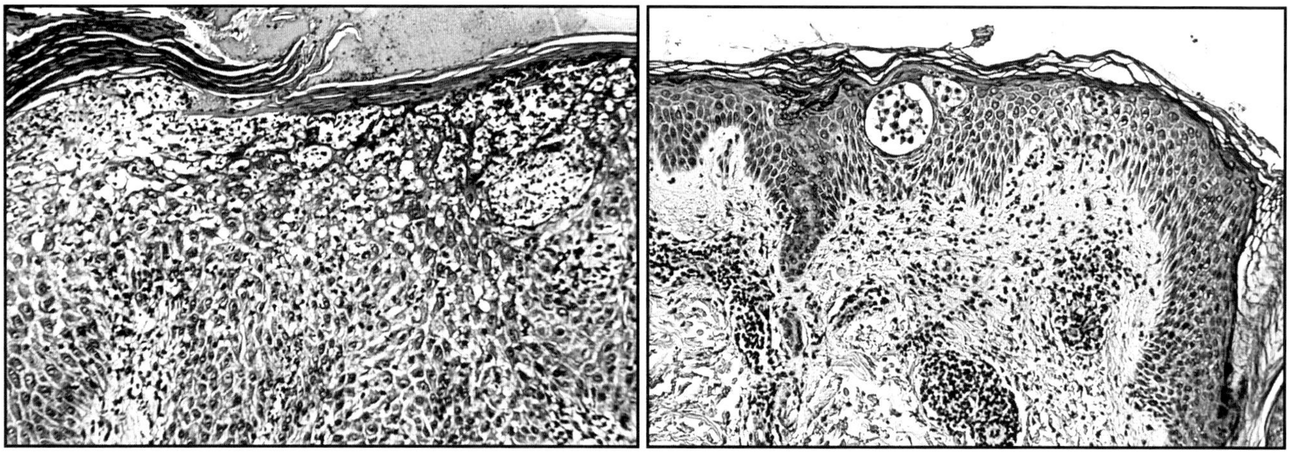

Fig. 5.13 Seborrheic dermatitis and pityriasis rosea. Note in the first lesion (*left*) the dense infiltration by neutrophils of the upper epidermis, the elongation of the rete ridges, and the patchy spongiosis. In the second lesion (*right*), there is mild but diffuse spongiosis along with a solitary epidermal vesicle. H&E ×100 o m

ridges with neutrophil infiltration seen in the lesion (Fig. 5.13, left) may bring psoriasis as an alternative diagnostic possibility. This consideration is excluded however, by the presence of spongiosis, categorically in favor of seborrheic dermatitis and against psoriasis.

Pityriasis rosea of Gibert is clinically characterized at its outcome, by a large, solitary plaque, the "*mother plaque*." This is followed later by smaller, itchy plaques disseminated all over the body in a characteristic "*Christmas tree distribution*." LM of the secondary lesions discloses areas of congestion and edema with scattered, extravasated red blood cells in papillary tips and diffuse spongiosis, often with a solitary vesicle, almost diagnostic of this condition [9] (Fig. 5.13, right).

In addition to the mentioned conditions, there are others, characterized by the spongiotic quality of their lesions, which the microscopist has to take into consideration when he or she faces the diagnosis of this type of lesions. One of these is infantile papular acrodermatitis, or Gianotti-Crosti syndrome, caused by *hepatitis B* virus, and another is hand-foot-and-mouth disease, due to a *Coxsackie virus*, both organisms belonging to the family of the *picornaviruses* (Fig. 5.2). These disorders are clinically characterized by vesicular eruptions, with histopathologic features reminiscent of pityriasis rosea of Gibert.

Necrotizing Lesions

Skin submitted to violent external agents may suffer sudden destruction, resulting in charring and loss of any former structural detail. Otherwise, it may go into coagulation necrosis, at the end stage of it, some cutaneous details may somehow be recognizable. Under steady unfavorable conditions, otherwise, the skin may die through a slow process of necrobiosis, to which enzymatic autolysis may be attributed.

According to the origin of the aggression that causes their necrosis, the lesions may be grouped as exogenous or endogenous. Table 5.3 presents a list of pathogenic agents of necrotizing lesions.

Necrotizing Lesions, Exogenous

Exogenous necrotizing lesions are frequently the result of violent aggressions by traumatic or physicochemical agents. They can also be the result of stings or bites caused by arthropod or other ectoparasites. In the latter case, trauma may be combined with the action of simultaneously secreted toxins to bring the tissues to the already mentioned stage of coagulation necrosis.

Figure 5.14, left, illustrates the intense effect of an electric discharge to the skin: the necrotic keratinocytes appear elongated and grouped as bundles which have been referred to as "*bunches of beans*." This deformation, caused by the loss of the cellular resistance, is not privative to external aggressions: it may also be noted as a result of internal processes, where it may be appraised as a sign of severe damage. The lesion to the right in the same figure shows a vertical section across the site of an arthropod aggression. In this case, the traumatic effect of the bite combined with the necrotizing effect of the toxins concomitantly released causes the immediate coagulation necrosis of the epidermis which is transformed into an "eschar" overlying a sharply delimited area of severe inflammatory changes in the dermis. When the eschar is shed, an area of the skin will remain *that is devoid of epidermis*. By definition, this is known as an "ulcer." In contrast to an ulcer, an area of the skin whose epidermis is only lacking its uppermost layers is defined as an "excoriation" [10]. The practical importance of the differentiation is that an excoriation heals without scarring, whereas ulcers leave a scar.

Figure 5.15 illustrates a lesion somewhat associated to the ones mentioned above. It differs in that it does not occur on living, but on an already dead tissue, in this case the thick horny layer of the sole of the foot (left). The central hole is the imprint of the mouth parts of a tick and remains unchanged after the piercing. Note the clear halo surrounding the hole, most probably the effect of toxins secreted by the tick at the time of the aggression (right). The culprit was found in the deepermost part of the biopsy.

Table 5.3 List of pathogenic agents of necrotizing lesions

Exogenous
UV radiation, intense
High and low temperatures
Basic and acid solutions
Ectoparasites
Endogenous
Viral agents
Microbial agents
Therapeutic agents
Neoplastic processes

Necrotizing Lesions, Endogenous

The Group of the endogenous necrotizing lesions is subgrouped as *superficial* and *massive* (Fig. 5.5). This separation is based on the fact that in the former case, the necrotic changes are limited to the upper epidermal layer, *while the germinal layer is left undisturbed*, whereas in the latter case, the entire epidermis, *including the germinal layer*, is involved in the process. Therefore, after the necrotizing process occurred, the lesions with superficial necrosis may undergo rapid regeneration, while the ones which underwent massive changes involving the germinal layer may not.

Necrotizing Lesions, Endogenous, Superficial

Superficial necrotizing lesions are caused in their great majority by microbial toxins. The most pertinent case is

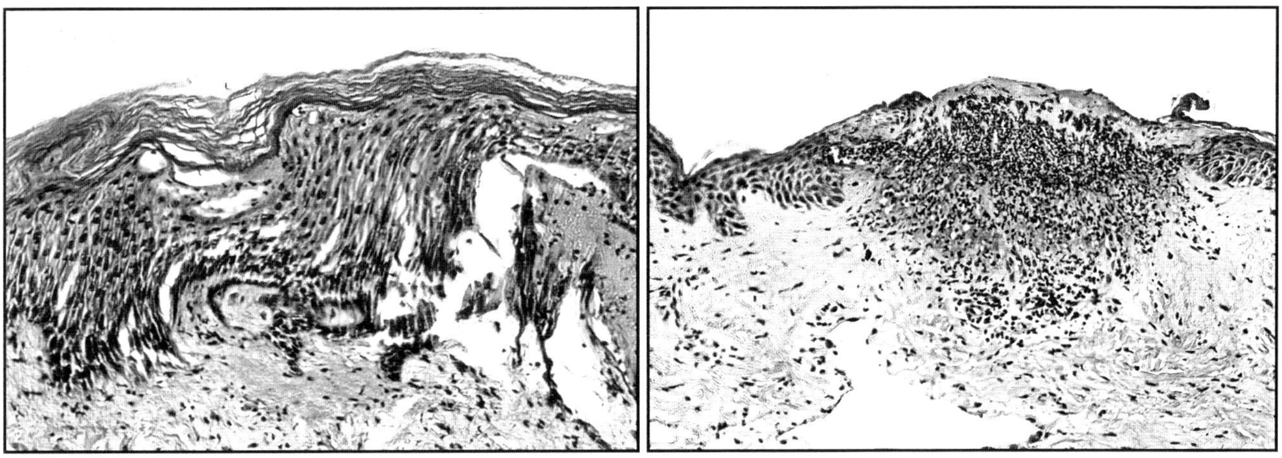

Fig. 5.14 Cutaneous necrosis due to electric discharge (*left*) and to arthropod aggression (*right*). See details in the text. H&E; ×100 o m

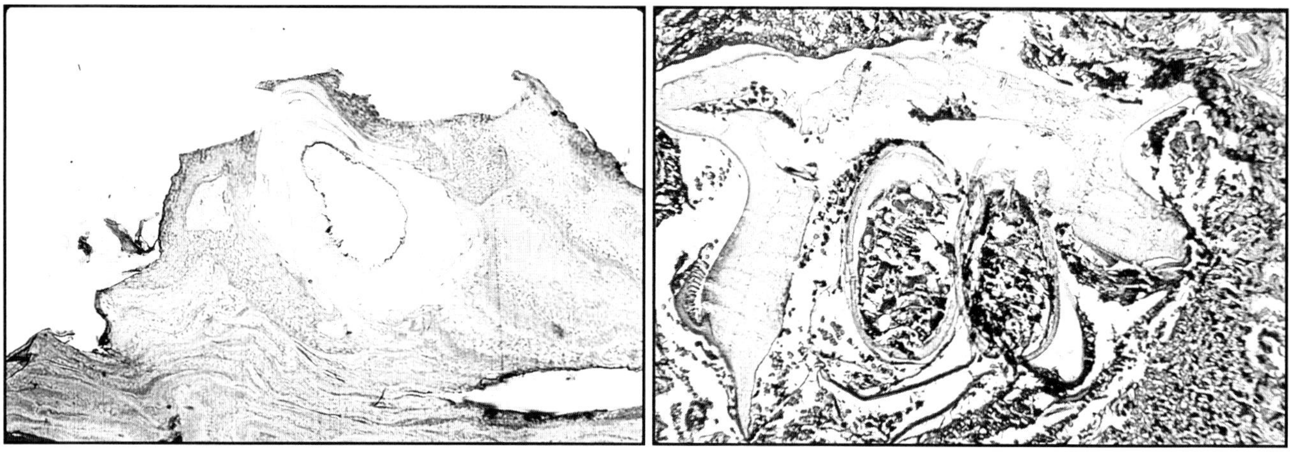

Fig. 5.15 (*Left*) Imprint of the mouth parts of a tick in the horny layer and (*right*) tick mouth parts in the deep dermis. See details in the text. H&E ×100; ×40 o m

staphylococcal scalded skin syndrome. This condition was described around 1850 by G. R. v. Rittershain, director of a pediatric hospital in Prague. It was considered to be a neonatal condition with a benign outcome which he called "dermatitis exfoliativa neonatorum." This disorder was introduced into the Anglo-American literature as "Ritter's disease." It was later called "scalded skin syndrome," abbreviated as "SSS," on account of the sloughing of the epidermis which made the patient look as if he or she had contacted boiling water. To the three S, a fourth was later added when the staphylococcal etiology of the condition was recognized.

SSSS follows rhinopharyngeal infections by *staphylococci phage group* II type 71 in lactating and young infants [11]. Exfoliatin, an exotoxin generated during the course of the infection, is selectively fixed on the uppermost epidermal layer, causing its sloughing as epidermal straps. The fact that the germinal layer is not affected allows generally a fast epidermal regeneration and the restitution of the skin to its normal conditions. For this reason, the prognosis of SSSS is frankly favorable.

Because SSSS patients usually seek medical assistance in the latter period of evolution, it is unusual to obtain samples of the lesion before the epidermal sloughing has occurred. However, a condition known as *bullous impetigo* exists, allowing the microscopist to examine a lesion similar to the one of SSSS in its early stage of development.

Bullous impetigo is a disease of children, although it usually affects patients of greater age. The lesion is caused by the same exotoxin active in SSSS although, instead of affecting the epidermis in a generalized way, it does so focally, resulting in isolated or confluent vesicles developed through the granular layer, as may be seen in Fig. 5.16.

The cavity in bullous impetigo (left) appears devoid of cellular elements: this detail, consistent with the one in SSSS, highlights its difference with impetigo contagiosa (right) – shown here for comparison – whose cavity is filled with neutrophils and cellular debris.

Post-scarlet fever desquamation is another example of a superficial epidermal necrosis very similar to the one of SSSS, although it is caused by totally different germs, that is, certain strains of *beta* hemolytic streptococci which generate a group of erythrogenic exotoxins. A few days after the infection which is generally localized on the tonsils or pharynx, a superficial necrosis of the upper epidermis ensues, followed by its massive desquamation, followed by epidermal regeneration to its normal conditions.

Glucagonoma syndrome, also known as necrolytic migratory erythema, is also a disorder characterized – at least in its initial phase – by superficial epidermal necrosis. The pathogenesis of these lesions is not related, as in the former cases, to microbial toxins but possibly to the lack of zinc and certain amino acids, associated in turn to the presence of a carcinoma of *alpha* cells of the pancreatic islets of Langerhans [12]. Microscopic examination of the lesion presents a devitalized upper epidermis, which appears as a pale pink, vacuolated band (Fig. 5.17). Its invasion by neutrophils contributes to the final degradation and elimination of this layer.

Necrotizing Lesions, Endogenous, Massive

A triad of disorders exists in which massive epidermal necrosis is brought about through a not totally well-understood process loosely qualified as a "*vascular reaction*." This leads through a succession of changes to a common end result, which is the necrosis and sloughing of the epidermis. These three disorders, hereby organized in order of increasing prognostic seriousness, are erythema multiforme (EMu), Stevens-Johnson syndrome (SJS), and toxic epidermolytic necrolysis (TEN).

Erythema multiforme is caused predominantly by *Mycoplasma pneumonia* and *herpesvirus* infections, whereas SJS and TEN result from the administration of particular

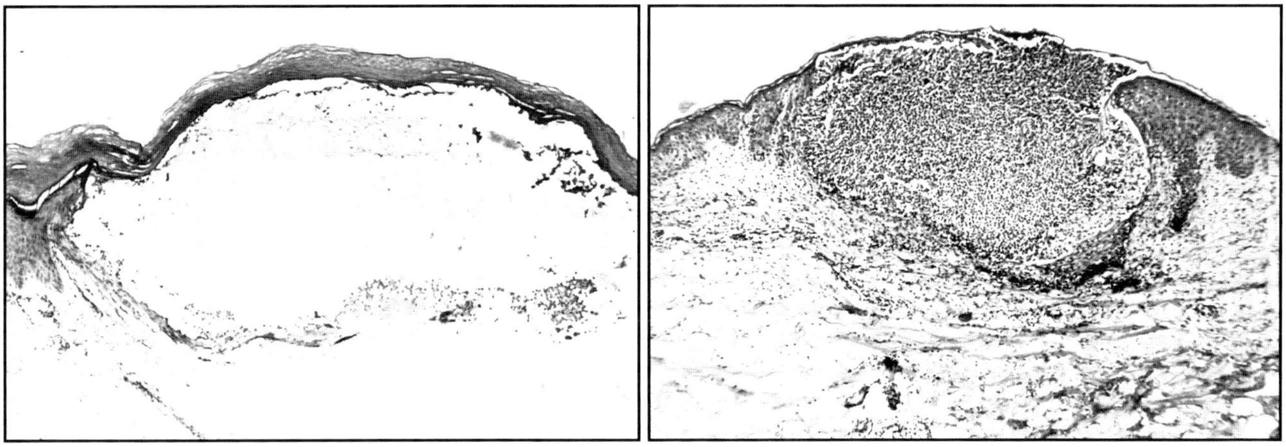

Fig. 5.16 Bullous impetigo and impetigo contagiosa. Note the acellular content of the cavity in bullous impetigo (*left*), formed in between the horny and the germinative layer of the epidermis. In impetigo contagiosa (*right*), a similar cavity appears filled with purulent material. H&E ×40

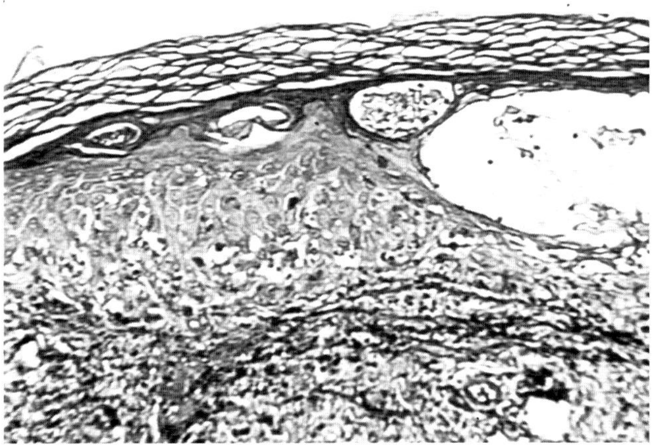

Fig. 5.17 Glucagonoma syndrome. Note the devitalized aspect of the epidermis (*left*). Advanced lesion with vacuolization and degradation of the epidermis (*right*). H&E ×100 o m

medications in the majority of the cases. Whereas it is conceivable that the implicated drugs may act directly in the production of SJS and TEN, the pathogenic mechanism in EMu appears to be more complex and is still motive for speculation.

The succession of histopathologic changes that leads to the common end result of *massive epidermal necrosis* in the three disorders may be summarized by those which occur in EMu.

Erythema multiforme was initially reported by F. v. Hebra, in 1860 [13]. This is a condition of young adults initially manifested by malaise, followed some days later by the appearance of plaques of congestion and edema. Afterward, patients develop characteristic concentric cutaneous lesions, with a necrotic center surrounded by an area of edema and a peripheral rim of congestion, forming so-called *target lesions*, or "*bull's-eye lesions*," etc. EMu may last for a couple of weeks, but its outcome is generally favorable.

Although the pathogenesis of EMu has yet to be clarified, it may be speculated that its sequence could be initiated by a vascular event, that is, the localized aggression to the endothelium by a circulating agent. This would increase vascular permeability, accounting for the *early prominent urticarial signs* in the patient. Later, the deposition of such agent on the skin surface would trigger the characteristic focal, necrotic lesions mentioned above [12].

The initial microscopic picture of EMu is dominated by strong edema associated with a flat and distended epidermis (Fig. 5.18, left). In more advanced stages, that image acquires a devitalized look, with a pale epidermis featuring loss of cellular details and vacuolization (Fig. 5.18, right).

In the final stage of the lesion, discontinuous clefts appear along the dermoepidermal junction. This clefting initiates the process of separation of the epidermis from the dermis, which at this point shows edema and an intense inflammatory infiltration (Fig. 5.19, left). In the final phase, the epidermis is reduced to an informal mass of necrotic tissue overlying a strongly edematous dermis. Note the similarity of the end stage of this picture with that of TEN (Fig. 5.19, right). In this latter case, the separation of the necrotic epidermis from the dermis has been completed, as shown by the presence of an irregular dermoepidermal space filled with serosanguinolent material.

Stevens-Johnson syndrome, a serious variant of EM, was reported several years after EMu. It begins with severe malaise and *selective mucosal involvement*, particularly of the oral and the conjunctival mucosae. LM examination of the lesion shows again diffuse epidermal necrosis, this time with abundant extravasated red blood cells.

Toxic epidermal necrolysis is the most serious of the three related disorders, ending most frequently with the patient's demise. When A. Lyell reported TEN in 1956, he arbitrarily enclosed SSSS in his description, considering the latter, – in spite of clear histopathologic differences – a minor form of

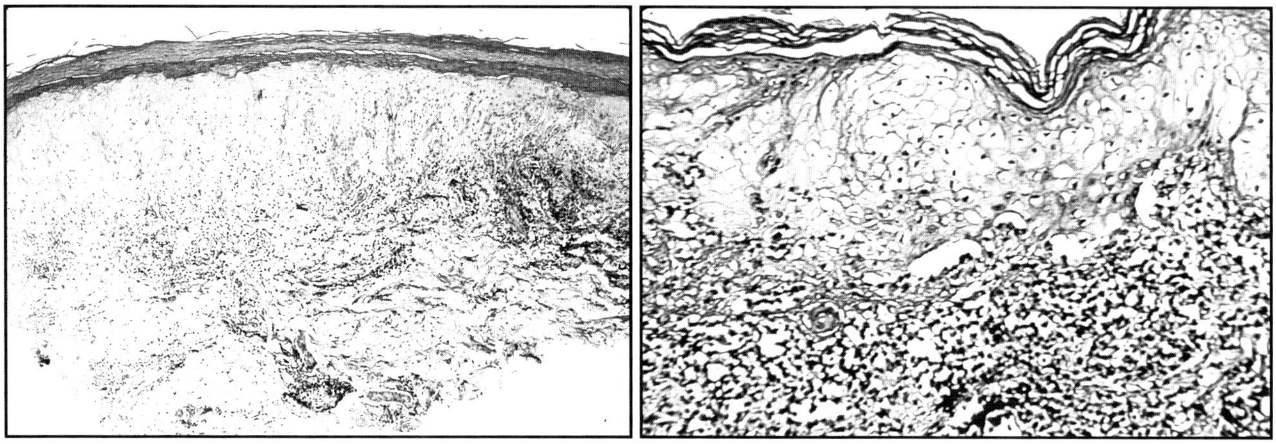

Fig. 5.18 Erythema multiforme, early (*left*) and advanced (*right*) phase. See the text for details. H&E; ×40; ×100 o m

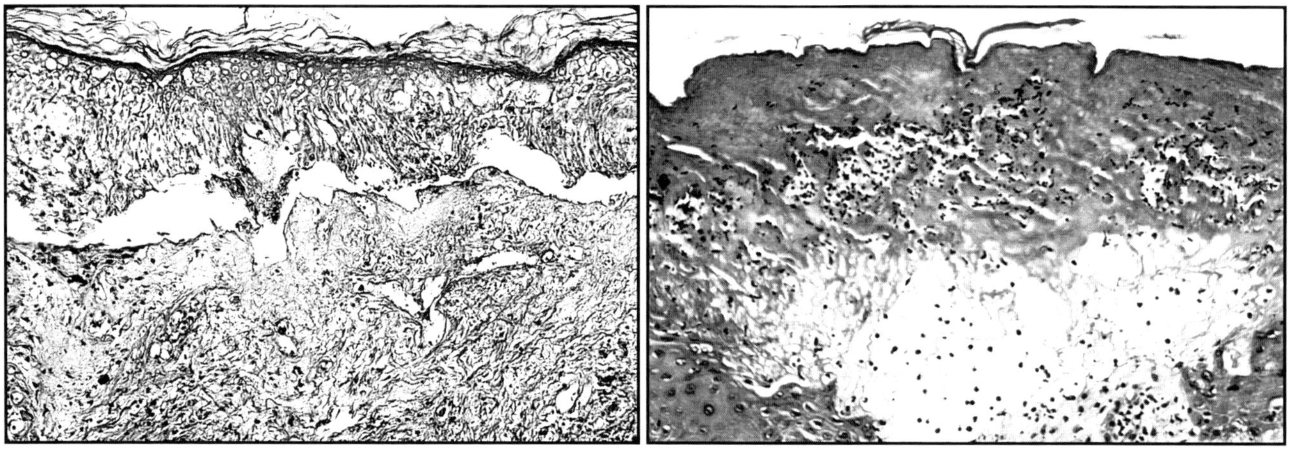

Fig. 5.19 Erythema multiforme, end phase (*left*), and toxic epidermolytic (*right*) necrolysis. See details in the text. H&E; ×40 o m

TEN: both conditions were called together "Lyell disease." [14] It was after years of confusion that the matter was clarified, and SSSS returned to have its own individuality, clearly different from the one of TEN. TEN occurs suddenly, causing a widespread epidermal necrosis of the worst prognosis, comparable to that found in patients with extensive burns. The seriousness of this condition can be appreciated by examining again the picture in Fig. 5.19, right, which shows the patient's skin in its entire thickness.

In discussing those entities whose lesions feature massive epidermal necrosis, another previously mentioned lesion pityriasis lichenoides et varioliformis acuta should be now reviewed.

Pityriasis lichenoides et varioliformis acuta (PLEVA), or Mucha-Habermann disease [15], is an already mentioned disorder of suspected viral etiology unrelated to any of the conditions studied above. PLEVA appears as discrete, disseminated crusted lesions on the body surface. This sequence of events is reminiscent of that occurring in varicella lesions. The qualificative "*varicelliform*" included in the designation "PLEVA" refers precisely to that clinical analogy, although microscopic examination fails to support it. The lesion in PLEVA, as in the other conditions belonging to this group of disorders, features under LM *massive epidermal necrosis* (Fig. 5.20), whereas the one of varicella, as it will be seen (p. 77), shows as its primary microscopic alteration *epidermolysis*, a totally different histopathologic feature. (See Fig. 5.28.)

Lesions with Inflammatory Infiltration

This fourth Subclass encloses lesions which present infiltration by acute inflammatory cells, overwhelmingly neutrophils, as their distinctive feature. The underlying stimulus, for the polynuclear mobilization, allows the separation of these processes – and consequently their lesions into two Groups: infectious and noninfectious (Fig. 5.5).

Lesions with Inflammatory Infiltration, Infectious

Impetigo contagiosa is a frequent lesion caused by pyogenic germs, particularly streptococci and staphylococci,

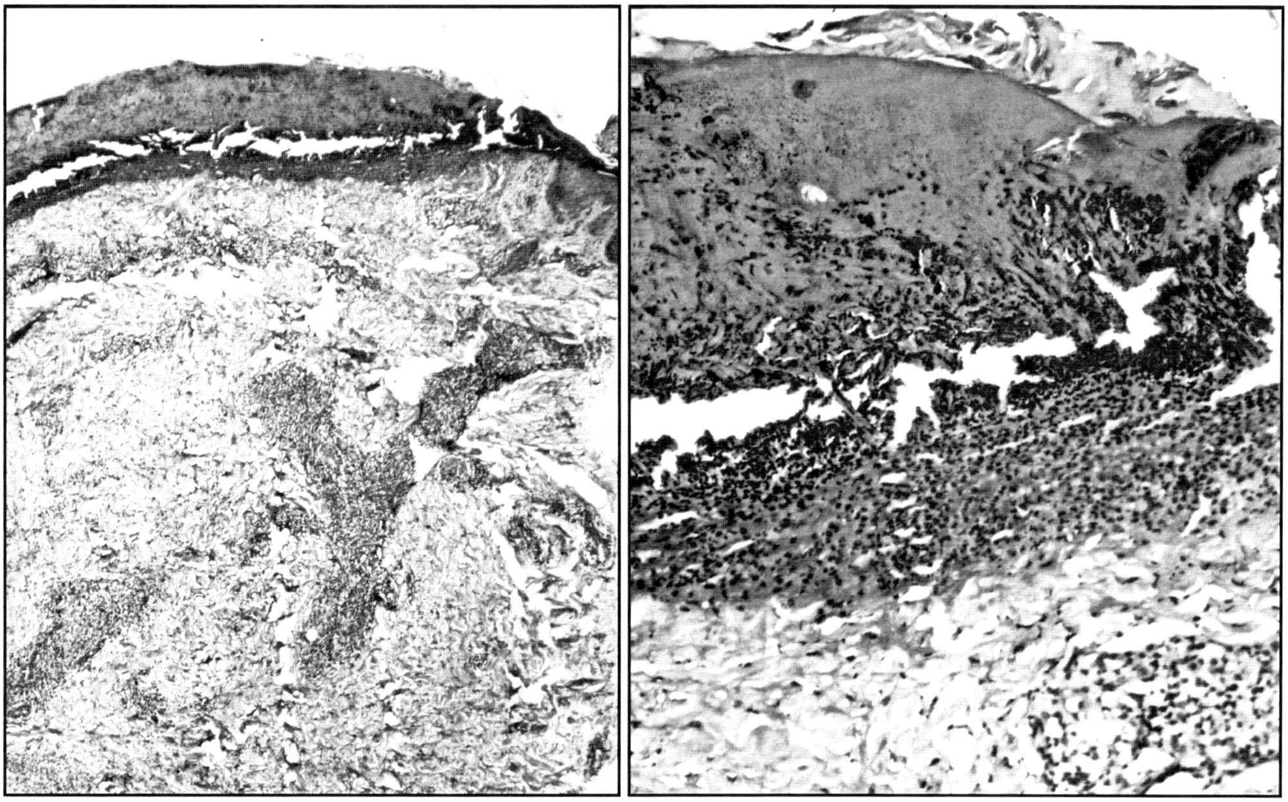

Fig. 5.20 Pityriasis lichenoides et varioliformis acuta. At low magnification (*left*), the lesion shows massive necrosis of the epidermis, which appears covered by a crust. The dermis of the specimen shows a dense inflammatory infiltrate forming thick perivascular cuffs. A high magnification shows details of the lesion (*right*). H&E; ×40; ×400 o m

introduced into the skin from the outside. The responsible agent causes a rapid inflammatory reaction with building up of highly infectious crusts. The histologic picture of these lesions is characterized by the separation of the epidermis at the level of the granular layer, with accumulation of purulent material within (Fig. 5.16, right). This sets this lesion clearly apart from the one of the previously discussed bullous impetigo (p. 70) (Fig. 5.21).

The invasion of the epidermis by *T. pallidum*, causal agent of syphilis, in individuals without previous contact with this organism, causes another lesion with acute inflammatory infiltration, the syphilitic chancre.

Syphilitic Chancre [16]: This is an indolent lesion of firm consistency. It has an eroded and oozing external surface. The lesion is surrounded by a rim of indurated tissue, presenting a swollen regional lymph node. The marked reactive acanthosis noted by LM in the first stage of the lesion usually prevents the total loss of its epithelial cover in such a way that in the majority of cases, the syphilitic chancre *is not an ulcer* but *an excoriation* (p. 73) (Fig. 5.22).

Secondary Syphilis: The gradual modification of the patient's defenses does not prevent the progression of the syphilitic infection into the secondary phase. This is exteriorized by the large repertoire of mucocutaneous lesions under which this stage of the infection may be manifested (Fig. 5.23 and 5.24). See also Fig. 5.46. Due to their strong epidermotrophism, spirochetae are found in high numbers in these secondary lesions. They are easily found via silver stains and several other available ancillary techniques (Fig. 5.23).

Figure 5.24 shows for comparison the cellular infiltrate in a primary and a secondary syphilitic lesion: in the first case (left), the infiltrate is formed by neutrophils pervading the epidermis, and in the second case (right), it is a mixture of plasmacytes with neutrophils admixed with mononuclear elements, localized in the dermis of the specimen.

Lesions with Inflammatory Infiltration, Noninfectious

Among the noninfectious lesions with inflammatory infiltrate, the most important and representative ones are those associated to psoriasis (*psor+iasis* [G] itch+condition). The pathogenesis of psoriasis is a topic not fully elucidated. It is still under speculation as to whether the primary cause of the characteristic neutrophilic epidermotrophism of this condition resides in the epidermis, the blood vessels, or the neutrophils themselves.

For working purposes in the laboratory, psoriasiform lesions may be divided into those associated to *psoriasis*

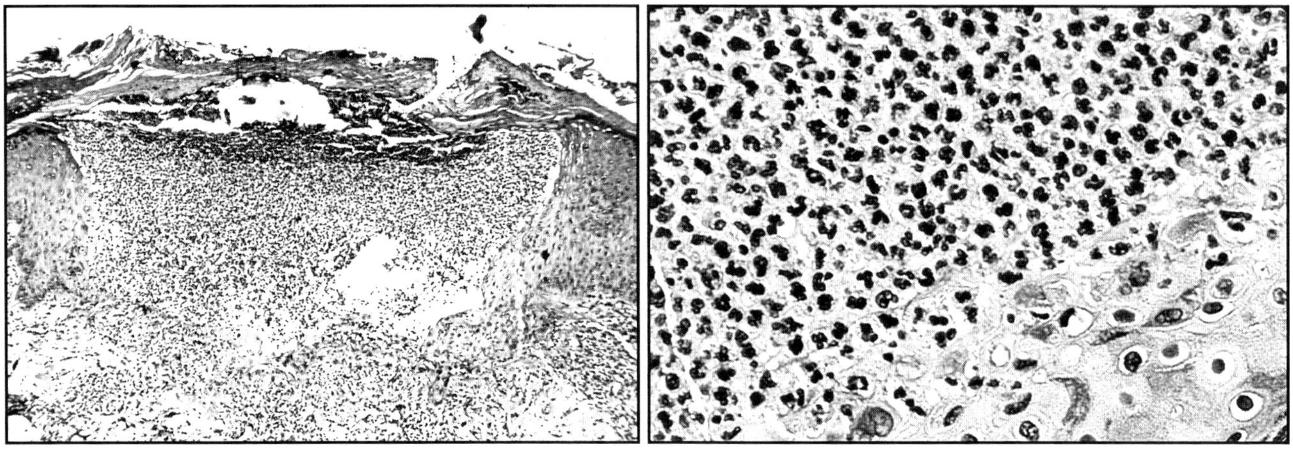

Fig. 5.21 Impetigo contagiosa. Note the well-circumscribed pocket of purulent material in a subcorneal position and overlaid by a crust (*left*). The picture to the right shows a higher magnification of the purulent content of the lesion, formed by neutrophils and cellular debris (*right*). H&E; ×40; ×400 o m

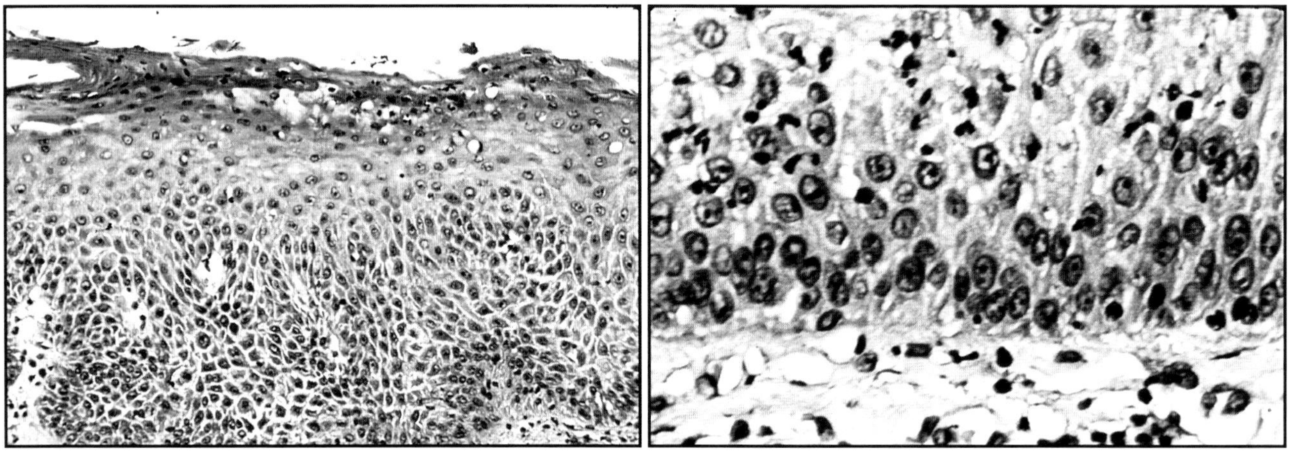

Fig. 5.22 Syphilitic chancre. The picture to the left offers an overview of the syphilitic chancre. Note the increased thickness of the crusted epidermis, infiltrated by neutrophils. These are drawn into the area by the presence of *T. pallida*. The picture to the right shows the active infiltration of the base of the lesion by neutrophils. H&E; ×40; ×400 o m

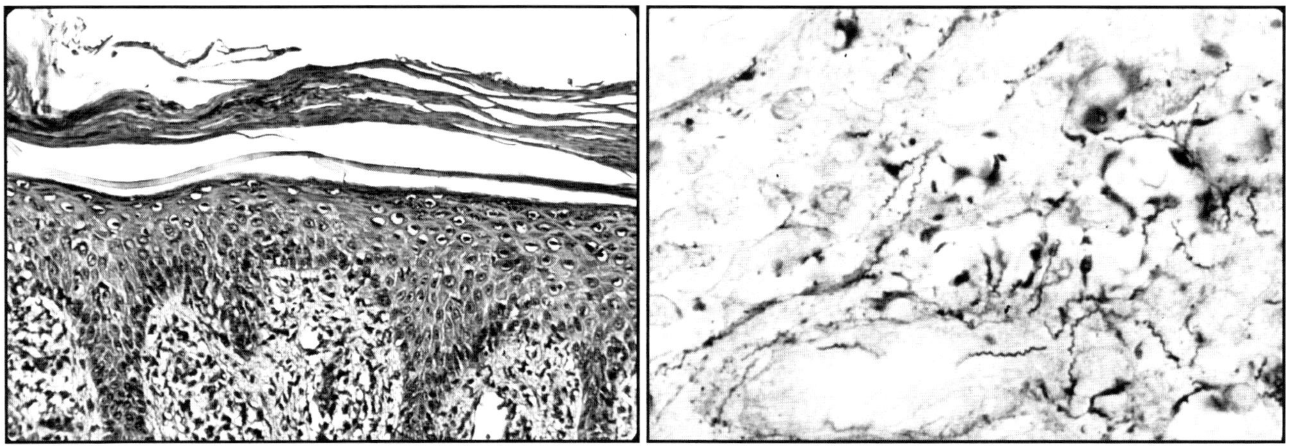

Fig. 5.23 Syphilis, secondary. (*Left*) The slightly spongiotic epidermis and the crusted horny layer are infiltrated by neutrophils. The dermis shows a dense infiltrate of plasma cells and neutrophils (*right*). The examination of silver-stained sections easily reveals the presence of the treponemata. WS ×1,000 o m

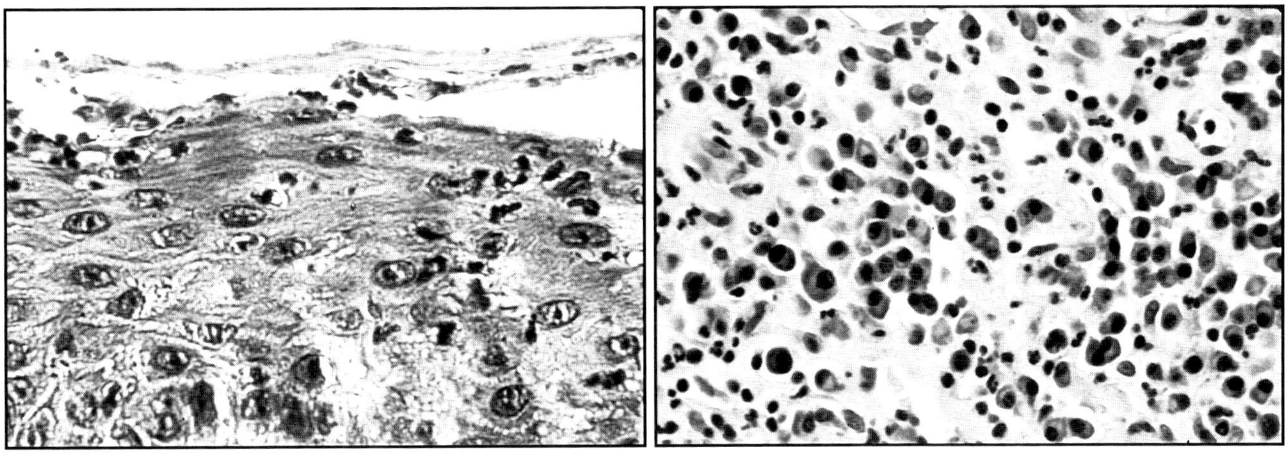

Fig. 5.24 Syphilis: cellular infiltrate in primary (*left*) and secondary lesion (*right*). See details in the text. H&E ×400 o m

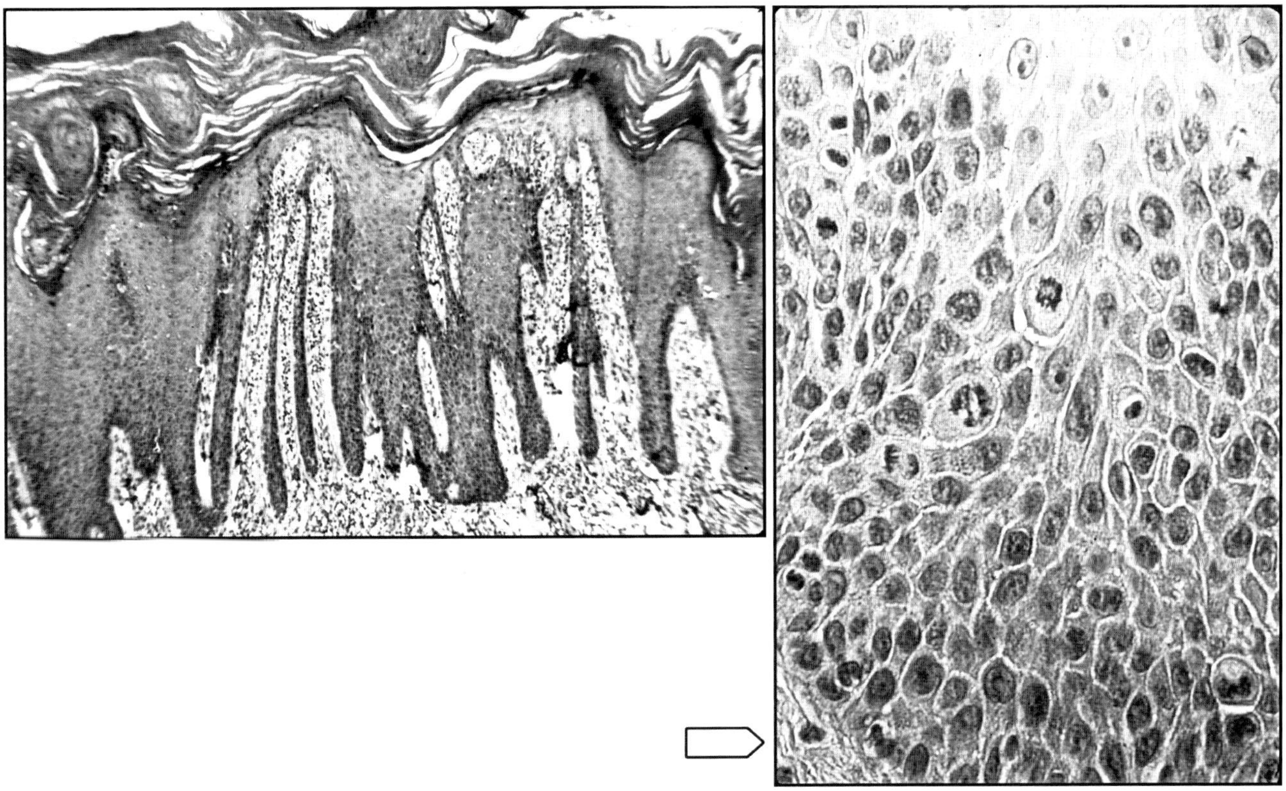

Fig. 5.25 Psoriasis vulgaris. (*Left*) Low magnification featuring the characteristic regularly elongated epidermal rete of the lesion. (*Right*) Numerous mitotic figures are noted in the midepidermis of the specimen. Note at the very left lower corner of the figure the germinal layer of the epidermis (*arrow*). H&E ×40; ×400 o m

vulgaris, to *pustular psoriasis*, or to any other clinical condition whose lesions microscopically resemble those of the two main varieties of this disorder.

Psoriasis vulgaris appears clinically as plaques with a dry, silvery surface, preferentially located on the extensor surfaces of the body. These lesions are associated with a microscopic image featuring a thickened, hyper- and parakeratotic epidermis with a thin and distorted granular layer. The epidermis shows an increased mitotic rate which, instead of being at the germinal layer as usually occurs, is more accentuated at midepidermal level (Fig. 5.25).

The dermal papillae of the specimen are infiltrated by neutrophils which emerge from tortuous capillaries running along their central axes (Fig. 5.26). They almost reach the papillary tips to deliver neutrophils, forming what were described by Pinkus as the "squirting papillae" in reference to the passage of neutrophils from them into the epidermis [17]. The neutrophils in the epidermis proceed further

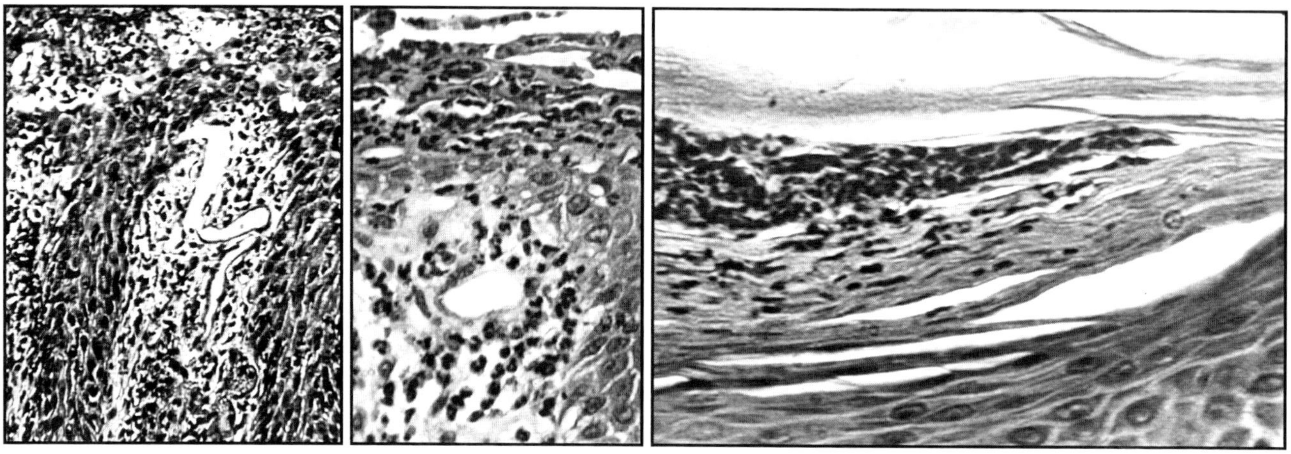

Fig. 5.26 Psoriasis vulgaris. (*Left*) A tortuous capillary is seen, ascending almost to the tip of a dermal papilla. (*Center*) Cross section of a capillary at the tip of a dermal papilla, with abundant neutrophils coming out from the vessel's lumen to invade the overlying epidermis. End stage of the neutrophil migration into the epidermis, forming the subcorneal Munro's microabscesses below the horny layer (*right*). H&E ×100; ×400; ×400 o m

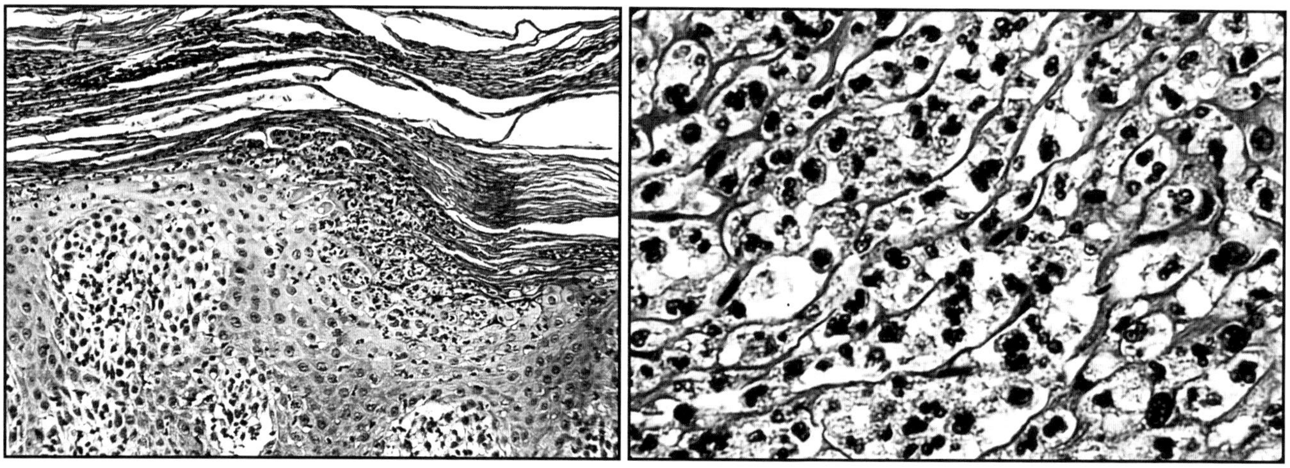

Fig. 5.27 Kogoj's spongiform pustule. (*Left*) Note the large number of neutrophils diffusely infiltrating the dermis and epidermis of the specimen. (*Right*) Neutrophils are held in the epidermis within a keratin mesh, forming a "Kogoj's spongiform pustule." H&E; ×40; ×400 o m

upward, ending up as dried subcorneal deposits, the so-called Munro's microabscesses [18], a pathognomonic element of the lesion in psoriasis vulgaris.

Due to the noted close vicinity of the papillary tips to the external surface, the curetting of a lesion in psoriasis vulgaris will damage the capillaries below, causing punctiform hemorrhages: this is the basis for the so-called Auspitz sign, characteristic of this lesion.

v. Zumbusch pustular psoriasis may be distinguished from psoriasis vulgaris by the former's more serious clinical picture and evolution. LM examination of its lesions discloses extensive dermoepidermal infiltrates filled with neutrophils, the Kogoj's spongiform pustules (Fig. 5.27), quite different from Munro's microabscesses (see above). Contrary to the latter, Kogoj's pustules are visible under naked eye inspection.

Impetigo herpetiformis is a condition which occurs in pregnant women, manifested by intensely pruritic papules. Due to its histopathology, this condition may be considered a variant of pustular psoriasis in pregnancy, characterized by the presence of Kogoj's spongiform pustules.

Hallopeau's Acrodermatitis Suppurativa: Because of its clinical features, this condition is often regarded as a variant of psoriasis vulgaris, although selectively localized at the finger tips. The histopathologic features of the lesion, though, are more in line with pustular psoriasis.

Reiter's disease is a condition whose cutaneous histopathology is totally superimposable to that of pustular psoriasis. The cutaneous lesion, however, occurs in a totally different setting, as a secondary feature – present only in about 30 % of Reiter's disease, that is, a symptomatic *triad of uveitis, urethritis, and arthritis*.

Sneddon-Wilkinson subcorneal pustular dermatosis deserves to be included in this section, too, since it is also a noninfectious, pustular condition. Sneddon-Wilkinson's disease is a chronic condition which appears as intertriginous blisters on the trunk and the base of the fingers. Under LM, its lesions appear as aseptic subcorneal blisters, totally unrelated to the histopathology of psoriasis vulgaris or pustular psoriasis. The nature of this condition is unknown, although it is suspected that it may be associated with a gammopathy.

Before ending this discussion, two further lesions of interest should be mentioned. These are eosinophilic spongiosis and eosinophilic abscesses, eventual precursors of pemphigus foliaceus and of bullous pemphigoid, respectively, characterized, as indicated by their names, by the presence of eosinophils in the epidermis.

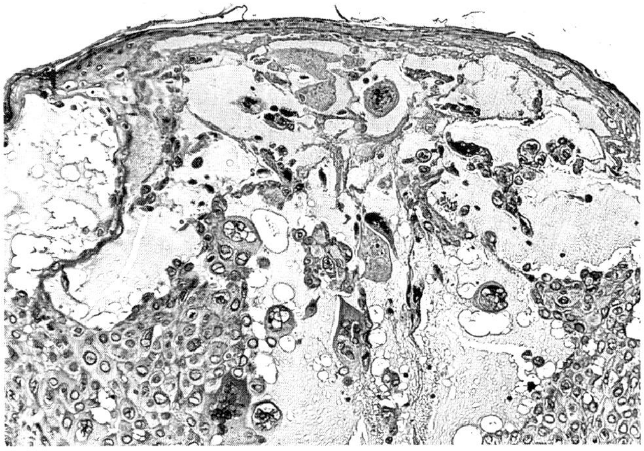

Fig. 5.28 Herpesvirus infection site. In the cavity formed as a result of the infection, the keratinocyte population appears as having almost totally disappeared. The space appears crossed by straps of necrotic cells, configuring the nonspecific picture of *reticular degeneration*

Epidermolytic Lesions

Epidermolytic lesions may result from the direct destruction of keratinocytes by epidermotrophic organisms or by the dissolution of their desmosomes during the course of autoimmune disorders. Therefore, these lesions may also be reasonably grouped as infectious and noninfectious.

Epidermolytic Lesions, Infectious

The agents responsible for this type of lesion are viruses of the *herpesviruses* family. These pertain to the double-stranded DNA viruses, which are medium sized and encapsulated (Fig. 5.1). The most important integrants of this family insofar as cutaneous pathology is concerned are the *herpesvirus simplex A and B* (HSV I and HSV II) and the *varicella-zoster virus* (VZV) [19].

The lesions caused by HSV I and HSV II may represent primary infections due to the direct implantation of the virus on the patient's skin or to reactivation of latent infections. Infections above the waist line are supposedly due to HSV I and infections below the waist line to HVS II. These two organisms are therefore called "herpes facialis" and "herpes genitalis," respectively.

Herpesvirus I and II Infections: The organisms responsible for these infections are directly implanted on the skin or mucosae by direct contact with an infected individual. After a period of latency, the infection is evidenced by a circumscribed exanthem which is later transformed into a crop of vesicles. These undergo crusting, disappearing within a week. Reactivations are manifested in a similar way as primary infections.

LM examination of recent lesion in both of these cases presents a picture which could be appropriately compared to the effects of an explosion within the epidermis (Fig. 5.28). The cellular elements of this layer have almost disappeared, leaving instead an almost empty space overlaid by scant keratin scales. The fact that in contrast with the epidermis, the dermis appears anatomically preserved in herpesvirus infection sites – although affected by a heavy, secondary inflammatory reaction – attests to the selective epidermotropism of the herpesvirus aggression (Fig. 5.28).

At this point, the diagnostic importance of Tzanck's smear should be emphasized. This fast technique allows the microscopist to find details such as multinucleated giant cells and intranuclear inclusion bodies (Fig. 5.29), which allows a rapid diagnosis of herpesvirus infection.

Varicella/zoster infections are acquired through the respiratory tract. After a period of latency of a few weeks, the virions undergo dissemination through the bloodstream. Their cutaneous localization is exteriorized in the form of vesicles which, upon external inspection, are found in diverse stages of evolution (asynergia).

Herpes Zoster Infection: At the time of the hematogenous dissemination, some virions reach the sensory dorsal root ganglia, where they remain inactive up to the moment of reactivation. At that point, they spread out centrifugally along the pertinent nerve toward the corresponding dermatome, invading the keratinocytes in this territory. Here, the lesions are manifested as itchy and painful vesicles (zoster or shingles) [20]. Viral reactivations may correspond to menstrual periods, solar exposures, infections, or to other circumstances. The microscopic picture in zoster is not significantly different from the one shown in Fig. 5.28 (Fig. 5.30).

In the context of infectious epidermolytic lesions, Grover's disease should finally be mentioned. This is done with reservation in view of its unconfirmed etiology. Grover's disease or transient acantholytic dermatosis (TAD) is a mild, itchy condition reported a few years ago [21], characterized under

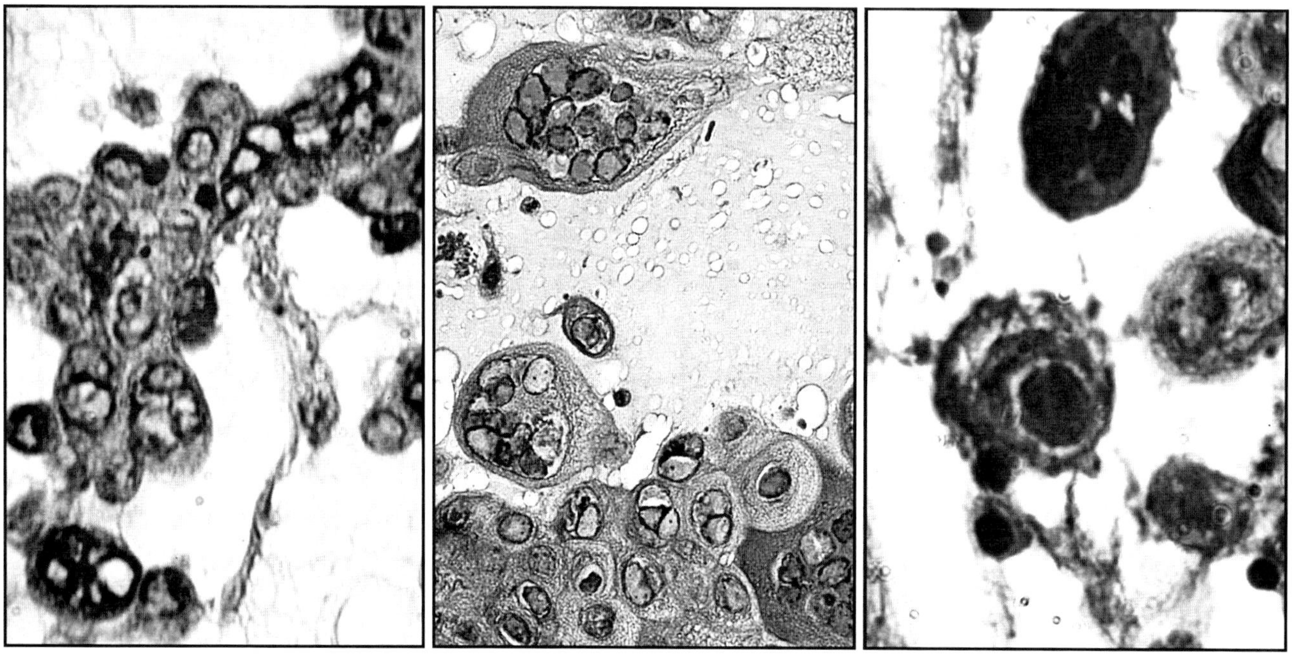

Fig. 5.29 Tzanck smear. (*Left*) Strap of necrotic keratinocytes. (*Center*) keratinocytes featuring globular degeneration. (*Right*) Keratinocytes with intranuclear inclusion bodies. Giemsa ×1,000 o m

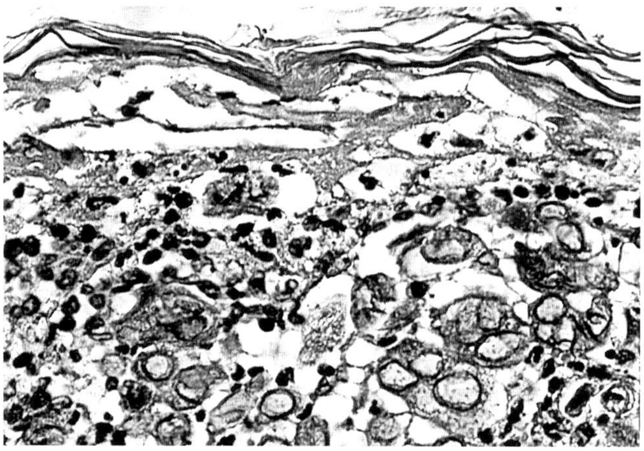

Fig. 5.30 Herpes zoster. Note the destruction of the epidermis and the globular degeneration of the keratinocytes. H&E ×100 o m

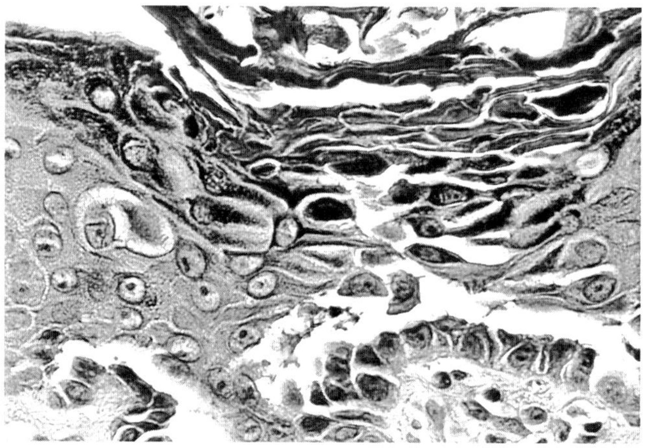

Fig. 5.31 Transient acantholytic dermatosis. Note the suprabasal acantholysis and the elements of benign dyskeratosis in the lesion. H&E; ×100 o m

the microscope by suprabasal acantholysis and benign dyskeratosis (Fig. 5.31). The transient character of TAD suggests a viral etiology, an assumption, still awaiting confirmation. TAD is worth being kept in mind by the microscopist, since it is not an infrequent condition among the material examined in the diagnostic laboratory.

It is of interest to note that TAD lesions, even being of inflammatory nature, present suprabasal acantholysis and benign dyskeratosis, features shared with the lesion of Darier's disease, a genodermatosis, and of warty dyskeratoma, a benign malformation. This fact, which brings up the diagnostic limitations of microscopy, also emphasizes the convenience of seeking clinical information to establish a clinico/pathologic correlations before rendering a final histopathologic report on a lesion under study. This situation is exemplified by Fig. 5.32.

If the microscopist had known in advance that the lesion in Fig. 5.32 top multiple and pertained to a patient suffering from Darier's disease, the diagnosis of that condition should obviously have been that. If the microscopist had been aware that the lesion in the center was solitary and had been sitting on the nape of neck of a patient for years, it would have put warty dyskeratoma first in the list of differential diagnoses. If on the other hand, he or she knew the lesion at the bottom was itchy and multiple and had only been present for some

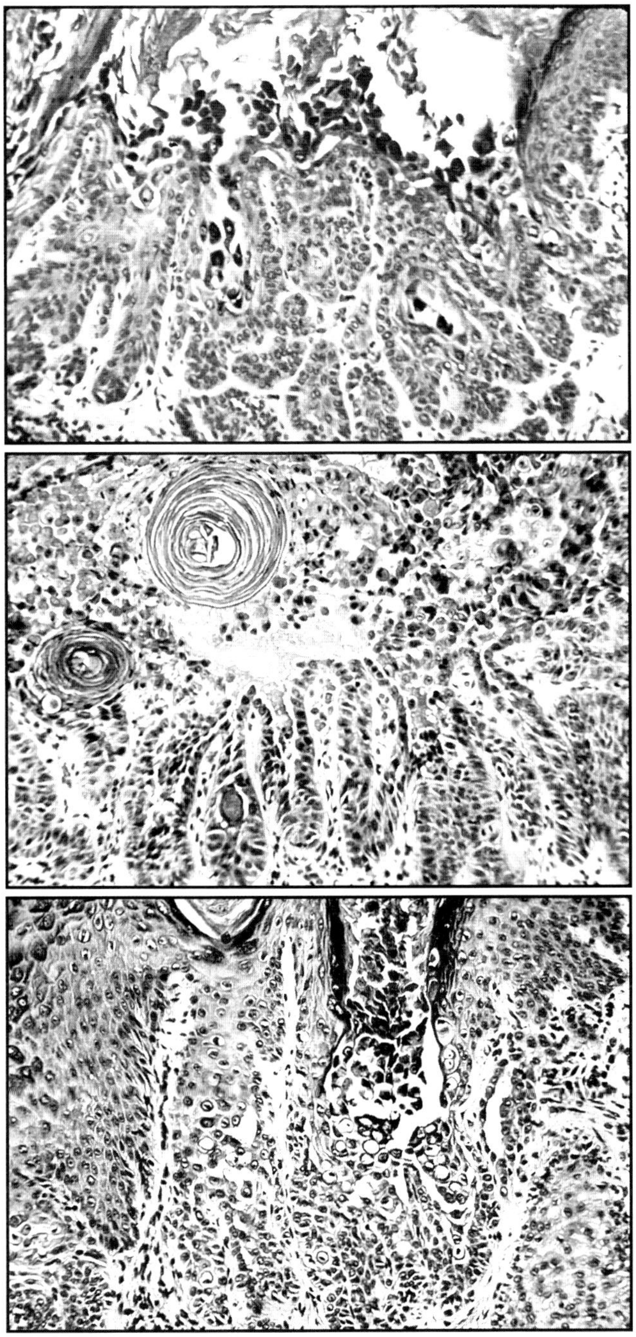

Fig. 5.32 Darier's disease, warty dyskeratoma, and Grover's disease (*top* to *bottom*). Note similar features, that is, suprabasal acantholysis and benign dyskeratosis in the three lesions. H&E ×40 o m

weeks, the first diagnostic choice would have been Grover's disease.

Epidermolytic Lesions, Noninfectious

The lesions discussed in this section are the result of aggressions to the skin by disorders recognized as being of autoimmune nature (p. 62). In the course of these conditions, grouped under the name of pemphigus (*pemphix* [G] a blister), circulating Abs raised against the epidermis for unknown reasons are fixed on the glycocalix coating keratinocytes, diminishing the cohesion among them and the physical strength of this layer, which tends to disintegrate spontaneously. There exist basically two types of pemphigus, pemphigus vulgaris and pemphigus foliaceus, each with some variations.

Pemphigus vulgaris (PV) [22] is a disease with a genetic profile characterized by the increased presence of HLA DR4 and DRW6: this disease shows a strong prevalence in the Jewish population. In the particular case of pemphigus vulgaris, circulating Abs directed against glycocalyx are diffusely deposited in the epidermal interstitial spaces. They activate proteolytic enzymes which destroy this substance and cause epidermal disintegration.

The clinical presentation of PV involves first of all, the skin. This organ shows evident fragility, as it undergoes disintegration upon slight external pressure. This phenomenon is elicited by the Nikolsky's sign, applying rotatory friction to restricted areas of the skin. The involvement of the oral mucosa in the form of eroded areas is an early and almost constant sign in the evolution of PV.

Blisters of flaccid quality are formed by the detachment from the dermis of the whole epidermis, with the exception of the germinal layer. These blisters easily lose their epidermal roof, leaving behind denuded areas of skin. Although in PV epidermal regeneration does occur, it does not match the high rate of loss of this layer. During the course of the disease, the condition therefore results in the increasing loss of epithelial coverage over the body surface. In turn, this leads to mounting losses of fluids and proteins, as well as increasing risk of infections, the two main problems the patient and doctor have to face in PV. The microscopic picture of an early lesion of PV (Fig. 5.33, left) already shows its acantholytic tendency, manifested by the appearance of a cleft above the germinal layer. Figure 5.33, right, exposes the spreading of a cleft, which appears as "dissecting" a hair follicle found in its path.

Figure 5.34 shows keratinocytes in the germinal layer at high magnification: these appear badly damaged but still attached to the basal lamina. That image was once romantically compared to *"disarranged tombstones in a neglected cemetery."* From this analogy derives the more technical expression "tombstone rows" [23] of common use in today's dermatopathology.

The fact that basal keratinocytes are not directly affected by the destructive process in PV, and do not become dislodged from the epidermis, may be possibly explained by the fact that the circulating Abs in PV are directed toward the glycocalyx, *which is not a component of hemidesmosomes.* These structures, which are responsible for the attachment of the basal keratinocytes to the dermis, are then still able to maintain a nexus to the dermis after the attack. For this

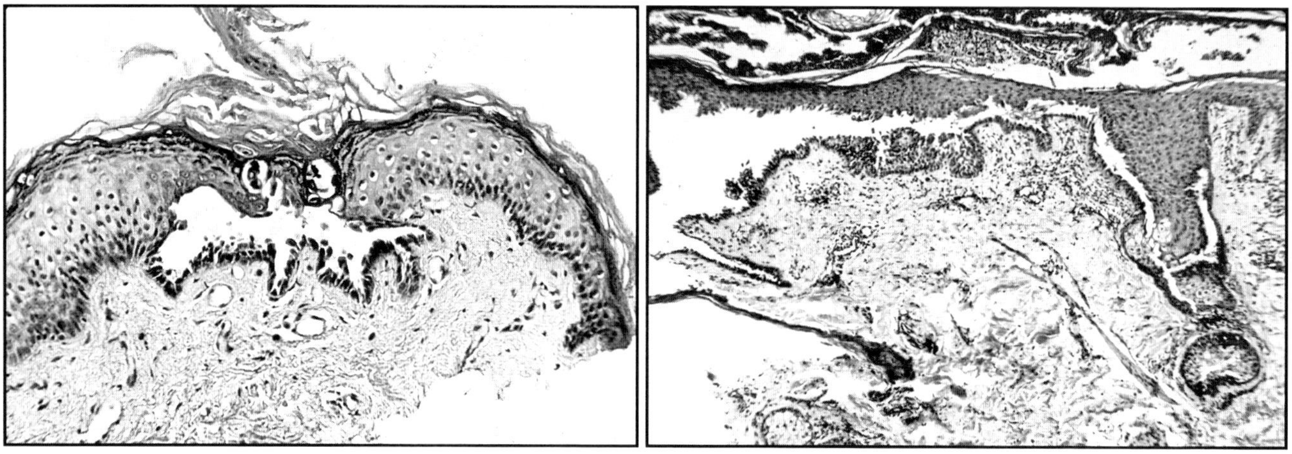

Fig. 5.33 Pemphigus vulgaris. Early and advanced clefting. See details in the text. H&E; ×40 o m

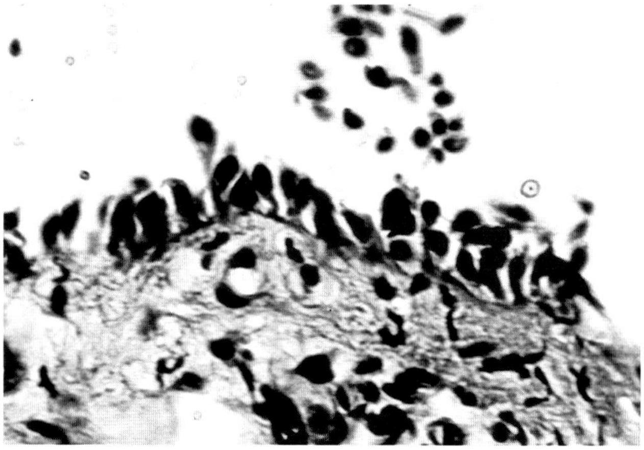

Fig. 5.34 Tombstones. See details in the text H&E ×400 o m

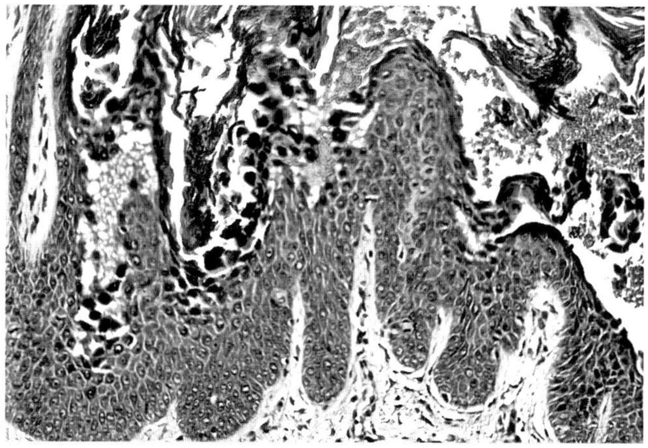

Fig. 5.35 Pemphigus foliaceus. In this condition, LM reveals a moderate disintegration along the granular layer. Note the preserved condition of the epidermis below, including the germinal layer, which appears unremarkable. H&E; ×100 o m

reason, they appear after the aggression, if not very healthy, still attached to the dermis, featuring the so-called tombstones figures (Fig. 5.34).

Pemphigus vegetans is a variant of PV. In this condition, the actual nature of the disorder is masked by the epidermal proliferation in the lesion, which sometimes takes away the microscopist from the correct diagnosis. In the long run, however, pemphigus vegetans reverts to PV, with all the implications the amended diagnosis carries.

Pemphigus foliaceus (PF) is a disorder with a genetic profile less accentuated than the one in PV. It does not have the marked predominance in the Jewish population that PV does. This is also a disorder caused by circulating Abs. Although under laboratory analysis these Abs present minimal differences to the ones of PV [24], they show a distinct tendency to be bound to keratinocytes below the granular layer. Due to this fact, PF results in moderate exfoliation with sparing of the low epidermic germinal layer, rather than causing the massive epidermal sloughing noted in PV. This facilitates epidermal regeneration after the immunoaggression and gives to PF a more benign prognosis than PV (Fig. 5.35).

Occasionally, before the clefting occurs, the epidermis in PF becomes infiltrated by scores of eosinophils, a phenomenon known as "eosinophilic spongiosis," noted with less frequency in PV and also in bullous pemphigoid.

Senear-Usher syndrome, also called "pemphigus erythematosus," is a variety of pemphigus foliaceus. It received the qualification of "erythematosus" not because of the pigmentation of its lesion but due to its distribution on the face and the thoracic V-shaped area of solar exposure, similar to that of LE.

Fogo selvagem or Brazilian pemphigus is a disorder closely similar in its clinicopathologic aspects to pemphigus erythematosus, which occurs in endemic form in the northeast region of Brazil.

Up until the antibiotics and corticoids era, PV diagnosis represented a death sentence for the patient. Pathologists were well aware of this fact and of the shortcomings of microscopy whenever they had to render the diagnosis of PV

Table 5.4 Content of subcorneal vesicles in four different disorders

Disorder	Bacteria	Polynuclears	Acantholytic cells
Bullous impetigo	No	No	No
Impetigo contagiosa	Strepto- and staphylococci	Neutrophils	No
Subcorneal pustular dermatosis	No	Neutrophils and eosinophils	No
Pemphigus foliaceus	No	Eosinophils	Yes

Table 5.5 Examples of bullous or blistering lesions

Associated nosologic entity	Here ditary	Structural defect	Pathogenic agent	Histopathology	Nosologic entity
Epidermolysis bullosa simplex	Yes	Yes	Trauma	Basement membrane destruction	Dermo separation
Herpes virus infection	No	No	Viral infection	Focal epidermo lysis	Focal epidermal destruction
Staphylococcal scalded skin syndrome	No	No	Microbial toxins	Superficial epidermal necrosis	Superficial epidermal loss
Toxic epidermal necrolysis	No	No	Toxins and immune reactants	Massive epidermal necrosis	Massive epidermal loss
Second degree burns	No	No	Heat	Massive epidermal necrosis	Massive epidermal loss

based just on their microscopic acumen. The situation changed however in 1964, when E.H. Beutner and R.E. Jordon, based on immunofluorescence studies, reported the existence of specific Abs against the epidermis in PV [25]. This discovery allowed the pathologist to diagnose PV with increased certainty, as well as to exclude cases of Hailey-Hailey- and other PV-alike conditions.

As a corollary to this section and as an introduction to the subepidermal bullae in the next one, four subcorneal vesicles which were mentioned in this discussion are comparatively presented and tabulated below (Table 5.4).

Lesions of Predominant Junctional Localization

The lesions enclosed in this class are the subepidermal bullae (SB). In this text, subepidermal bulla is a lesion featuring dermoepidermal separation as the result from the almost invariable immunomediated destruction of the basement membrane (BM). In contrast, the term "bulla" without further specification is loosely used here as macroscopic designation for a lesion which, from the outside looks "a bleb" (Table 5.5).

In a very simplistic way, following the level at which the dermoepidermal separation occurs, two subclasses of SB may be recognized: the ones developed above the lamina densa (LD) or below it. According to the class of immunoglobulin (Ig) predominantly involved in the destructive process, the lesions in each of these subclasses may be further grouped as mainly IgG- or IgA-mediated (Fig. 5.36).

SB are associated in their pathogenesis to the bullous disorders, a large and still not totally settled group of entities. The most representative of these are posted on the left column in Table 5.6 following the same scheme proposed in Fig. 5.36. The horizontal double line in the table separates

Fig. 5.36 Subepidermal bullae: subclasses and groups

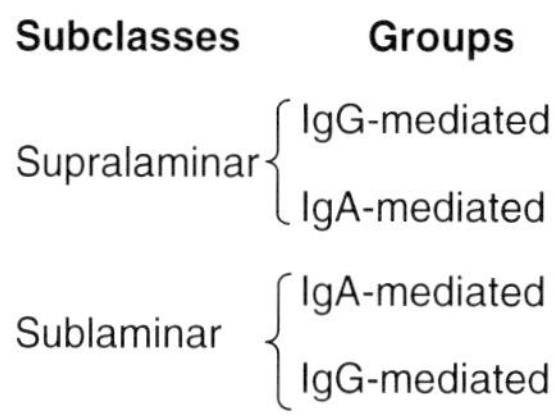

the bullous disorders occurring above the LD from the ones taking place below. The dotted lines separate the bullous disorders in each of these groups according to the Ig involved in the pathogenesis of the pertinent SB. The most significant features of the SB are found in the columns to the right of the corresponding disorder.

The frequency with which the elements mentioned in the table are found is expressed by a scale going from 0+ when they are absent to 5+ when present in 100 % of the cases, with increases of 20 % for each +.

Subepidermal Bullae, Supralaminar

In consideration of the Ig involved in the destructive process, supralaminar SB may be grouped as IgG- and IgA-mediated (Table 5.6).

Subepidermal Bullae, Supralaminar, IgG-Mediated

The disorder heading this group bullous pemphigoid (BP) was identified by W.F. Lever in 1953 on the basis of microscopic studies [26]. This author recognized it as a *bullous* condition whose lesions were characterized by dermoepidermal separation. Since the floor of the bulla lacked the "tombstone rows" characteristic of PV, Lever called the condition "*bullous pemphigoid*" to distinguish it from the former.

Table 5.6 Bullous conditions: genotypes and prevalent nosologic associations, immunoreactants, lesional, extralesional, and circulating

Clinical entity	Prevalent HLA genotype	Clinical associations	Immunoreactants lesional	localization	circulating
Bullous pemphigoid	None	Nonsignificant	IgG 4+ C3-5+	Basal keratinocytes and lamina lucida	IgG-anti BMZ-4+
Pemphigoid cicatricial	DR3-4+ DR3/DR4-2+	Pregnancy & postpartum 5+	IgG 2+ C3-5+	Basal keratinocytes and lamina lucida	HG-factor 4+
Herpes gestationis	None	Nonsignificant	IgG 4+ C3-4+	Basal keratinocytes	IgG-anti BMZ-4+
Linear IgA Dermatosis	B8-1+		IgA 4+ C3-2+	Lamina lucida or sublamina densa	IgG-anti BMZ 4+
Chronic bullous disorders of childhood	B8-1+ C3-2+		IgA 4+	Lamina lucida or sublamina densa	IgG-anti BMZ 4+
Dermatitis herpetiformis	B8/DR3 4+	Gluten-sensitive enteropathy 5+ other autoimmune disorders	IgA-FS 5+ C3 2+	Sublamina densa granular	IgA-anti BMZ 2+
Epidermolysis bullosa acquisita	DR2 3+	Systemic LE Crohn disease diabetes	IgG 3+ C33+	Lamina densa or sublamina densa	IgG-anti BMZ 4+
Porphyria cutanea tarda	None		IgG 3+ C33+	Sublamina densa	

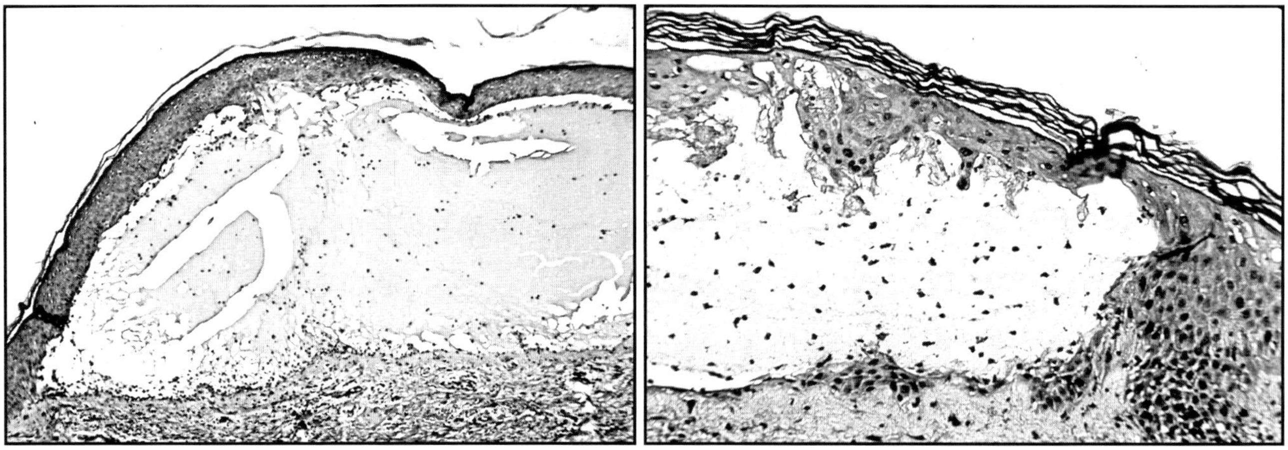

Fig. 5.37 Bullous pemphigoid. Initial lesion (*left*). Note the clean separation of the dermis from the epidermis, whose microscopic details are preserved. Advanced lesion (*right*). Observe the deteriorated condition of the epidermis, as well as the epithelial tongue of regenerated epithelium advancing over the base of the lesion from the right toward its central region. H&E; ×40 o m

Bullous pemphigoid appears in general in adults over 60 years old, without any particular association to a HLA or any nosologic condition. Initially, BP manifests itself by tense, itchy vesicles which appear either on normal or inflamed skin. Microscopically, the initial lesion of bullous pemphigoid (Fig. 5.37) shows a clean dermoepidermal separation with formation of a well-delimited cavity. The epidermis forming the roof of the cavity displays a remarkable degree of preservation. The dermis underneath features an inflammatory reaction of variable intensity, depending on the area of the skin from which the lesion was removed: whereas lesions derived from normal skin present just a moderate reaction, the ones removed from an area of inflamed skin show intense edema and heavy infiltration by inflammatory cells, with a striking proportion of eosinophils. Eosinophils are indeed, characteristic of BP and may be found in any of its lesions, either in the tissues or in the cavity of the bulla. The presence of eosinophils is quite important for the differentiation of BP from dermatitis herpetiformis, in which the characteristic cell is the neutrophil.

The beginning of a reparative process is frequently noted under the microscope in the form of epithelial tongues at the periphery of more advanced lesions. These tongues, sliding over the base of the lesion, meet at the center of the lesion with similar ones advancing from the opposite side and thereby completing the regenerative process of the epidermis. This eventually transforms the bulla from its initial subepidermal position into an intraepidermal, located between the old and the regenerated epithelial layer.

Patients affected by BP present circulating IgG against the BM (Table 5.6). After confirmation of the initial suspicion that these Abs were raised against "self" components of the patient transformed into "nonself," BP became recognized as an autoimmune disorder. Since BP Abs are fixed – along with C3 – forming a smooth band above the LD, it was assumed that the Ag resided in the lamina lucida (LL). This assumption was modified after new studies identified BPAg with laminin, an integrant of the hemidesmosome. Laminin has actually two components of 240kD and 180kD, localized respectively within the basal keratinocyte and the lamina lucida.

The development of the BP is an example of the cytotoxic, type II hypersensitivity which occurs upon fixation of circulating Abs on the BM. This event activates the C system, giving rise to a local inflammatory process which involves liberation of anaphylotoxins. These in turn attract eosinophils to the lesion which upon disintegration liberate proteolytic enzymes responsible for the destruction of the LL. The end result of this process is the dermoepidermal separation and the formation of the subepidermal bulla.

Cicatricial Pemphigoid: In contrast to BP which although prolonged is generally an autolimited condition, cicatricial pemphigoid is a chronic cicatricial process. It affects the mucosae selectively, particularly the ocular one. It can produce severe ocular damage and even cause the loss of sight in a patient [21]. Clinically, it is very easily distinguished from BP, although not by its histopathologic features.

Herpes gestationis (HG), the third disorder in this group, has a close clinicopathological resemblance to BP, except for its elective occurrence in pregnant and puerperal women, for which reason it was called "bullous pemphigoid of pregnancy" [27].

Significant differences between HG and BP are also the former's more intense itching and its association with HLA DR3, either alone or in a DR3/DR4 combination, something not found in the case of BP. Another important difference between the two conditions is that the course of HG is strictly limited to the pregnancy and postpartum period, whereas BP may show a protracted evolution. On the other hand, HG displays a combination of fixed and circulating immunoreactants closely similar to those seen in BP (Table 5.6). HG-factor, a circulating element in HG patients, has recently been identified as an IgG. The histopathologic picture of HG (Fig. 5.38) shows more acute damage than in BP but essentially no major differences that would allow a differential diagnosis between both conditions.

Subepidermal Bullae, Supralaminar, IgA-Mediated

Linear IgA Dermatosis: In 1979 T.P. Chorelski and S. Jablonska recognized via IF studies two new bullous conditions, associated this time to the presence of IgA above the LD. One of these, featuring a granular IgA band, was later identified as a variety of dermatitis herpetiformis, whereas the other was recognized as a new entity, linear IgA dermatosis (L-IgA-D) [28]. Although the microscopic image of this condition is not conclusive, its smooth supralaminar IgA band is very characteristic. Besides, the circulating Abs in L-IgA-D seem to be associated to a particular Ag, a 97KD peptide. Furthermore, the lesion in L-IgA-D includes the presence of sublaminar Abs whose importance is presently unknown. Upon completing the immunoaggression in L-IgA-D, a cleft appears along the LL.

Chronic Bullous Disease of Childhood (CBDCh): In connection with the L-IgA-D, mention should also be made of another chronic bullous disease of childhood (CBDCh). This condition is probably a variant of L-IgA-D. Indeed, except for its incidence in youth, the features of both overlap (Table 5.6).

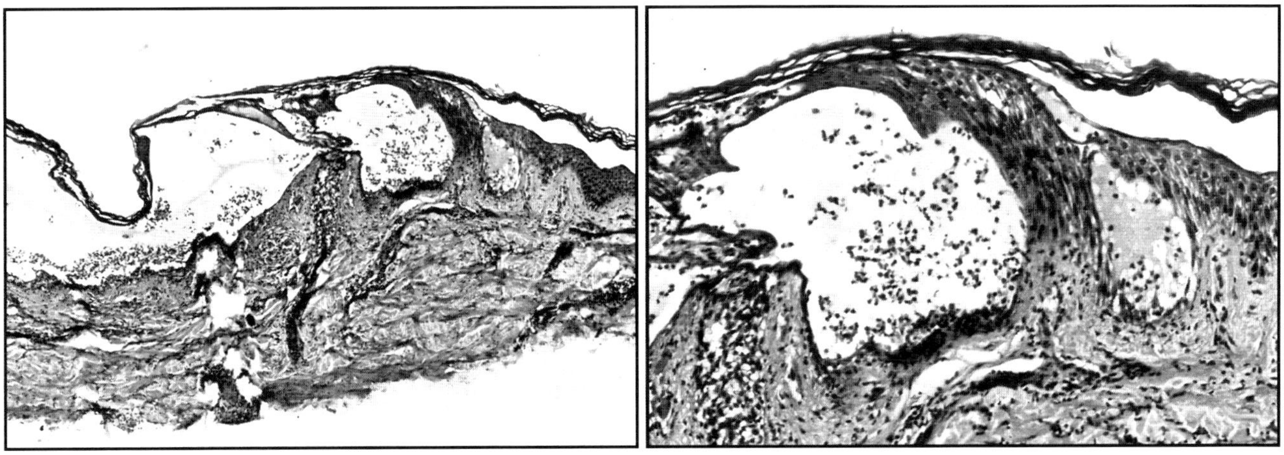

Fig. 5.38 Herpes gestationis. (*Left*) Note the severe epidermal destruction in the lesion, (*right*) and the subepidermal bulla crossed by straps of necrotic epithelium. H&E; ×40; ×100 o m

Subepidermal Bullae, Sublaminar

The conditions covered in this Subclass may be grouped according to the class of the Ig predominantly involved in their immunoreactions. These are either IgA or IgG.

Subepidermal Bullae, Sublaminar, IgA-Mediated

The only, although prototypic, condition enclosed in this group is dermatitis herpetiformis. DH is also the senior member among the SB since it was already reported in 1884 by L.A. Duhring [29]. Dermatitis herpetiformis, also called Duhring's disease, is a disorder of middle-aged patients, with a clear male predominance. Clinically, this condition appears as intensely pruritic plaques and crops of vesicles distributed in extension surfaces of the limbs and on the chest and trunk. DH presents a close association with HLA DR3/DR4 and with a gluten-sensitive enteropathy. It is also associated to several autoimmune disorders (Table 5.6).

The role of the enteropathy in the pathogenesis of DH has still not been fully clarified. It is however known with certainty that in DH, the intestinal mucosa is the source of IgA. IgA molecules pass through the intestinal mucosa as dimers, joined by an FS-chain upon entering blood circulation. They reach the skin, being fixed on papillary tips below the LD. Then, they combine with C and eventually, by virtue of cross antigenicity, bind on fibers of the elastic plexus. The binding of the complexes induces an acute in situ inflammatory reaction with strong influx of neutrophils, forming the characteristic papillary abscesses, with narrow clefts separating these from the epidermis (Fig. 5.39, left). In a more advanced phase, there is a coalescence of the isolated cleft giving way to extensive dermoepidermal separations on a background of strong, acute reactions with heavy inflammatory infiltrates (Fig. 5.39, right).

The fact that IgA, the same effector as in DH, is involved in the pathogenesis of L-IgA-D and CBDCh forces the question of whether those two nosologic entities could somehow be associated to DH. The fact that in these two latter conditions the lesions are supralaminar, whereas in DH, they are infralaminar would in itself be dismissive of that possibility. The comparative features shown in Table 5.6 are not supportive of that assumption either. Indeed, the B8/DR3 HLA combination of DH does not indicate any association of this condition with L-IgA-D and CBDCh. Besides, the two last mentioned disorders do not display the gluten-sensitivity characteristic of DH at all. Moreover, the circulating IgA in DH is combined with the FS-chain, indicating its intestinal origin, whereas the IgA in L-IgA-D and CBDCh does not show that chain, which points toward their extraintestinal origin.

Subepidermal Bullae, Sublaminar, IgG-Mediated

In connection to sublaminar bullae with IgG deposition, epidermolysis bullosa acquisita should be mentioned.

Epidermolysis Bullosa Acquisita (EBA): The bulla formation in this condition, as in EBC is trauma-associated. It is probably for this reason that when R Kablitz reported it in 1904 [30], he deliberately called it "*acquisita*" to emphasize its difference with the "*congenita*" type of this disorder. Only a few years ago, it was realized that EBA fits also as an autoimmune disorder. This finding resulted upon discovery that in EBA patients, IgG can be found circulating or fixed below the LD. A high incidence of HLE DR2, and an array of autoimmune disorders such as diabetes, Crohn's disease, SLE etc, were also associated with this condition. The clinical similarities between EBA and pemphigus, plus the fact that both conditions are of autoimmune nature and contain circulating Abs of the IgG class, allowed the supposition that these may be different clinical forms of a same disease. The LM studies did not support that assumption since they failed to reveal in EBC the characteristic epidermolytic features of PV. Further studies confirmed these findings insofar as in

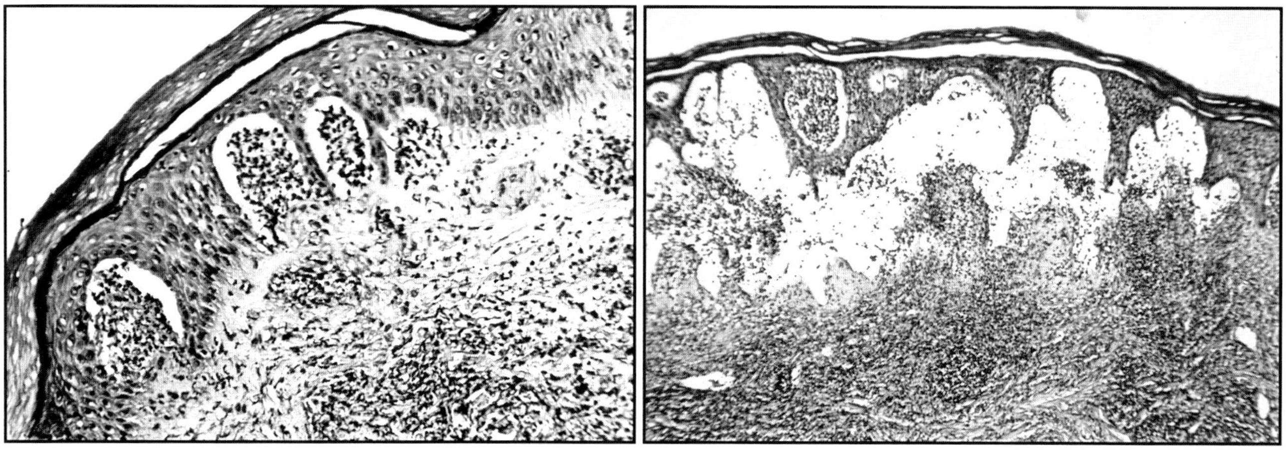

Fig. 5.39 Dermatitis herpetiformis. (*Left*) Papillary abscesses; (*right*) dermoepidermal separation with intense acute inflammatory reaction. H&E; ×100; ×40 o m

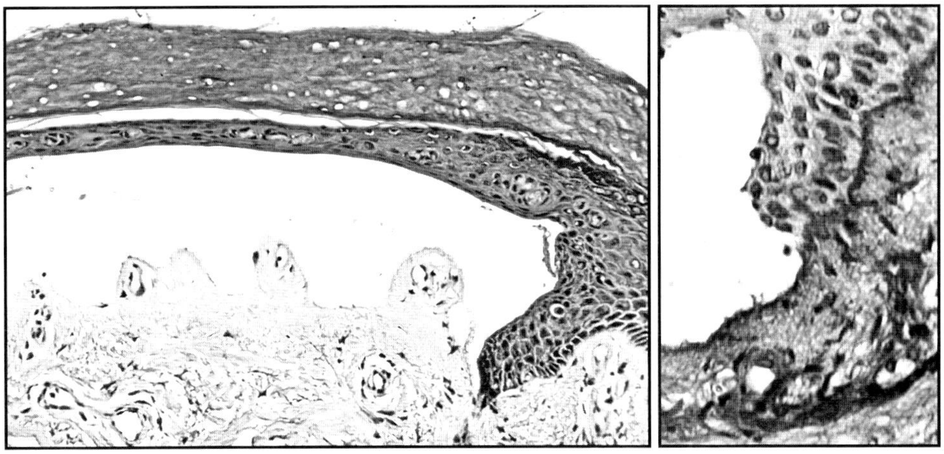

Fig. 5.40 Subepidermal bulla of porphyria cutanea tarda. (*Left*) The lesion shows a clean dermoepidermal separation, with papillae ascending from the bottom into the cavity, a feature attributed to the rigidity of the tissues, infiltrated by a PAS-positive material. (*Right*) Special stained sections reveal thickening of vessel walls and BM due to the deposits of an amorphous, PAS-positive substance. See more details in the text. H&E; ×40; PAS; ×400

EBA IgG was not found in an epidermal position but in a sub-LD band, totally different from the epidermal "chicken wire pattern" in which ABs appear in PV 85. Moreover, it was also found that in EBC, IgG is bound to the anchoring fibrils in the dermis, contrary to what happens in PV, where IgG are bound to the glycocalyx in the interstitial spaces.

In concluding this review of subepidermal bullae, a reference to porphyrias is warranted. These conditions, already discussed in the section of HEwCR, present various manifestations on the skin, among which the bullae are the most characteristic. The pathogenesis of these bullae is not Ig-associated but is related to the presence of abnormal metabolites of the hem-cycle deposited in close vicinity to the BM. Upon returning to the base state after being UV-irradiated, these metabolites emit secondary longer-wave radiation with irreversible damage to tissues within their range. A characteristic feature of the microscopic picture of porphyria bulla is that *it lacks any sign of inflammatory reaction* (Fig. 5.40), in contrast to what happens with the rest of the subepidermal bullae.

Some studies reveal the presence of IgG and C3 in the lesion, but it is believed that these elements are drawn into the lesion secondarily, not being, therefore, directly involved in its pathogenesis of the bulla.

In concluding this section, it should be stated that the obvious morphological differences between the lesions of DH, BP, and other conditions may give the microscopist the erroneous idea that LM examination is infallible when trying to identify unknown bullous disorders. This is not so: in practice, there exist variants and intermediate forms of these disorders, as well as other blistering conditions still not well identified, such as the pruritic conditions of pregnancy and the bullous conditions of childhood, affections which may become very problematic to diagnose, even upon applying the most advanced analytical techniques. For this reason, clinicopathologic correlations must be considered of primary importance for the diagnosis of the bullous conditions.

Subclasses	Groups	Subgroups
Of prevalent vascular character	Capillaritis	Allergic Non allergic Miscellaneous
	Venulitis	
Of prevalent cellular character	Perivascular	
	Periadnexal	
	Band-like	
	Granulomas	Foreign body Palisading Sarcoidal Tuberculoid
	Diffuse	Non infectious Infectious

Fig. 5.41 Evolutive inflammatory lesions of predominant dermal localization: subclasses, groups, and subgroups

Lesions of Predominantly Dermal Localization

As already mentioned, the dermis is a well-vascularized and innervated mesenchymatous structure with numerous potentially reactive cellular elements. Although inflammatory reactions result from the combined activity of all the elements present in the area, due to the preponderant participation of one or other sector, the resulting lesions may be subclassified as of a prevalent vascular or cellular character (Fig. 5.41).

Lesions of Predominantly Dermal Localization and Prevalent Vascular Character

In this subclass are studied lesions originated in capillaries and the thinnest venules that follow these. The capillaries of the lymphatic network at this level are devoid of pathogenic importance, and, therefore, there is no need to consider them here. Lesions on lymphatics of wider caliber are more conveniently discussed along with lesions which occur in the deep dermis and the subcutaneous tissue.

Capillaritides are translated in the practice as "urticarial reactions" and venulitides as "vasculitides."

Capillaritis (Urticarial Reactions)

In its initial phase, capillaritis implies minimal and reversible alterations of capillary walls, with retraction of endothelial cells. This allows leakage of fluid from the intravascular to the interstitial space and as a result, the buildup of edema. These events are reflected in the clinic by the appearance of itchy and evanescent wheals and plaques, a phenomenon referred in general terms as "urticarial reaction" (*urtica+aria* [L] a stinging weed + a condition).

The most significant histopathologic feature of edema is the paleness of the dermis and the lack of formed elements, displaced from the microscopic field by the fluid accumulated in the tissues (Fig. 5.42). The presence of red blood cells in edema hints toward a damaged endothelium, which allows the passage of these elements, normally contained by the vascular wall. Chronic urticaria musters, in addition to edema, a faint inflammatory infiltrate; the presence of eosinophils in it pictures an indication of the probable allergic nature of the process (Fig. 5.42). The extension of the edema to subcutaneous tissue, GI tract, and other internal organs is reason enough to change the name of the condition from "edema" to "angioedema."

As it has been already discussed, urticarial reactions are considered the result of IgE-mediated mast cell degranulation in the course of the allergic, type I hypersensitivity reactions. It must be kept in mind however that there is a group of substances, which include aspirin, codein, acetilcholine, etc., which after binding to specific receptors on the surface of the mast cells, are able to induce directly, *without IgE intervention*, mast cell degranulation, and urticarial reactions similar to the already described. Therefore, urticarial reactions may be considered allergic when they are IgE-mediated and nonallergic when they are not. A third subgroup of miscellaneous urticarial reactions may be also mentioned here, not associated at all with mast cell degranulation (Table 5.7).

Urticarial Reactions, Allergic

Allergic urticarial reactions are not infrequent findings in the clinic as the result of food or drug intolerance; they proceed along the already discussed pathway of type I hypersensitivity, with IgE fixation on the mast cell and following already discussed events.

Urticarial Reactions, Nonallergic

In these cases, mast cell degranulation is provoked by the binding of the pertinent substance, without IgE intervention onto specific receptors on the mast cell surface. This triggers the known chain of events which end up with the cutaneous manifestations of the reaction.

In regard to the nonallergic urticarial reactions, acetylcholine is of special relevance. This substance is a neurotransmissor constantly liberated and metabolized at the synapses of the peripheral nerve without causing any problem. Under determined circumstances, however, physical stimuli like

Table 5.7 Urticarial reactions, subgroups, and examples

Allergic
Food intolerance
Drug intolerance
Arthropod bites
Nonallergic
Cold related
Heat related
Vibratory
Dermographism
Miscellaneous
Hereditary angioedema Polymorphous light eruption Systemic lupus erythematosus

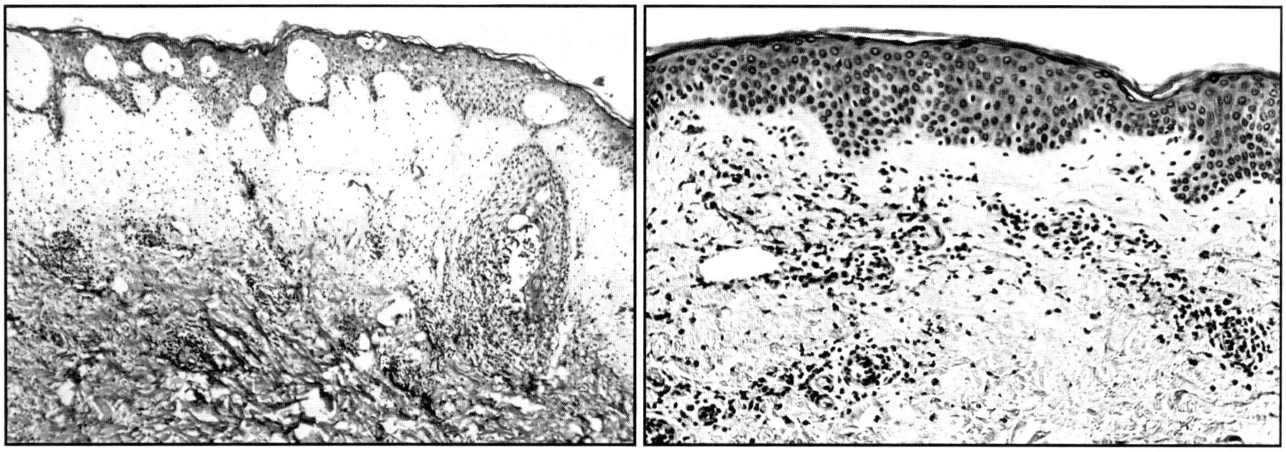

Fig. 5.42 Urticaria acute and chronic. In contrast to acute urticaria (*left*), chronic urticaria (*right*) shows in addition to edema a faint inflammatory infiltrate. The overlying epidermis appears uninvolved in both cases. H&E ×40 o m

UV exposure, high or low temperatures, traumas, or vibrations may induce sudden acetylcholine discharges able to trigger urticarial reactions, frequently manifested as numerous tiny itchy papules. These reactions are called in general terms "cholinergic urticarias." [31] Particular examples of them are cold urticaria and heat urticaria, mechanic urticaria and vibratory urticaria, etc. An example of a mechanic urticaria is dermographism. This underlies Lewis's triple response [32] upon linear scratching on the skin. Pruritic disorders of pregnancy, whose pathogenic mechanism has not been totally clarified, have also an urticarial component which may be eventually related to mast cell degranulation.

Urticarial Reactions, Miscellaneous

Hereditary angioedema is also an urticarial reaction. This disorder is an HDCwCR characterized by the congenital lack of the natural inhibitor of activated C1. In the absence of its physiologic control, the activation of C1 fraction may lead to the sudden and untoward activation of the whole C cascade, with generalized liberation of vasoactive substances, which cause diffuse edema. If this involves the air passage, this may lead to fatal consequences.

Erysipelas (*erysi+pelas* [G] red+skin): Although this is an infectious condition caused by *beta hemolytic group A streptococci*, erysipelas deserves to be included in this Subgroup because of the prominent edema characteristic of its clinical presentation. Under the microscope, the lesion appears to be mainly localized to the superficial levels of the dermis, featuring capillary and lymphatic dilatation with prominent edema; a diffuse, though mild infiltration by neutrophils; and the presence of the causative microorganisms if a gram stain is performed. When the lesion tends to spread down involving the subcutaneous fat, the process may be more conveniently called "cellulitis."

Polymorphous light eruption is the expression of an abnormal form of light hypersensivity frequently associated to strong dermal edema. This may be a reason for including it into this Subgroup but, since its lesions also display strong perivascular cuffs of mononuclear cells, it was found more adequate to deal with it along with perivascular dermatitides.

Due to the prominent edema which accompanies some of its cutaneous lesions, systemic lupus erythematosus (SLE) also deserves to be quoted in this section (Fig. 5.43).

Lupus Erythematosus: At the beginning of the nineteenth century, L. Biett sketched out a condition, presumedly lupus erythematosus to which his name was attached. P. Cazenave, three decades later on clinical grounds, was able to separate from Biett disease another condition known since the Middle Ages by the name of "lupus" (*lupus* [L] the wolff). That condition carried severe facial lesions which in the popular imagination appeared as caused by wolves chewing and gnawing on the patients' face. Impressed by the similar appearance of the lesions in lupus and the new condition he was studying, Cazenave postulated a relationship between them. Due, however, to the reddish discoloration that the lesions in the new entity displayed, he called it "lupus erythematosus," in opposition to the old one, renamed "lupus vulgaris." R. Koch was able to demonstrate in 1907 the presence of *M. tuberculosis* in the lesions of lupus vulgaris, considered since then a cutaneous form of tuberculosis.

Lupus erythematosus (LE) is the result of a profound disorder of the immunogenic system which results into a variegated group of circulating auto-Abs as well as of clones of cells programmed for the destruction of tissues of their own organism. This is reflected by the wide spectrum of presentation forms of LE. In a simplified approach, the microscopic features of two polar forms of that spectrum, systemic and cutaneous, shall be shortly discussed.

The lesions of systemic LE feature edema and collagen degeneration as outstanding histopathologic features (Fig. 5.43). For this reason, these lesions were already mentioned above, among other edematous conditions. The lesions of the cutaneous form of LE (DLE), intimately connected to the skin, present a destructive quality along with a

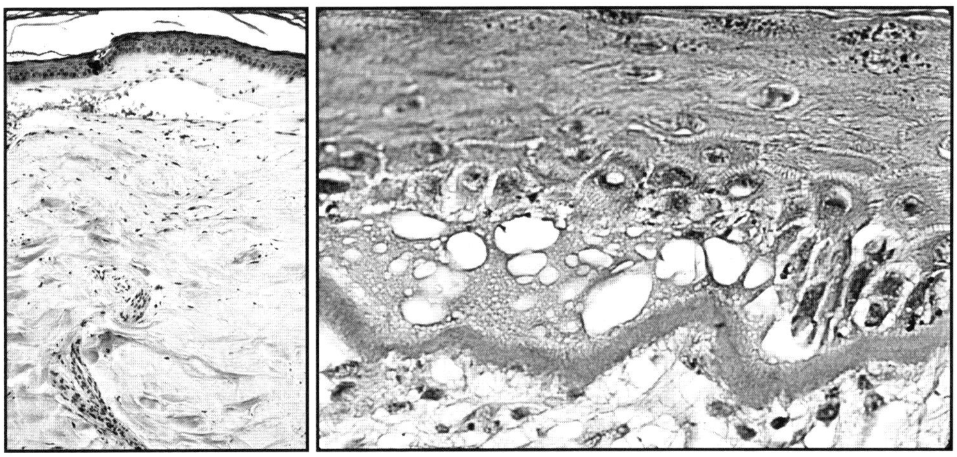

Fig. 5.43 Lupus erythematosus, systemic. (*Left*) At low magnification, the lesion reveals a flat epidermis overlying a strongly edematous dermis featuring faintly eosinophilic areas of structureless stroma with dilated lymphatics. (*Right*) At higher magnification, the germinal layer of the lesion appears strongly deteriorated, with marked vacuolar degeneration and separated from the basal membrane zone by a band of vacuolated fluid. H&E ×40; ×400 o m

characteristic patchy round cell infiltrate as their main microscopic alterations. These lesions will be dealt with later on, along other cellular lesions of predominant dermal localization.

Venulitis (Vasculitis)

Venulitis forms the second Group of vascular lesions of prevalent dermal localization (Fig. 5.41). These lesions, known as "vasculitis," respond to type III, immunocomplex-mediated hypersensitivity. Immunocomplexes (IC) may be formed in the bloodstream by the direct combination of drugs or other chemicals with Abs raised against them. ICs can appear in the organism in response to a long-term systemic administration of these substances. Otherwise, IC may be generated during the course of infectious disorders such as syphilis or leprosy, or of systemic disorders such as LE, rheumatoid arthritis, or allergic granulomatosis. ICs are usually promptly and efficiently removed from circulation by the reticuloendothelial system (RES). Increased IC levels in blood may respond to their exaggerated production in response to any of the mentioned situations, although they may also reflect an RES failure to remove them. At any rate, when ICs are present in the blood at increased levels, they tend to be deposited in the lumen of the thinnest venules, those *immediately following* the capillaries, due to blood flow turbulence or other hemodynamic reasons. The IC deposition causes C activation, and the inflammatory response, a reaction conventionally called "*vasculitis*" in immunopathology [33]. The primordial LM manifestation of vasculitis is *fibrinoid degeneration* of the wall of the involved venule. This shows a smudginess of its contour, with subsequent loss of its histologic details (Fig. 5.44). To this picture may be added in variable and inconstant proportions extravasated red blood cells, eosinophils, edema, and neutrophils with "nuclear dust," derived from nuclear fragmentation. It is only this last feature, the *presence of nuclear dust*, that justifies calling a vasculitis "*leucocytoclastic*." Otherwise, according to the predominance of one or the other mentioned element, the lesions may be qualified as "purpuric," "allergic," or "urticarial vasculitis."

Lesions of Predominant Dermal Localization and Prevailing Cellular Character

The lesions of prevalent cellular character may appear under several patterns in the dermis, that is, as perivascular-, periadnexal-, or band-like infiltrates, as granulomas, or in a granulomatous, diffuse distribution (Fig. 5.41).

Perivascular Infiltrates

"Perivascular infiltrates" is a descriptive term for collections of elements previously defined as "*mononuclear*" (p. 63), disposed as cuffs or sleeves around small veins in the superficial and deep dermis (Fig. 5.45).

Perivascular infiltrates are formed by inconspicuous mononuclear elements devoid of mitotic activity or any other particular feature and disposed as cuffs in the lax perivascular sheath, offering a nondiagnostic picture. If the microscopic examination of lesions with perivascular infiltrates discloses any other histopathologic feature – present in a significant proportion – that feature will take prevalence in its designation over "perivascular." For instance, if the image of a perivascular infiltrate also shows spongiosis or edema, that lesion may be then categorized to as "spongiotic" or "edematous" rather than to a perivascular dermatitis.

Perivascular infiltrates are a frequent finding in the laboratory. They quite often are the microscopic substrate of exanthems, the clinical conditions characterized by a reddening of the skin. Exanthems are, in turn, symptomatic components of widely different nosologic conditions. In fact, the information the laboratorist may gather about the circumstances

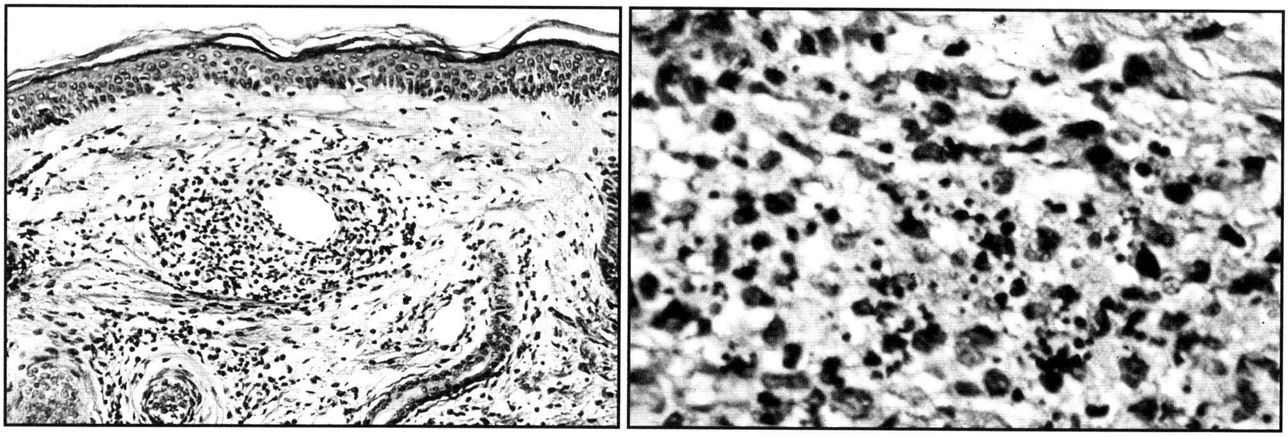

Fig. 5.44 Leucoclastic vasculitis. Note the central damaged venule surrounded by inflammatory elements (*left*). At higher magnification, these appear to be mostly neutrophils and nuclear dust (*right*). H&E; ×40; ×100 o m

under which an exanthem developed may be much more contributory to the correct diagnosis of a lesion under study than its exhaustive microscopic examination.

As far as the diagnostic workout of a perivascular dermatitis is concerned, it is important for the microscopist to know if from the outside, the exanthem to which the perivascular lesion being examined is associated, displays linear contours, being then called a "figurate exanthem," or if it is otherwise a "diffuse" exanthem. Examples of both types of exanthems are shown in Table 5.8.

Postprimary syphilitic lesions – the syphilides – are mentioned here for illustrative purposes because of the extraordinary guise of exanthems, cyclic, arcuate, spiral, etc., under which they may appear (Fig. 5.46).

In actuality, though, syphilides are translated in histopathologic terms as thick infiltrates which frequently display plasma cells and neutrophils showing a tendency to expand into a diffuse pattern.

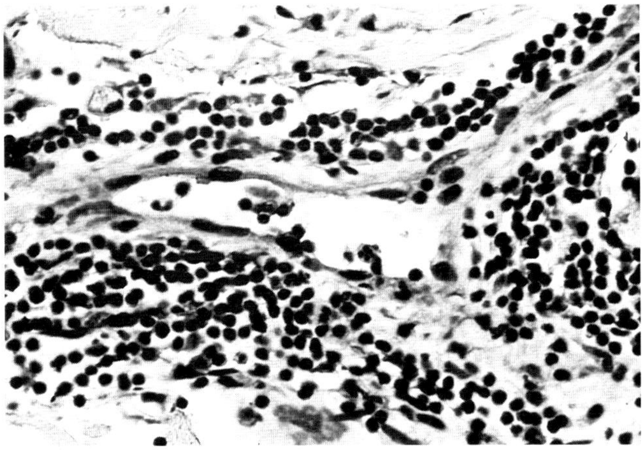

Fig. 5.45 Perivascular infiltrate. Note the uniform mononuclear cells around a capillary. H&E; ×400 o m

Table 5.8 Exanthems associated to perivascular infiltrates

Figurate exanthems	Diffuse exanthems
Erythema annulare centrifugum	Measles exanthem
Erythema marginatum	Toxic exanthem
Erythema chronicum migrans	Luminic eruptions
Postprimary syphilis	Delayed reactions to arthropod aggressions
Erythema gyratum repens	Systemic lupus erythematosus

Conditions Associated to Figurate Exanthems

Erythema annulare centrifugum should be mentioned first in this context because it is the exanthem most frequently seen in the clinic (Table 5.8). Externally, this lesion is characterized by a typical linear, arciform exanthem, which may help the microscopist in his or her final diagnosis (Fig. 5.46). Under the microscope, it is characterized by thick coat-sleeve perivascular deposits of mononuclear cells distributed in the superficial and deep dermis, without affecting the overlying epidermis.

It should be mentioned, incidentally, that erythema annulare centrifugum has been repeatedly associated to cases of malignant neoplasias from the breast, lung, and GI tract: this circumstance would make this condition a *cutaneous marker* for internal neoplasias, comparable to several others already reported (Fig. 5.47).

Erythema Marginatum (Table 5.8): This exanthem presents an inconspicuous microscopic aspect closely similar to the one of erythema annulare centrifugum, which would not allow any diagnostic conclusion. However, since erythema marginatum represents a first-class component of the symptomatic picture of rheumatic fever [34], if the microscopist is aware of the fact that the patient is affected by this condition, he or she

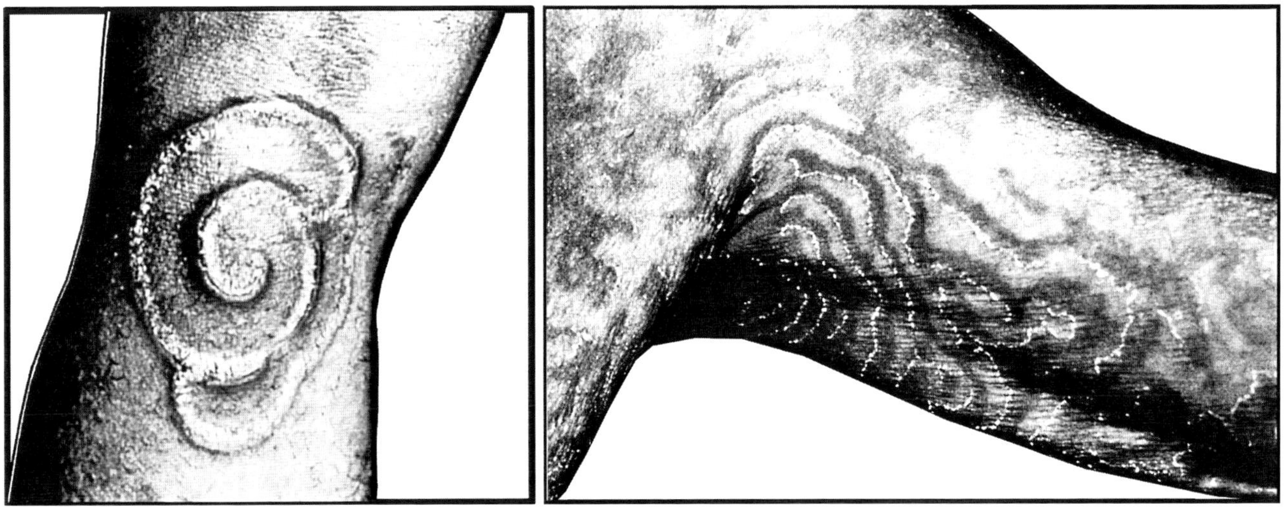

Fig. 5.46 Examples of figurate exanthems. Syphilide (*left*). Erythema gyratum repens (*right*) (Courtesy of H. Shatin, M.D.)

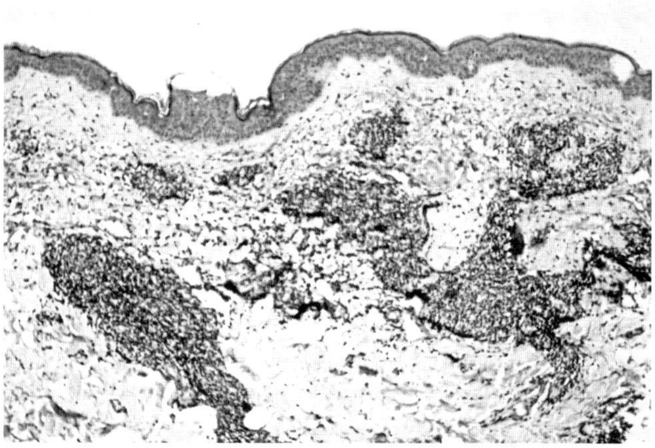

Fig. 5.47 Erythema annulare centrifugum. Note the thick perivascular cuffs of mononuclear cells and the lack of further significant details in the lesion. H&E ×40 o m

may confortably render the diagnosis of "erythema marginatum" on this lesion of otherwise "nondiagnostic" features.

Erythema chronicum migrans offers again under LM examination an inconspicuous perivascular pattern. Its nature, as has been stated above, may be clarified, not so much through its microscopic examination but by knowing the patient's whereabouts. Indeed, being aware that the patient has been the victim of a tick bite, the vector of *B. burgdorferi* (the agent of Lyme disease), the microscopic image may be, at least tentatively, interpreted as corresponding to that condition, a diagnosis that may be further strenghtened by finding the causative *borrelia* in silver-stained tissue sections.

Erythema gyratum repens is a quite rare exanthem of sudden apparition, considered almost invariably a paraneoplastic sign of malignant tumors of the lung, breast, etc. The lesion, which tends to be regional in its distribution, appears as advancing waves of linear streaks distributed in a peculiar way, somehow resembling the grain of a wooden log (Fig. 5.46). It is amazing to realize that the microscopic substrate of such an intricate pattern is just an inconspicuous perivascular infiltrate!

Conditions Associated to Diffuse Exanthems

In contrast to the figurate exanthems, diffuse exanthems appear as papules or plaques of variable extension and unprecise contours, the so-called morbilliform exanthems (*morbili+form* (L] resembling measles) (Table 5.8). This group of exanthems is associated, besides measles, to infectious mononucleosis, rubella, fifth disease, and other viral infections. Eventually, when these lesions are examined under the microscope, they may show next to inconspicuous perivascular infiltrates the presence of multinucleated giant cells, which may suggest a viral etiology.

Toxic Erythema: The term "toxic erythema" was coined by Pinkus to describe *diffuse exanthems* which, among their responsible agents, included food or drug intolerance [35]. The microscopic examination of these lesions reveals patchy mononuclear infiltrates sprinkled with eosinophils and neutrophils, in the absence of any noticeable epidermal or vascular participation (Fig. 5.48).

Delayed Arthropod Reactions: The presence of neutrophils and eosinophils in a perivascular infiltrate associated with diffuse exanthem brings food and drug intolerance as first diagnostic consideration. The introduction of epithelioid histiocytes to the picture should add delayed arthropod reaction to the list of differential possibilities. This is quite important because in these lesions, prominent histiocytic proliferations of unusual features are not uncommon (Fig. 5.49), suggesting to an uninformed observer the possibility of an ongoing lymphoproliferative process instead of an inflammatory reaction of fully benign nature.

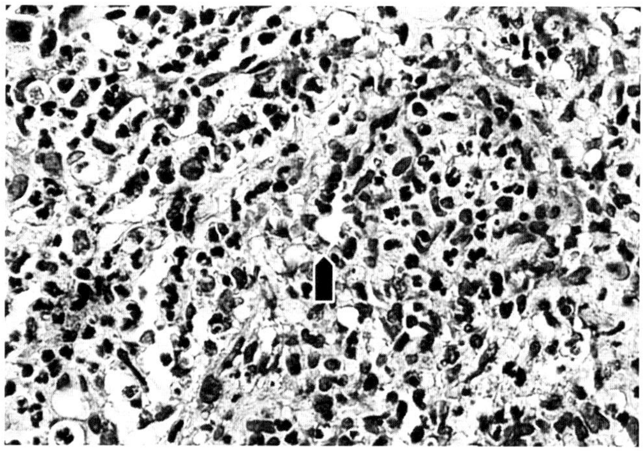

Fig. 5.48 Toxic erythema. The heavy presence of neutrophils and eosinophils in the infiltrate masks the presence of an uninvolved vessel (*arrow*) in the lesion. H&E; ×400 o m

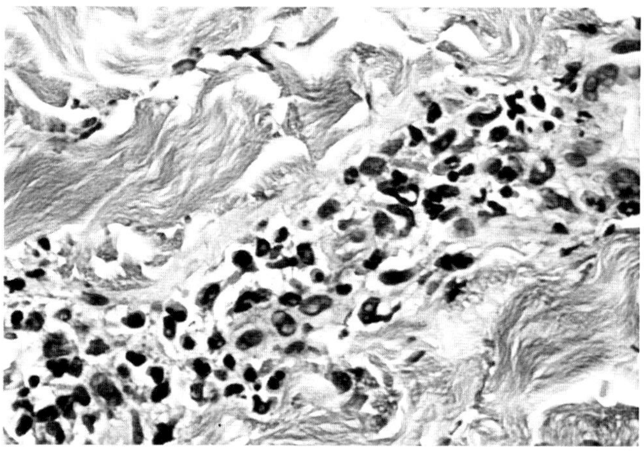

Fig. 5.49 Delayed arthropod reaction. Note in the thick perivascular cuff the presence of eosinophils admixed to the epithelioid population of the lesion. H&E ×400 o m

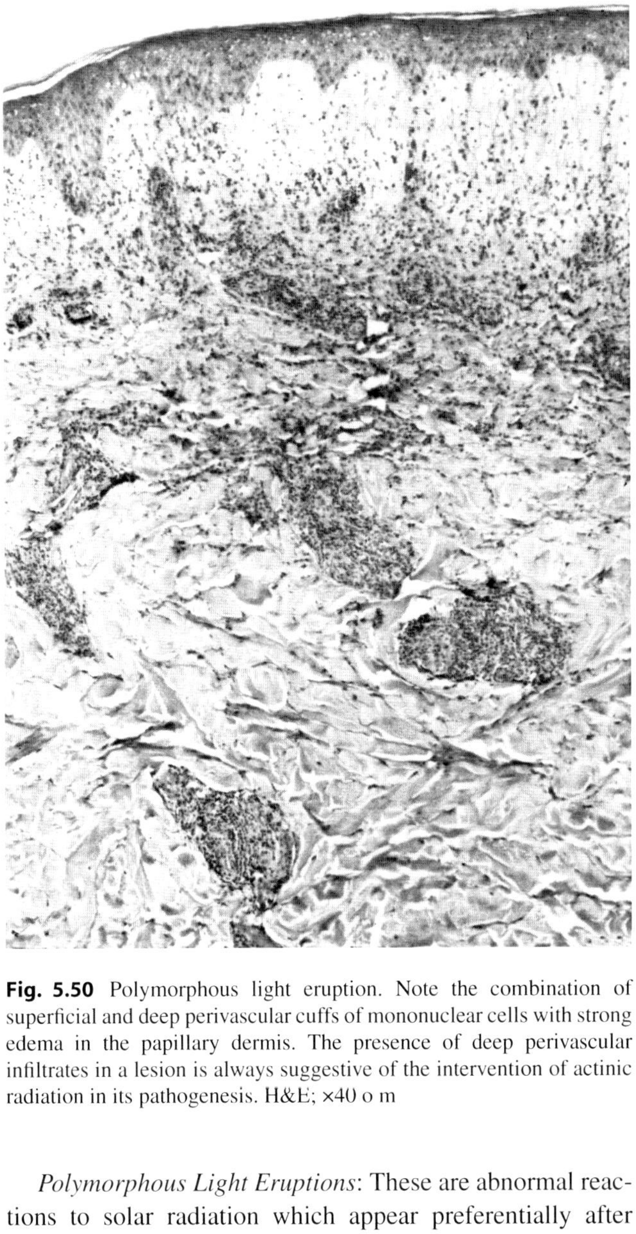

Fig. 5.50 Polymorphous light eruption. Note the combination of superficial and deep perivascular cuffs of mononuclear cells with strong edema in the papillary dermis. The presence of deep perivascular infiltrates in a lesion is always suggestive of the intervention of actinic radiation in its pathogenesis. H&E; ×40 o m

Polymorphous Light Eruptions: These are abnormal reactions to solar radiation which appear preferentially after puberty and are exteriorized by a series of diffuse exanthems. From these, the *plaque-like type* has been hereby selected for a short discussion. The perivascular infiltrates in this condition are characterized by their clear tendency to involve, along with the superficial, the deep vascular plexus of the dermis: this distribution, combined to a strong edema of the superficial dermis, creates an almost pathognomonic picture (Fig. 5.50) which allows the LM identification of this condition.

Periadnexal Infiltrates

Jessner lymphocytic infiltration of the skin is the most fitting example of a periadnexal infiltrate. This lesion features patchy, angulated, and sharply delimited collections of mononuclear elements, tightly disposed around hair follicles frequently devoid of the sebaceous component (Fig. 5.51). This description covers also the characteristic infiltrates of *discoid lupus erythematosus* (DLE). In fact, Jessner lymphocytic infiltration is considered *a precursor* of DLE, as long as the diagnostic details of the last condition such as hydropic degeneration or the BM are absent from the microscopic picture. The appearance of these elements (see below) justifies the change of diagnosis of the lesion, from Jessner lymphocytic infiltration to DLE.

Discoid Lupus Erythematosus (DLE): In the simplified approach previously proposed, SLE was discussed along with cutaneous lesions of predominant edematous character. In this section, the lesions of DLE will be described. These lesions are intimately associated to the affected skin, featuring dense infiltrates that have sharp, angulated contours. The lesions are also closely associated with atrophic changes of the epidermis and pilosebaceous complexes, the latter often devoid of their sebaceous component and surrounded by dense collections of mononuclear cells. The so-called liquefaction or hydropic degeneration of the BM is an important sign in favor of DLE. Figure 5.52 illustrates some of these histologic details.

Band-Like Infiltrates

Band-like infiltrates of the superficial dermis are found under LM examination in a group of clinical conditions, of which the prototypic example is *lichen planus* (Table 5.9).

Lichen planus [36] (LP) (*leichen*[*G*]+*planus*[*L*] a flat lichen-like eruption) is usually an intensely pruritic lesion which appears as solitary or multiple papules, eventually clustered or in a linear arrangement, depending on the direction in which the patient rubs the lesion (Koebner phenomenon). This spreading, "koebnerization," is not privative of LP, however, being found in psoriasis, verrucae, etc. The predominant localizations of LP are the flexion areas of the arms, the legs, and the bucal mucosa.

LP is considered a type IV, immunocellular autoaggression process directed against the epidermis. This is evidenced primarily by the dense, "band-like" infiltrate in the superficial dermis, "hugging" the overlying epidermis, as it is frequently described. As a clear sign of distress, the dermoepidermal junction loses its natural waviness, adopting instead an angulated profile classically compared to that of the dentated edge of a tooth saw. This profile may be blurred by the dense band-like infiltrate, but on the other hand, it may be enhanced by narrow clefts caused by the vacuolar degeneration of the interphase, the Max-Joseph spaces (Fig. 5.53).

Another important feature of LP is the presence of Civatte's bodies, that is, keratinocytes in the elimination process of apoptosis (p. 193) which drop them from the epidermis into

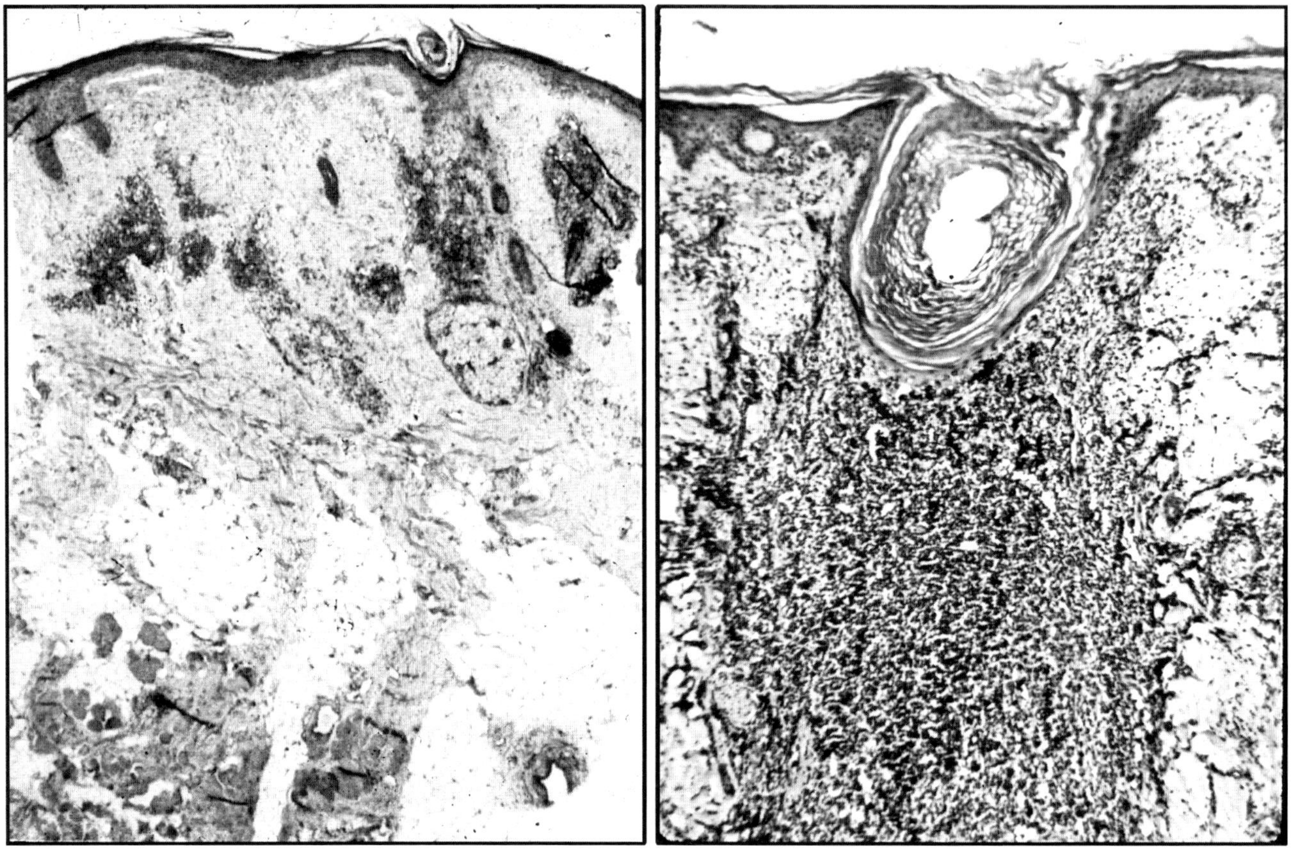

Fig. 5.51 Jessner lymphocytic infiltration of the skin. Note the patchy, angulated, and sharply delimited collections of mononuclear cells, some distributed around hair follicles at low (*left*) and high magnification (*right*). H&E; 40×; 400× o m

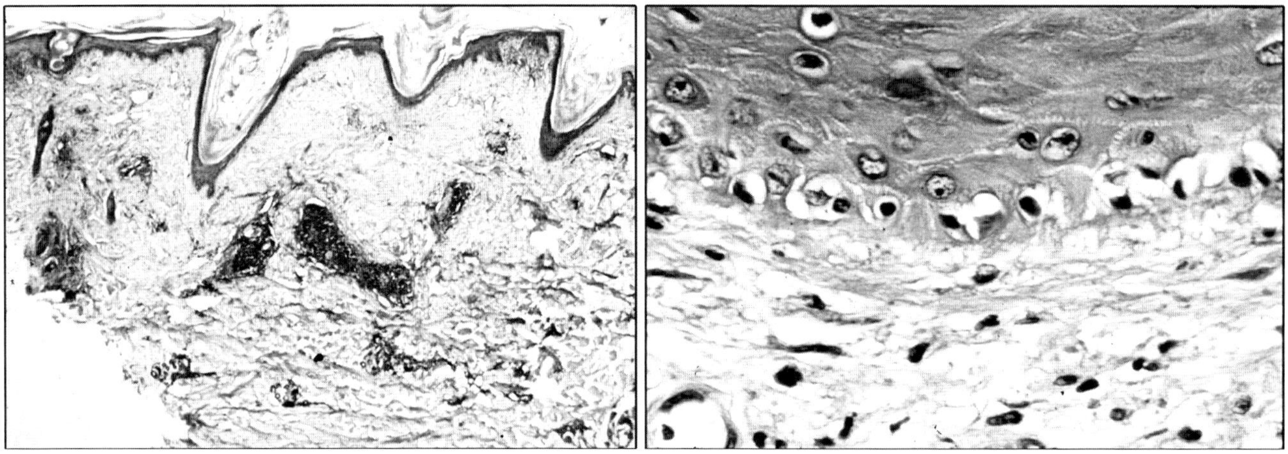

Fig. 5.52 Discoid lupus erythematosus. (*Left*) Note the thinned out epidermis with atrophic follicular infundibuli and the dense patchy mononuclear cell infiltrate underneath. (*Right*) Observe the vacuolar changes (hydropic degeneration) in the interphase. H&E; ×40; ×400 o m

the dermis. The widening of the Max-Joseph spaces leads to the clinical form of bullous LP (Fig. 5.54).

The details provided up to now take place at the lower level of the lesion, which is the battle ground of LP. The epidermis, however, also manifests very important details concerning the diagnosis of LP. The first, and a most significant one, *is the compactness of the horny layer* and its *lack of parakeratosis*. Another highly characteristic feature of this lesion is the "beading of the granular layer," caused by its alternating thickening and thinning (Fig. 5.55).

Lichen Nitidus [37]: The microscopic picture of this lesion is characteristic. It shows a neat papule formed by a mass of mononuclear cells which in its central part shows some granulomatous elements. The lesion appears crusted and parakeratotic, being surrounded by elongated ridges which tend to meet at its base "as if they were the claws of a bird of prey" (Fig. 5.56).

This picture of lichen nitidus, convincingly as it may look, is insufficient, however, to secure its diagnosis since it skips the most important clinical feature on the lesion, that is, its *plurality*. Indeed, lichen nitidus appears clinically as a diffuse eruption of numerous pinhead papules, frequently on the male genital areas. If the lesion put under the microscope is a *solitary one*, it cannot be diagnostic of lichen nitidus, as much as the histologic picture may suggest. Indeed, this is another example of the importance for the microscopist to be provided with clinical information about a lesion prior to rendering its diagnosis.

Table 5.9 Clinical conditions associated to lichenoid lesions

Lichen planus
Lichen nitidus
Halo nevus
Graft vs. host reaction
Pigmented purpuric dermatitis
Stasis dermatitis
Drug and food intolerance
Lichenoid dermatitis, nonspecific

Halo nevus [38] is also known by its patronymic name of "Sutton nevus" as well as by leukodermia centrifuga acquisita. It was already mentioned as a special form of nevocytic nevus undergoing an autoimmune aggression, akin to that which occurs in LP. In the case of halo nevus, though, the reaction is directed toward a nevocytic nevus rather than against the epidermis. Halo nevus presents a dynamic character, appearing initially on the body surface as a pigmented mole surrounded by a halo of depigmentation. The latter advances in a matter of days toward the center as the mole disappears simultaneously, leaving a depigmented spot in its place. This unusual and characteristic set of events would make a biopsy unnecessary in

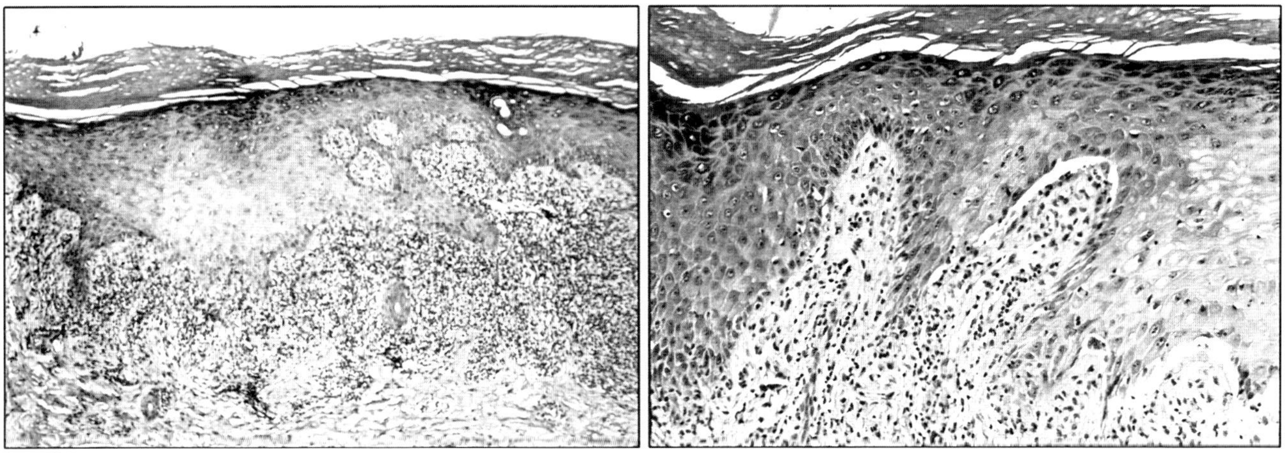

Fig. 5.53 Lichen planus. (*Left*) Observe the band-like infiltrate of the dermis, the main feature of LP. (*Right*) The "sawtooth" profile of the rete ridges is outlined by Max-Joseph spaces. H&E; ×40; ×100 o m

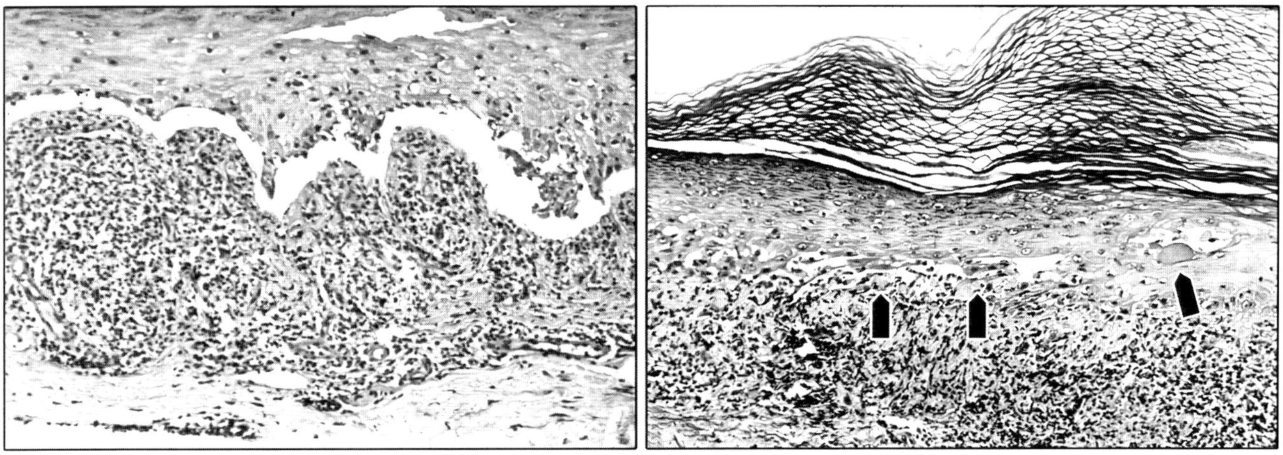

Fig. 5.54 Bullous lichen planus and Civatte's bodies. Note the wide separation between the heavily infiltrated dermis and the devitalized overlying epidermis (*left*). Civatte's bodies are noted dropping from the epidermis into the dermis (*arrows*) (*right*). H&E ×100 o m

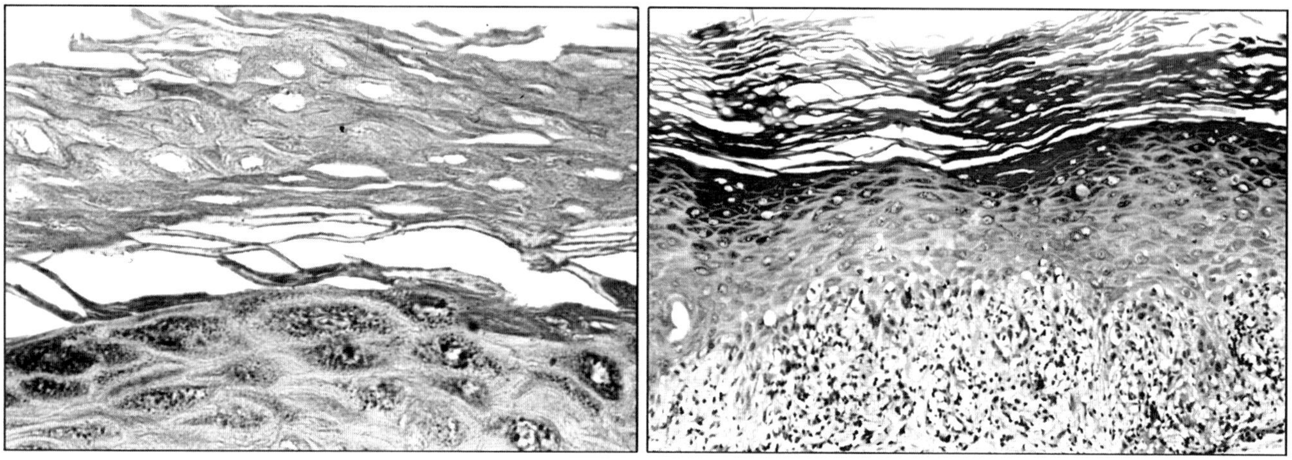

Fig. 5.55 Lichen planus. Note the compactness of the horny layer and its lack of parakeratosis. (*left*). This picture shows the "beading" of the horny layer (*right*). H&E; ×40; ×400 o m

Fig. 5.56 Lichen nitidus. See details in the text. H&E ×40 o m

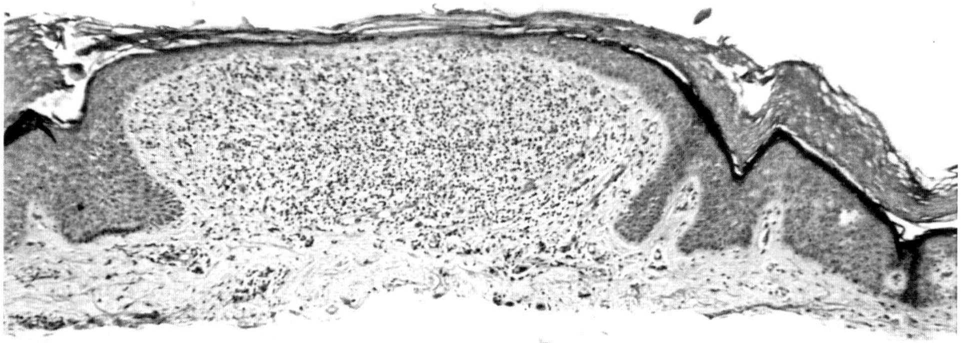

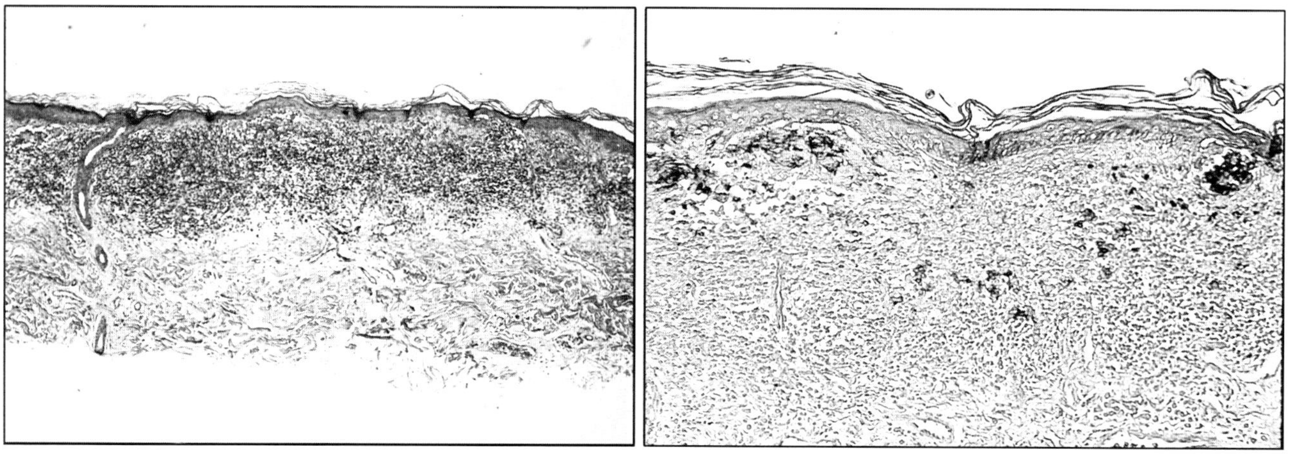

Fig. 5.57 Halo nevus. (*Left*) The lesion presents a dense band-like infiltrate occupying the superficial dermis. (*Right*) The study of silver-stained sections reveals the presence of melanin-containing debris in the infiltrate. H&E ×40; FM ×100 o m

order to render the diagnosis of halo nevus. Regardless, if the clinician were to take a biopsy, its microscopic examination would simply reveal a densely cellular band occupying the superficial dermis of the lesion. The examination of silver-stained sections would reveal in the lesion the presence of melanin-containing remains of nevocytes (Fig. 5.57).

Graft-versus-host reaction is another instance of cellular aggression in which a lichenoid infiltrate may occur. It happens upon the introduction of immunocompetent

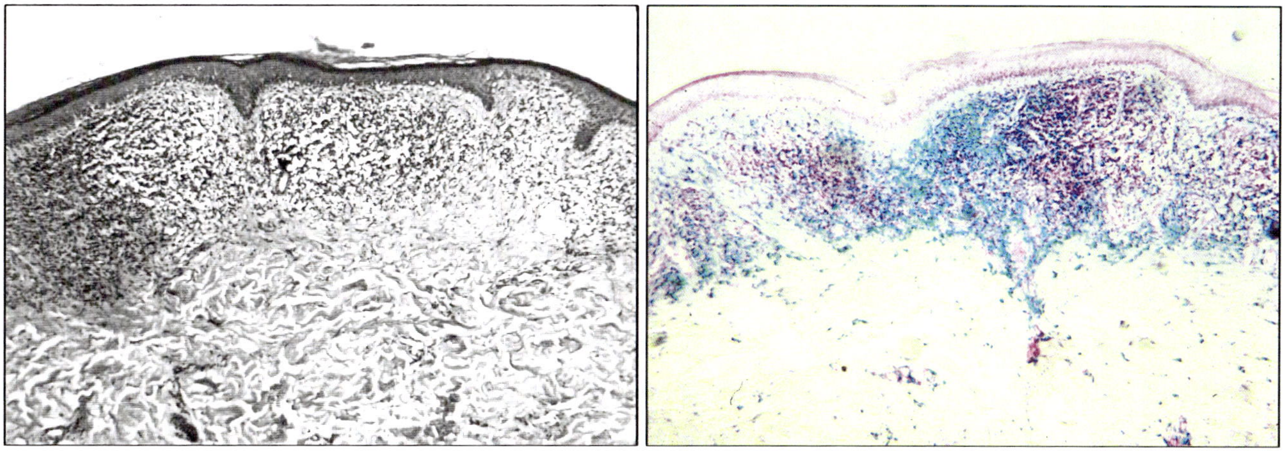

Fig. 5.58 Pigmented purpuric dermatitis. (*Left*) The examination of the lesion at low magnification shows a band of mononuclear cells in the superficial dermis overlaid by a flat and distended epidermis. (*Right*) The application of a special stain reveals an overload of blue-stained hemosiderin granules in the dermis of the specimen. H&E ×40; M/P ×100 o m

lymphocytes, usually within a bone marrow graft, into an immunodeficient patient. Under this condition, the lymphocytes are able to mount an aggression against the host. This is mainly manifested in the GI tract, the liver, and the skin, the last one shown as an ill-defined macular exanthem in the patient. The microscopic examination of the lesion in the skin reveals a lichenoid infiltrate in the superficial dermis spreading out into the epidermis. This layer, in turn, shows a marked paleness with vacuolization, along with necrotic keratinocytes. These are frequently surrounded by lymphocytes, forming a pattern known as "necrosis with satellitosis."

Pigmented purpuric dermatitis (PPD) also known as "purpura pigmentosa chronica" [39] covers a group of conditions mainly localized on the lower legs that have a common pathogenic mechanism. This is based on the chronic sweeping of erythrocytes across a deteriorated endothelium. For this reason, hemosiderin granules derived from the red cell decomposition are noted in the band-like infiltrate of these lesions. These granules may not be easily visualized on H&E-stained sections but are easily evidenced after a special hemosiderin staining of the section (Fig. 5.58).

The differential diagnosis among the principal forms of PPD, Majocchi's disease, Schamberg's disease, and purpura annularis teleangiectoides, relies on their clinical characteristics, since their microscopic pictures are similar. Stasis dermatitis is slightly different from the PPD because it is specifically localized on the patient's ankles and also because the LM examination presents characteristic thick-walled vessels.

Lichenoid infiltrate, a nonspecific term, is the ultimate designation for lesions featuring band-like infiltrates garnered with neutrophils, eosinophils, and parakeratin. These may suggest intolerance to drugs, such as gold, hydralazine, or even certain foods, but otherwise do not show features supportive of the diagnosis of any particular condition.

Granulomas

Granulomas (Fig. 5.41) are hereby defined as discrete and compact masses of histiocytes, activated by the presence of an irritant. "Activated" or "irritated" histiocytes change their shape from spindled to flattened, forming sheets of epithelioid cells closely apposed to each other, giving the appearance of layers of *epithelial* tissue (from where the term "epithelioid" derives). Epithelioid cells are *the first components of granulomas*. Activated histiocytes meanwhile increase their tendency to stick to and ingest surrounding solid elements, thus transforming themselves into "macrophages," *the second component of granulomas*. Due to their activated status, histiocytes show a tendency to merge with one another, thereby forming multinucleated giant cells, *the third component of granulomas*. According to additional histopathologic features, granulomas are separated in this text as *foreign body*, *palisading*, *sarcoidal*, and *tuberculoid*.

Foreign Body Granulomas

Under microscopic examination, foreign body (FB) granulomas frequently disclose the responsible element of the reaction, either incorporated into, or surrounded by macrophages if because of their size, the latter are unable to phagositize them. The presence of a FB in a granuloma may be enhanced by use of *polarized light*, if the FB posesses the appropriate structure. Under this circumstance, the optic phenomenon of double refringency will be generated, thus revealing the FBs as bright spots against a black background (Fig. 5.59).

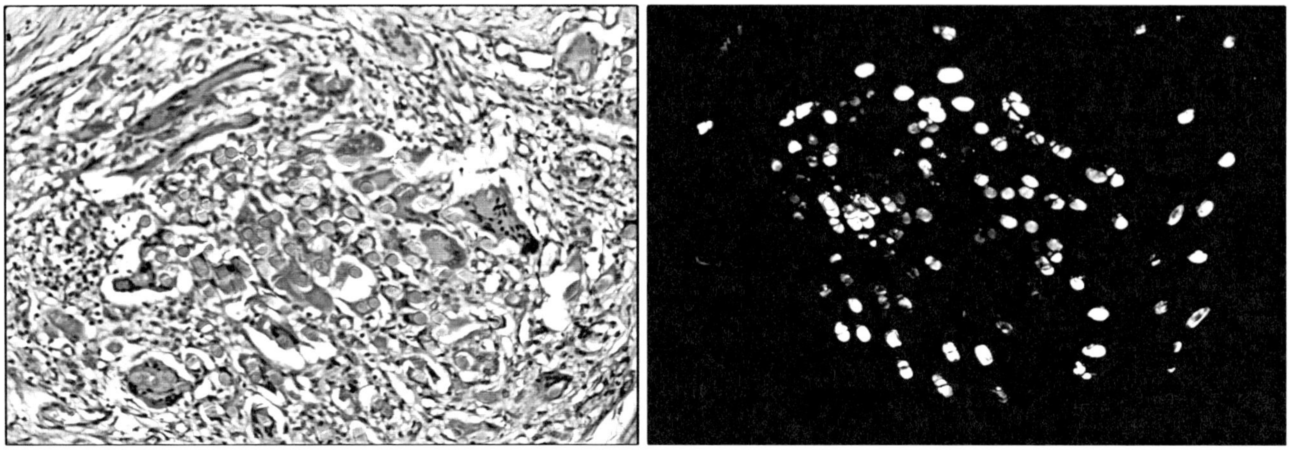

Fig. 5.59 Suture granuloma under natural and polarized light. (*Left*) The direct examination of H&E-stained sections reveals irritated macrophages surrounding not very evident suture threads. (*Right*) Through the use of polarized light, the suture threads appear as bright spots against a black background. H&E ×100; polarized light ×100 o m

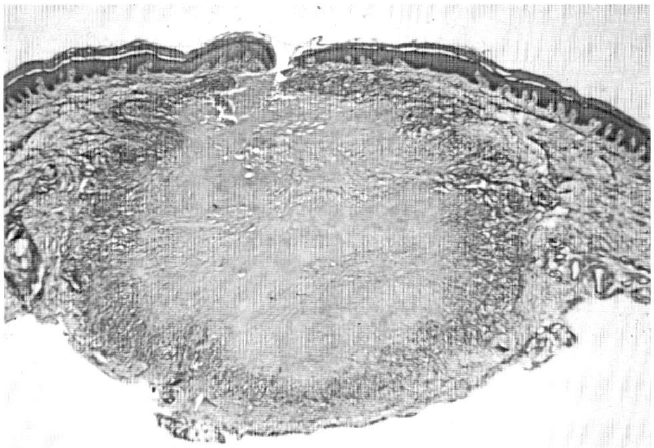

Fig. 5.60 Granuloma annulare. See details in the text. H&E ×40 o m

Palisading Granulomas

Palisading granulomas refer to granulomas in which a central mass appears surrounded by histiocytes. These, being unable to penetrate this mass, are disposed in a palisading pattern around it.

Granuloma annulare (GA), a typical example of palisading granuloma, appears on the skin as rings raised above the epidermis. These rings undergo a centrifugal expansion: they are frequently found on the dorsum of the hand and around the knuckles. The cause of this lesion has not been conclusively established, although suspicion exists that it may be the expression of a necrobiotic process, eventually of ischemic nature. Its microscopic examination reveals a central area of necrosis surrounded by histiocytes disposed in a palisading pattern. The particular lesion shown in this picture presents a break in the surrounding capsule, through which necrotic material is being extruded to the exterior (Fig. 5.60).

Rheumatoid nodule is another pertinent example of palisading granuloma. The fact that this lesion is of a larger size, has a deep localization, is painful, and is associated to rheumatoid arthritis contributes to its differentiation from GA, in spite of its microscopic similarity.

Sarcoidal Granulomas

Sarcoidosis [40] is a systemic disease of unknown cause, manifested by sarcoidal granulomas in the liver, spleen, lungs and other internal organs, and skin. Frequently, these are multiple structures in close approximation to each other, formed by tightly apposed epithelioid histiocytes. Due to their lack of any external coverage, they are nicknamed "naked granulomas," in contrast to tuberculoid granulomas, which are surrounded by a mantle of lymphocytes (see below). Sarcoidal granulomas do not show "*caseosis*" either, the peculiar type of necrosis seen in tuberculous lesions, reason for which they are also called "noncaseating granulomas" rather than "caseating granulomas" as their counterpart, the tuberculoid granuloma, – which show caseosis – is called. In sarcoidal granuloma, other peculiar elements are frequently noted, even though they are not pathognomonic of it: they are the "asteroid bodies." The meaning of these structures has not been clarified, but under LM, they appear to be formed by clusters of intracytoplasmic droplets occupying the cytoplasm of histiocytes (Fig. 5.61). Another element frequently found in the sarcoidal granuloma are Schaumann bodies, probably formed by debris of intracellular structures within multinucleated giant cells.

The presence of a sarcoidal granuloma elicits first of all the diagnosis of sarcoidosis. Tuberculoid leprosy, which under the microscope appears just as a sarcoidal granuloma,

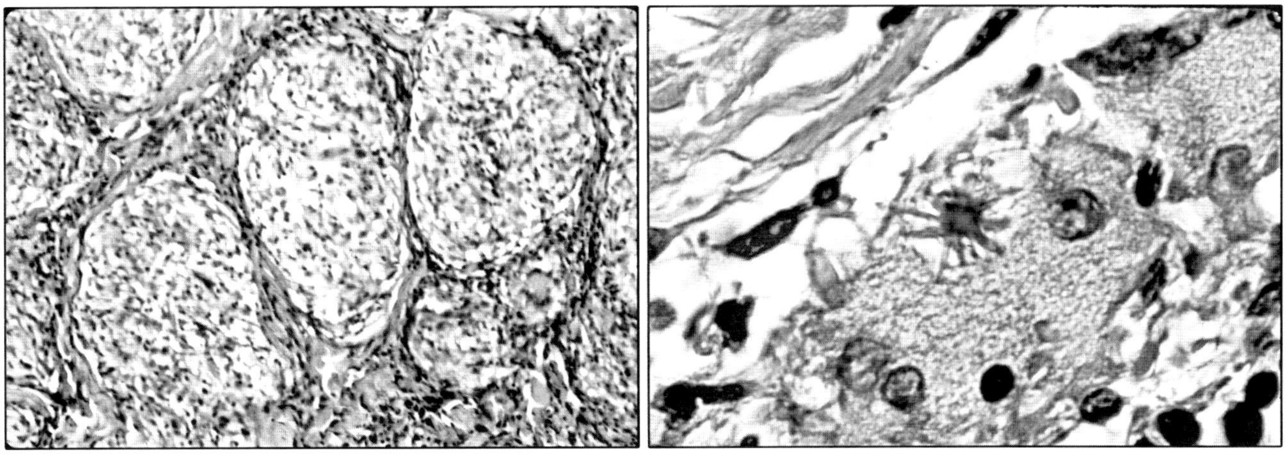

Fig. 5.61 Sarcoidal granuloma. (*Left*) Several sarcoidal granulomas are found, tightly apposed to each other, but preserving their individual limits. Observe their lack of encapsulation and their composition of epithelioid cells with multinucleated elements. To the right, an asteroid body in the cytoplasm of a macrophage is seen. H&E ×40; ×400 o m

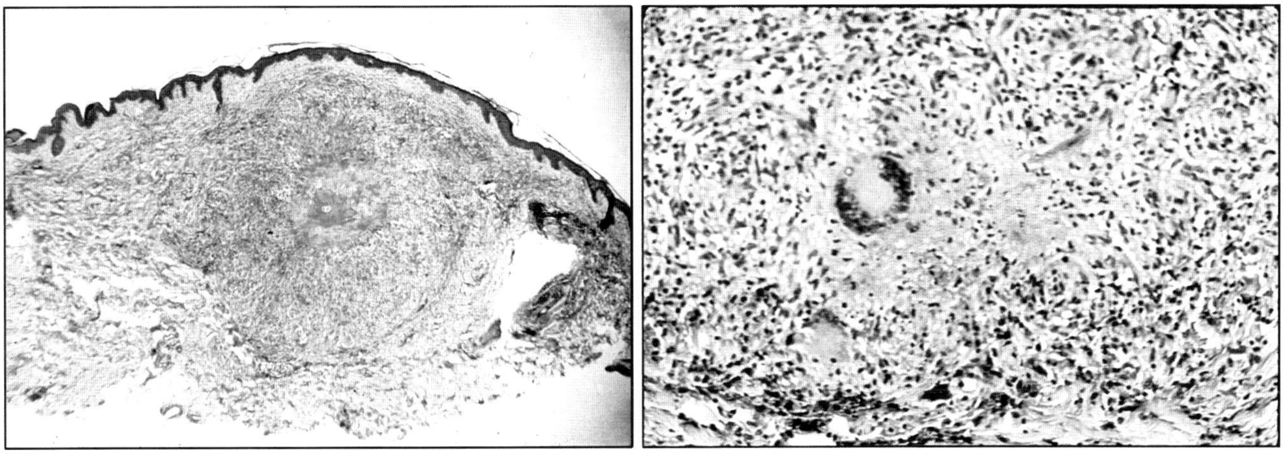

Fig. 5.62 Fish tank granuloma. (*Left*) This lesion involves the dermis and subcutaneous tissue of the specimen but is not spreading to the overlying epidermis. (*Right*) At higher magnification, it presents a center of caseosis surrounded by a mantle of lymphohistiocytes. A multinucleated Langhans giant cell, characteristic of the tuberculoid granuloma, is seen. H&E ×40; ×100 o m

puts this condition as the first alternative diagnostic possibility to sarcoidosis. Other types of sarcoidal granulomas to be mentioned are circonium, berylium, and barium granuloma. In contrast with the two former ones, barium granuloma shows up under polarized bright particles of the mentioned metal.

Tuberculoid Granulomas

The etiology of the tuberculoid granuloma seen in daily dermatopathology practice has shifted from *M. tuberculosis* to less aggressive forms of *atypical mycobacteria*, of which *M. balneomarinum* is one of the most important. This is responsible for the swimming pool and the fish tank granuloma. These are primary cutaneous TB infections acquired by people associated with activities related to those mentioned in the stated lesions. Contrary to sarcoidal granuloma, tuberculoid granuloma presents a core of caseosis (*caseum* [L] cheese), the peculiar type of necrobiosis associated to tuberculous infections, with scattered Langhans multinucleated giant cells surrounded by a mantle of lymphohistiocytes. Figure 5.62 presents a fish tank granuloma as an example of tuberculoid granuloma.

Diffuse Dermal Infiltrates

The lesions enclosed in this Group present a granulomatous character, but contrary to the granulomas reviewed in the previous section, they do not show recognizable limits, having on the contrary a tendency to expand into neighbor structures. Two Subgroups of these lesions may be recognized: the noninfectious and the infectious.

Diffuse Dermal Infiltrates, Noninfectious

Granuloma faciale (GF) is the first condition to be mentioned in this subgroup. It is important to note that the name of this lesion "*granuloma faciale*" is of clinical origin and does not refer to its histopathologic features. GF is a solitary lesion of not infrequent incidence. It primordially affects the face of male patients and runs a chronic course. The lesion, for which no pathogenic agent has been identified, may represent a delayed arthropod reaction modified by unknown circumstances. It may begin by the perivascular accumulation of neutrophils and eosinophils which instead of undergoing purulent degeneration, changes progressively to an almost exclusively histiocytic one. The hallmark of the lesion is an acellular band interposed between the epidermis and the lesion, the "grenz zone" (Fig. 5.63).

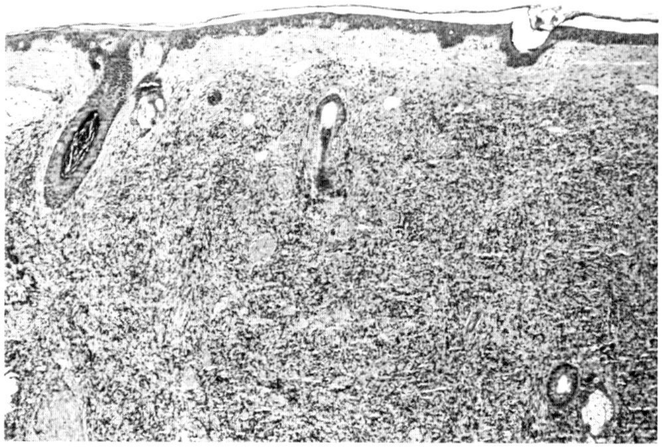

Fig. 5.63 Granuloma faciale. See details in the text. H&E ×40 o m

Erythema Elevatum Diutinum (EED): Upon approaching EED, it is a good policy to keep in mind the English translation of the lesion "elevated and persistent erythema." This definition highlights EED's main characters, which are its bulkiness and its tendency to chronicity (*diutinum* [L] persistent). EED resembles GF in its evolution and its histologic composition – with the exception of the grenz zone – to the point that a relationship between both has been suggested. EED differs significantly from GF, however, in several other aspects. In the first place, it is a much less frequent lesion, and in the second place, it has an acral and symmetric distribution instead of a facial localization as GF does. EED may be somehow associated to midsized vessels in its pathogenesis but appears very unconvincingly to be the result of a vasculitic process, as it is often considered. Its microscopic features are grossly superimposable to the ones of GF.

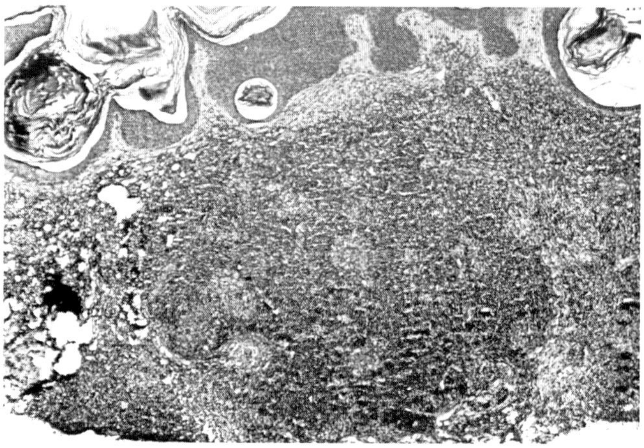

Fig. 5.64 Spiegler-Fendt pseudolymphoma. Note the dense cellular infiltration spreading down from the dermoepidermal junction, without involving the epidermis. Observe the well-formed germinal nodules in the lesion. H&E ×40 o m

Spiegler-Fendt pseudolymphoma may also be incorporated into this subgroup of diffuse, noninfectious infiltrates. This lesion appears as curtains of mononuclear cells of unremarkable features which descend from an unremarkable epidermis into the deep dermis. It has embedded germinal centers which interrupt their uniformity (Fig. 5.64). In spite of the germinal centers, which may suggest a lymphoproliferative nature for this lesion – from where its name actually derives – Spiegler-Fendt pseudolymphoma seems to be a reactive inflammatory condition, for which the alternative name of "lymphocytoma cutis" has been proposed. That denomination does not help, however, in dispelling the idea that this lesion may be a lymphoproliferative process.

Necrobiosis lipoidica diabeticorum is a necrobiotic process of possible ischemic nature, whose name was shortened to "necrobiosis lipoidica" once realized that it was not privative to diabetic patients as initially thought. It occurs on the shins of adults. Under the microscope, the lesion shows alternating layers of palisading histiocytes with multinucleated giant cells, alternating with necrotic tissue. In a way it resembles GA but in a flat disposition instead of forming granulomas (Fig. 5.65).

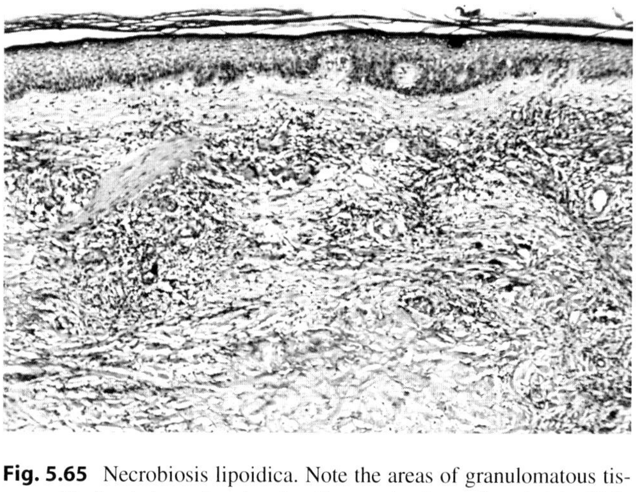

Fig. 5.65 Necrobiosis lipoidica. Note the areas of granulomatous tissue with the intervening bands of necrotic tissue "sandwiched" in between. H&E ×40, o m

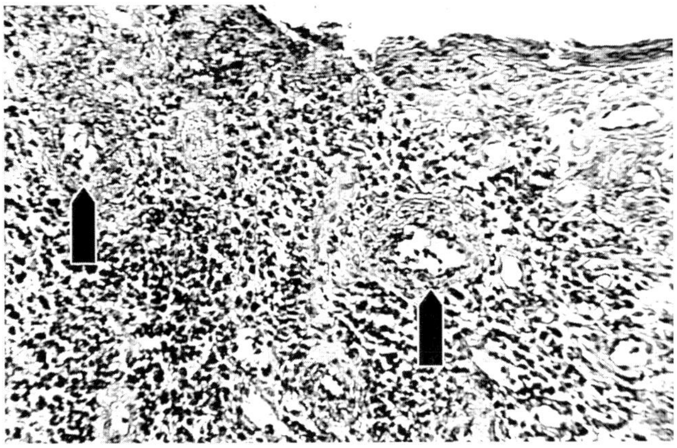

Fig. 5.66 Postprimary syphilis. Note the dense cellular infiltration and ulceration of the lesion, which also shows two cross-sectioned vessels in the dermis with vasculitic changes (*arrows*). H&E ×100 o m

Diffuse Dermal Infiltrates, Infectious

These infiltrates are distinguished by their strong granulomatous and frequently necrotizing character. As a result of their infiltrating activity, they end up as torpide processes involving in addition to the dermis, subcutaneous fat, and often osteotendinous structures.

Postprimary Syphilis: The *clinical* manifestations, that is, the exanthems to which these lesions are associated, have already been reviewed (p. 89). The tendency of these infiltrates to spread out, along with their mixed composition, with abundant plasmacytes and neutrophils, has also been brought up. Other important features of these lesions are their frequent ulceration and the concomitant presence of vasculitis (Fig. 5.66). Examination of the specimens by appropriate techniques often reveals abundant *T. pallida*.

With regard to the presence of *T. pallida* in the tissues, the Jarisch-Herxheimer reaction should be mentioned. This reaction may occasionally be seen when starting a patient whose tissues have a high treponema tenor, on a penicillin treatment: the liberation of massive amounts of toxic products derived from the sudden destruction of these organisms by the antibiotic may cause severe adverse effects in the patient. These effects are known by the stated name.

Cutaneous tuberculosis is due primordially to infections by *M. tuberculosis*. For the study of cutaneous tuberculosis, this text distinguishes the forms caused by *external inoculation* from those caused by *internal contamination*. The first ones may occur as *primary infections* in subjects formerly free of tb infection, or as *reinfections* in those individuals previously infected. Regarding internal contaminations, these may be the result of *hematogenous disseminations* from distant foci, or from cutaneous *contaminations by contiguity* from nearby foci. Table 5.10 offers examples of all these infective modalities. Tuberculides are not included in that list, since they are unconfirmed cases of tb infections.

Table 5.10 Forms of cutaneous tuberculosis

From external inoculation
Primary
Tuberculous chancre
Reinfection
Prosector nodule
From internal dissemination
Hematogenous disseminations
Lupus vulgaris
Miliar tuberculosis
Contaminations
Orificial tuberculosis
Scrofuloderma

The primary tb infection of the skin in the form of tuberculous chancre is a rare event these days. This lesion appears as a complex formed by an ulceronecrotic nodule combined with a regional lymphadenitis. Tuberculosis verrucosa in contrast to the former is no such an infrequent event, representing an external reinfection in individuals with a moderate level of defense. This lesion, of which the prosector nodule or the butcher nodule are particular examples, is generally found on the hands, knees, and other points of external contact and appears as a verrucous nodule. Under the microscope, the lesion exhibits acanthosis and a purulent papillomatosis in which the presence of *M. tuberculosis* may eventually be demonstrated.

Among the forms of internal contamination of tb, lupus vulgaris is the most pertinent example. This condition corresponds to the hematogenous dissemination of the tb bacillus from a primary visceral site to the skin and has an elective localization in head and neck. The lesion offers the microscopic image of a granulomatous inflammation in the dermis with disseminated areas of caseation. It also affects the epidermis, which appears atrophic and frequently ulcerated. The demonstration of *M. tuberculosis* is not frequent in these cases (Fig. 5.67).

Leprosy [41] is caused by *Mycobacterium leprae* or *Hansen's bacillum*. The status of the patient's defenses combined with the finding of bacteriology and pathology allows the classification of this condition, also called "Hansen disease" into six clinical types. They occur in a continuous spectrum ranging from the extreme of tuberculoid leprosy, which appears when the patient has a high level of defense, to that of lepromatous leprosy, when the patient is in anergic condition, at which point he or she cannot resist the ongoing infection.

For the sake of simplification, the clinical manifestations of the intermediate forms of the spectrum of leprosy will hereby be left aside. Instead, the two extreme forms will be brought briefly into discussion. Those are the *tuberculoid* and the *lepromatous* forms. The former is clinically characterized by the presence of asymmetric, hypopigmented, and scaly spots (*leprae* [G] scale), whereas the latter features

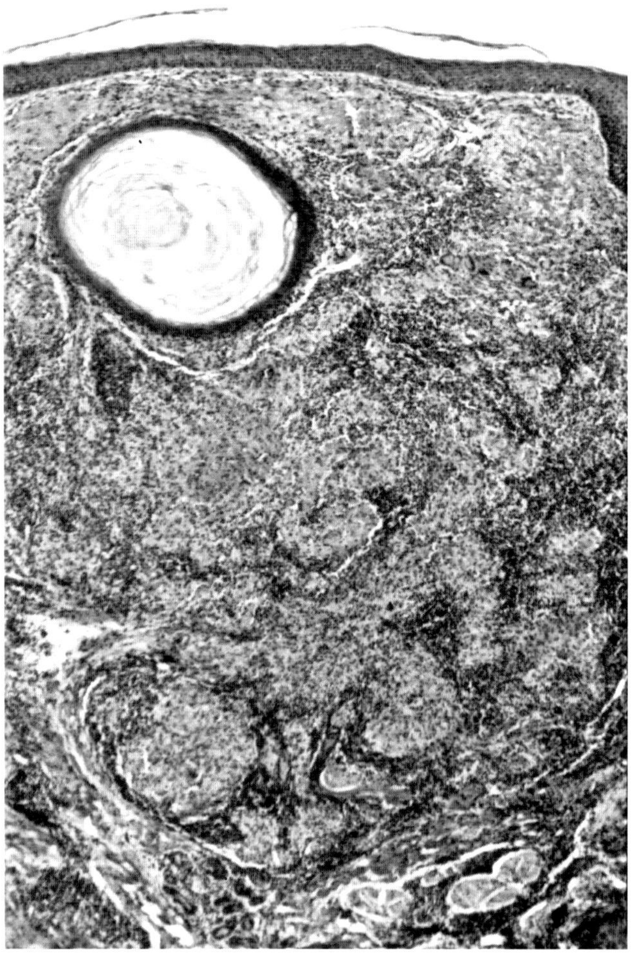

Fig. 5.67 Lupus vulgaris. Note the confluent granulomatous nodules with central caseation and the intervening streams of lymphocytes. An atrophic follicular cyst is also found in this lesion, which is overlaid by a strongly atrophic epidermis. H&E ×40 o m

succulent symmetric plaques such as the ones forming the "facies leonina" of lepromatous patients.

Regarding the histopathology of tuberculoid leprosy, its typical form is a sarcoidal granuloma, closely similar to the one already described for *sarcoidosis* (p. 96). *M. leprae*, whose presence would settle the discussion about the etiology of the granuloma, is hardly ever demonstrated in this condition. Nevertheless, a microscopic differentiation from sarcoidosis may be reached based on the recognized tendency of Hansen disease, but not of sarcoidosis, of developing around peripheral nerves.

Lepromatous leprosy, in contrast to its tuberculoid counterpart, features a profuse granulomatous reaction teaming with acid-fast bacilli, mainly along thin peripheral nerves. The hallmark of this lesion is the presence of foamy histiocytes, "Virchow's cells," enclosing large amounts of *M. leprae* bacilli (Fig. 5.68).

Histioid leprosy is a special type of lepromatous leprosy. From the outside, it features the dome-shaped aspect of a benign fibrohistiocytoma (p. 159). Upon microscopic examination, the Virchow's cells appear replaced by spindle-shaped elements. These are heavily loaded with *M. leprae* bacilli, easily demonstrable by LM after appropriate staining procedures (Fig. 5.69).

Deep fungal infections [42] feature prototypic examples of heavy granulomatous lesions. Due to the character of the text, only a restricted list of agents of these lesions will be presented in Table 5.11.

The frequency with which fungal agents enter the body through the respiratory tract (*R*) or the skin (S) is expressed by a scale ranging from 0+ if this event never happens to 4+ if it occurs in 100 % of the cases, with 25 % increments representing each "+".

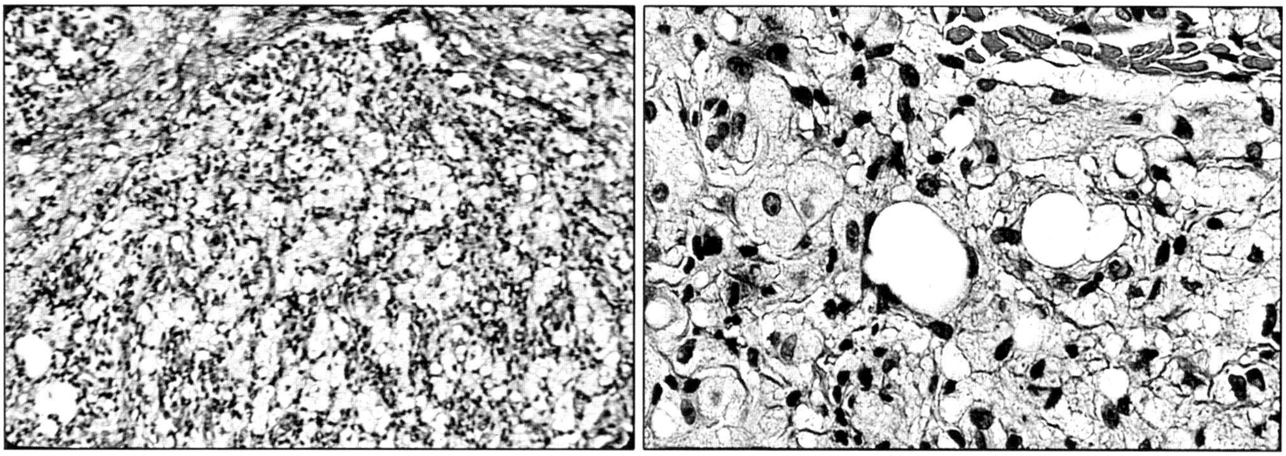

Fig. 5.68 Lepromatous leprosy. (*Left*) Note the diffuse inflammatory reaction which makes the original anatomical elements of the site irrecognizable. (*Right*) Observe at high magnification the large amounts of foamy histiocytes, that is, Virchow's cells in the lesion. H&E ×40; ×400 o m

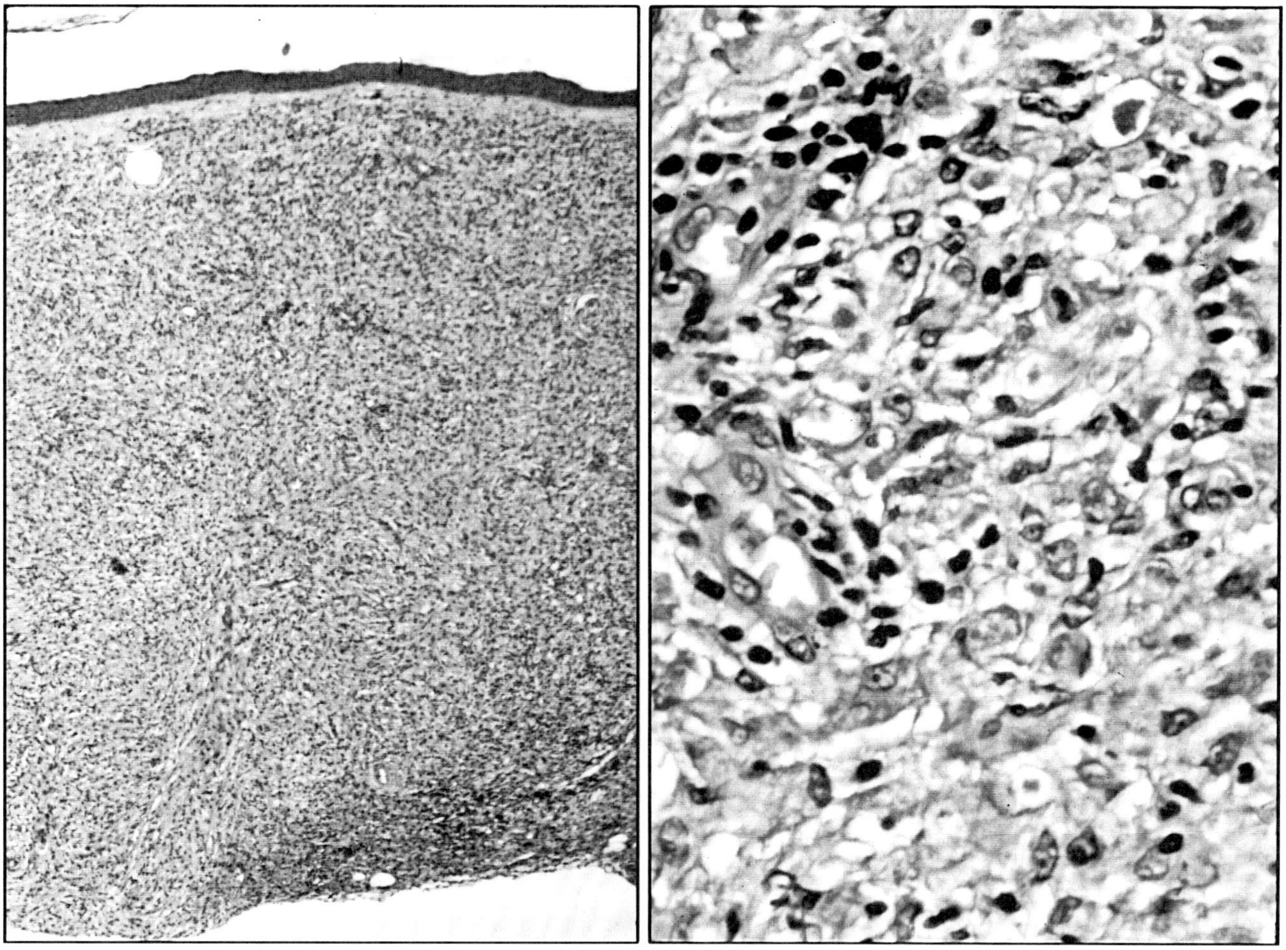

Fig. 5.69 Histioid leprosy. (*Left*) The lesion presents a compact appearance. (*Right*) It is formed by bundles and whorls of spindle-shaped elements. H&E ×40; ×400 (Compare this picture with that of lepromatous leprosy in Fig. 5.68)

A glance at Table 5.11 reveals that the histopathology of the posted deep fungal infections, although frequently of a more purulent character, is similar to the granulomatous type present described in general terms, for the lesions in the previous Subgroup (p. 97). These pictures are impressive and may striking characters, as shown before, although in the absence of the responsible agent, they are nonspecific.

The diagnosis of a suspected dermatomycosis relies on the presence of the etiologic agent in the lesion. This may be achieved by simple LM inspection of tissue sections stained by the standard H&E technique or other staining modalities (Figs. 5.70 and 5.71), by culture of material derived from the lesions or by other, more sophisticated techniques (Figs. 5.72 and 5.73).

Mycetoma, also known by the general name "pie de Madura," is a torpid process appearing on the feet of barefoot-walking people. It is characterized under the microscope by a heavy, deep-seated granulomatous reaction with destruction of osteotendinous tissue and abscess formation. Mycelial clumps or "*grains*" are found in the lesion and discharged through fistulous tracts (Fig. 5.74).

Mycetomas may be caused by true fungi such as *M. mycetomatis* and *P. boydii* or by filamentous bacteria, most commonly *N. brasiliensis* and *S. somaliensis*. In the first case, the lesion is specifically called "eumycetoma" and in the second, "pseudomycetoma." The difference has important implications because pseudomycetomas are amenable to antibiotic and other medical treatment, whereas eumycetomas are not, requiring radical surgery as the only effective therapeutic approach [43].

After considering the evolutive inflammatory lesions with predominant dermal localization, the ones with predominant subcutaneous tissue should now be considered.

Lesions of Predominant Subcutaneous Localization

Following the general approach, lesions in the subcutaneous tissue may be subclassified as of prevalent vascular or cellular character (Fig. 5.75).

Table 5.11 Some agents responsible for deep fungal infections: name of the condition, etiologic agent, port of entry, and histopathology

Disease	Agent	Port of entry R	Port of entry C	Histopathology
Cryptococcosis	*C. neoformans*	4+	0+	Granulomatous infiltrate with histiocytes, giant cells, abscesses, necrosis, and fibrosis
South-American blastomycosis	*P. brasiliensis*	4+	0+	Mixed acute and granulomatous infiltrates. Abscesses, Steering wheel figures
Coccidioido mycosis	*C. immitis*	3+	1+	Mixed infiltrate with predominant neutrophilic component, multinuceated giant cells and epidermal hyperplasia
North-American Blastomycosis	*B. dermatitides*	3+	1+	Verrucous lesions with pseudo carcinomatous hyperplasia and ulcers. Abundant neutrophils and abscesses
Histoplasmosis infiltrates and necrosis	*H. capsulatum*	3+	1+	Ulcerated lesions with granulomatous inflamation
Chromomycosis	*F. pedrosi* and other sapro phytic fungi	3+	1+	Mixed acute and granulomatous infiltrates with abscess formation giant cells and abscesses "Cooper coin Spores"
Sporotrichosis	*S. schenki*	0+	4+	Mixed acute and granulomatous infiltrates with abscess formation and ulceration

Port of entry: *R* respiratory, *C* cutaneous

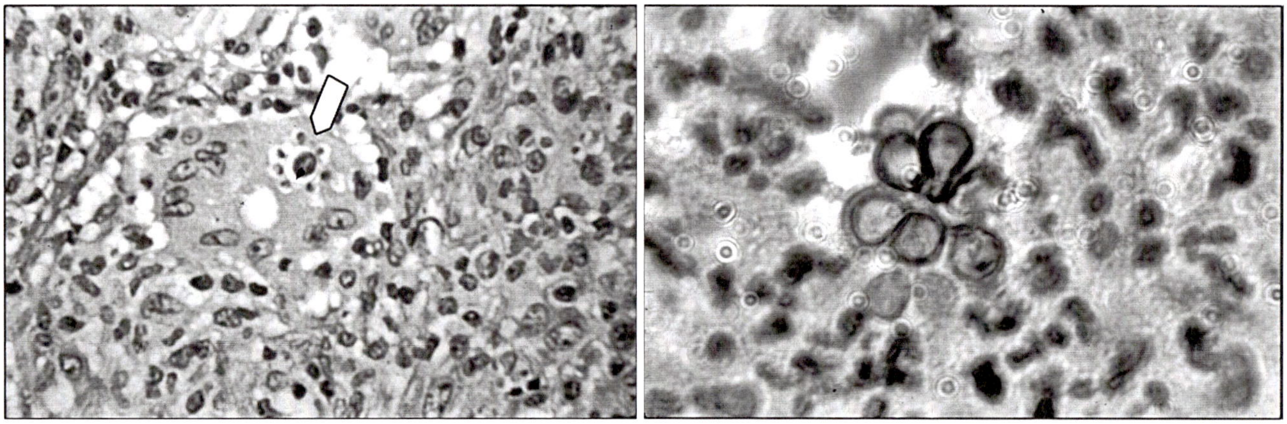

Fig. 5.70 South-American blastomycosis and chromomycosis. In South-American blastomycosis (*left*), a spore with several peripheral buds configurating a "steering wheel picture" is seen (*arrow*), within a multinucleated giant cell. In chromomycosis (*right*), a cluster of so-called copper coin spores is noted, surrounded by poly- and mononuclear cells. H&E ×400; ×1,000

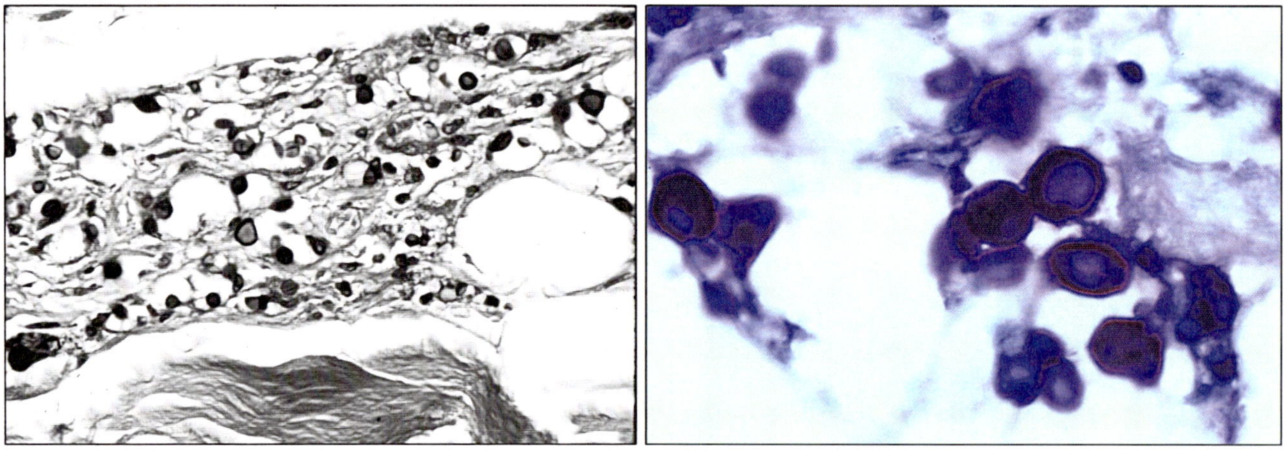

Fig. 5.71 *Cryptococcus neoformans* in an HIV case. (*Left*) Note the fungal organisms invading the adipose panniculus of an HIV patient without eliciting any inflammatory reaction. (*Right*) The spores surrounded by the gelatinous capsule are seen at higher magnification. MC ×100; ×1,000

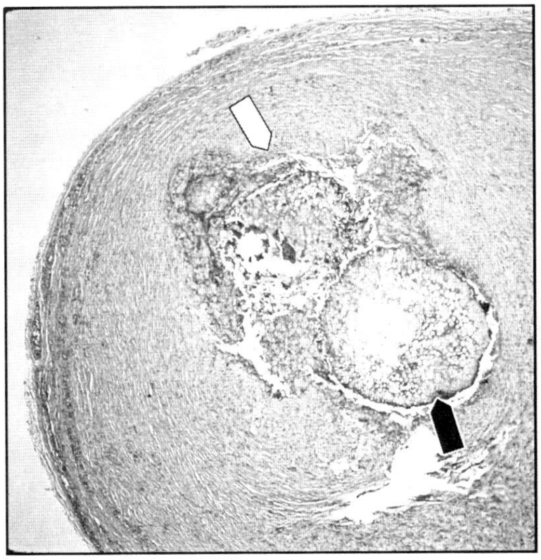

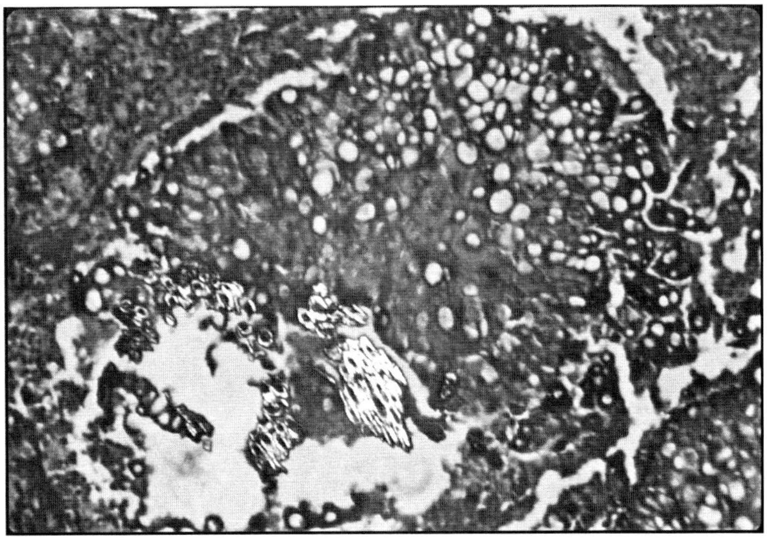

Fig. 5.72 Aspergillus colony on a wooden splinter. On the left, the aspergillus colony is indicated by the *white arrow* and the cross section of the splinter by the *black arrow*. On the right, the colony is seen at higher magnification under polarized light. Small pieces of wood feature double refringency. H&E ×40; polarized light ×400

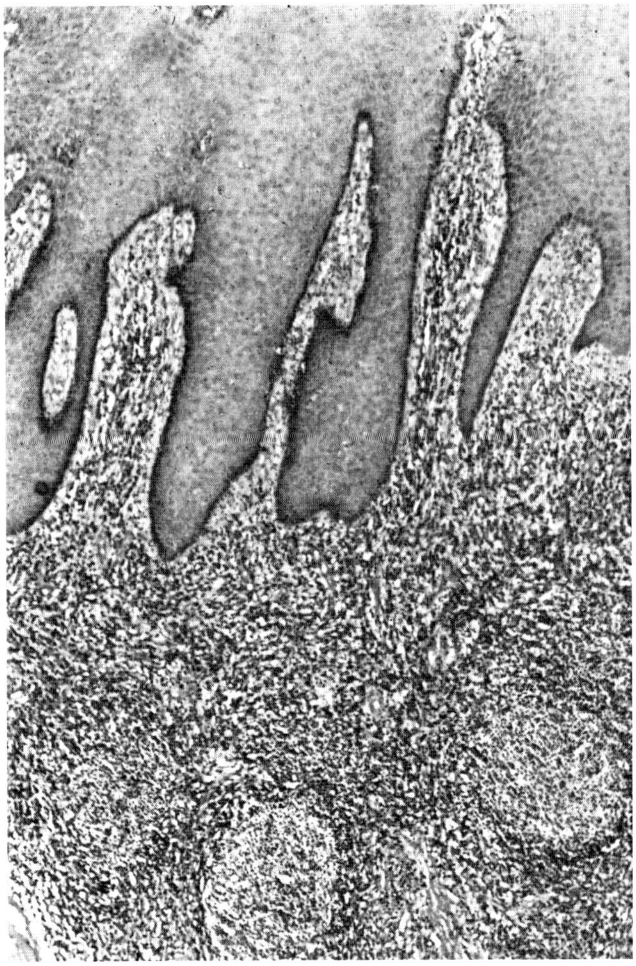

Fig. 5.73 Coccidioidomycosis. Note the striking reactive pseudocarcinomatous hyperplasia, with a profuse granulomatous reaction and germinal center formation. H&E ×40. The etiology of this particular lesion was established via cultures. H&E ×100 o m

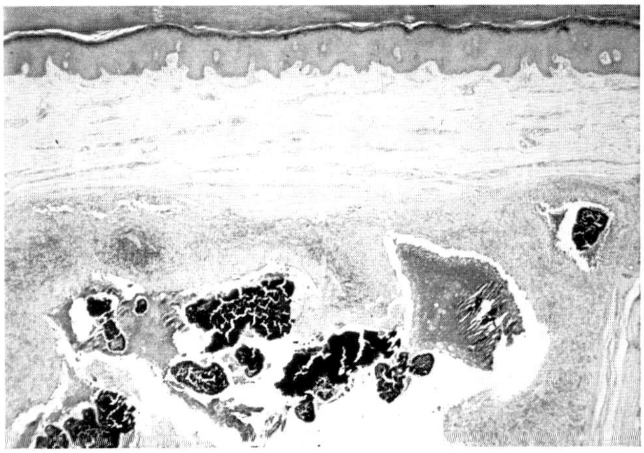

Fig. 5.74 Mycetoma. Note the "grains" within a fistula. H&E ×20

Lesions with Prevailing Vascular Character

The Subclass of vascular lesions featured in Fig. 5.75 contains, in addition to arteritis and phlebitis, a new group of entities, that is, the one of the lymphangitides. Indeed, the lymphatic vessels, having reached a sizable caliber in the subcutaneous tissue, display nosologic processes worthy of discussion.

Arteritis

Erythema Nodosum Arteritis: In this group, the first lesion to be considered is the vessel associated to erythema nodosum, the erythema nodosum arteritis [44]. This is, as a rule, a mid-sized artery running through the fibrous interlobular septae of the adipose tissue. The interruption of its flow, due to its damage and thrombosis, leads to the ischemic necrosis of its

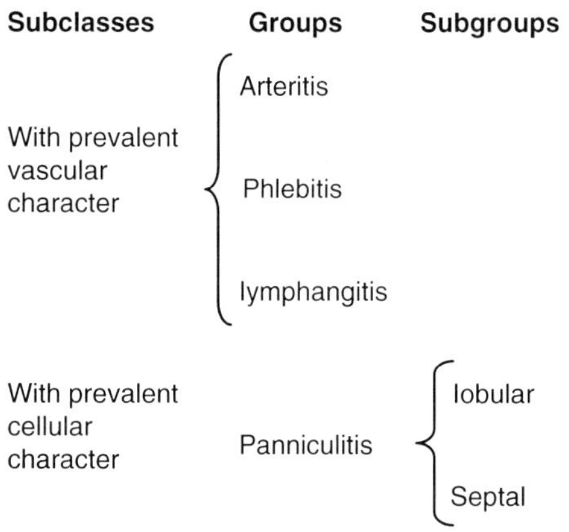

Fig. 5.75 Evolutive inflammatory lesions of predominantly subcutaneous localization: subclasses, groups, and subgroups

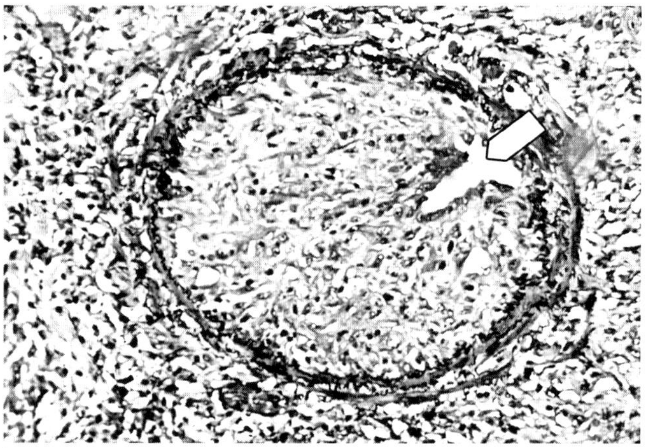

Fig. 5.76 Arteritis in erythema nodosum. Note the thrombosed and rechannelized vessel (*arrow*). EvG ×100 o m

tributary territory. (See erythema nodosum, next Subclass of lesions.) As for the cause of the vessel's damage, several agents of widely different nature have been suspected: infections, mainly by *M. pneumonia* and *herpesvirus*, drug intolerance, sarcoidosis, type III hypersensitivity reactions, and others. The microscopic study of the lesion reveals a heavily damaged and thrombosed midsized vessel in an area of acute or chronic inflammatory reaction, with or without multinucleated giant cells, depending on the evolutive stage of the lesion (Fig. 5.76).

Giant cell arteritis [45] is another nosologic process involving midsized arteries, although through a totally different pathogenic mechanism. The presumption exists that the close proximity of the vessels to the external surface of the body and the inadequate protection offered to them by the scant subcutaneous tissue in the area allows external physical agents, mainly *trauma* and *cold*, to affect them. LM examination of the lesion reveals a destructive granulomatous process surrounding a midsized artery. The most pertinent example of this type of lesion is *temporal arteritis*.

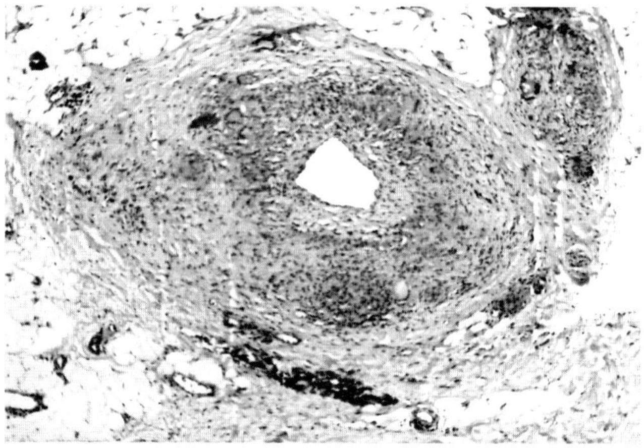

Fig. 5.77 Temporal arteritis. Note the intense granulomatous reaction with abundant multinucleated giant cells surrounding the heavily damaged vessel. H&E ×100 o m

Temporal arteritis appears as a painful, reddened area in the temporal region, in which the contour of the affected vessel can be recognized from the outside. Under LM, a severe granulomatous reaction involving the affected vessel is noted, with abundant multinucleated giant cells (Fig. 5.77). In the particular case of temporal arteritis, the treating doctor must be aware of the potential complication which may ensue if the lesion spreads from its original localization along the homolateral optic artery, an event that may lead to ipsilateral blindness.

Another example of giant cell arteritis is occipital arteritis. In this case, a superficial position comparable to that of temporal arteritis makes this vessel liable to the same aggressive agents. It may be said in passing that *external trauma* and *cold* – claimed as a frequent pathogenic agent in these lesions – have been proven to be a highly damaging combination for other anatomic element in close proximity to the external surface of the skin, the ear cartilage, as shall be discussed below (p. 111).

Phlebitis

Phlebitis and thrombophlebitis are processes within the realms of internal medicine. Among the cases where these conditions may present an interest in dermatology, migratory thrombophlebitis should be mentioned as a prime example. This process, also known by the name of Trousseau's sign [46] occurs in cases of internal malignancies, particularly pancreatic cancer, along the saphenous vein of the left leg.

Lymphangitis

Among the midcaliber lymphatics which run through the subcutaneous tissue, two nosologic conditions deserve a short comment. Acute bacterial lymphangitis is the first. This is usually a trivial infection running along the vessel wall, usually ending at the regional lymphatic node. The second is a specific condition, sporotrichotic lymphangitis, caused by inoculation

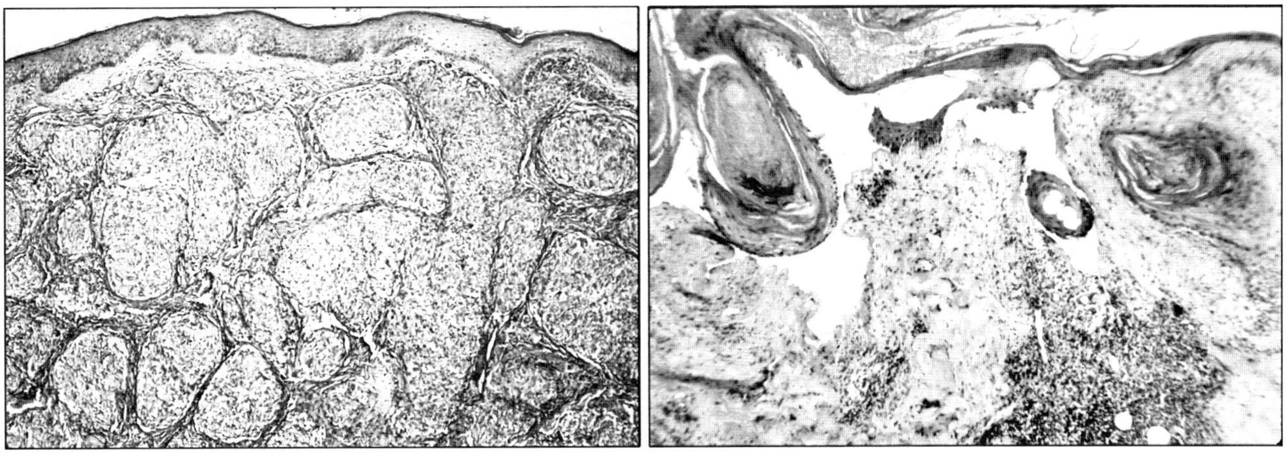

Fig. 5.78 Subcutaneous sarcoidosis and lupus profundus. In the first case (*left*), the characteristic sarcoidal nodules are spreading downward from the dermoepidermal junction, totally occupying the dermis and massively invading the subcutaneous tissue. In the second case (*right*), dense, angulated, and sharply delimited patches of mononuclear cells pertaining to a case of DLE are found in the subcutaneous tissue. H&E ×40

of the fungus *S. schenkii* into wounds, most frequently on the hands of gardeners and people in contact with rotten wood and earth. The infection is manifested along the lymphatic vessels by discrete nodules, which have a mixed structure, purulent in their central area and granulomatous at the periphery.

Lesions of Prevailing Cellular Character

The subcutaneous tissue is formed by faintly encapsulated fat lobules, with intervening fibrous septae through which the elements responsible for their irrigation and innervation run. Fatty tissue is extremely labile and cannot mount any defensive reaction, undergoing instead diffuse necrosis after any aggression, with collapse of their reticulin network. The inflammatory processes of the subcutaneous tissue are called "*panniculitis*."

Panniculitis may directly follow the aggression to the fatty lobules by a pathogenic agent, or may occur indirectly, after the damage of an artery and interruption of blood flow into its tributary fat lobules. Direct panniculitis are called "*lobular panniculitis*" and indirect ones, "*septal panniculitis*."

Lobular Panniculitis

Cytosteatonecrosis is the most pertinent example of a direct aggression to the fatty tissue, causing a lobular panniculitis. It occurs in cases of acute pancreatitis, when the pancreatic lipases liberated during the acute inflammatory process attack the adipose tissue, and saponification and combination with Ca occurs, resulting into white chalky spots easily visible at the unaided examination against the background of the fatty tissue.

Weber-Christian disease or nodular febrile nonsuppurative recurrent panniculitis [47] is a disease of unknown cause, associated to focal areas of necrosis in the subcutaneous tissue resembling the ones in cytosteatonecrosis. This condition, however, displays a systemic character evident in internal organs as well. Its cutaneous lesions offer a microscopic picture of necrotic fatty tissue, but this has the distinguishing pathognomonic feature of abundant "*foamy cells*" that are lipid-loaded histiocytes, derived from necrosis of fatty tissue. These are reminiscent of the ones in *histiocytic cytophagic panniculitis*, a condition which will be reviewed with the transitional inflammatory lesions (p. 113).

The presence of sarcoidal nodules or the patchy LE infiltrates in the subcutaneous tissue may be also regarded as cases of lobular panniculitis. The first condition is called "sarcoidal panniculitis" and the second "lupus profundus" (Fig. 5.78).

Septal Panniculitides

Erythema nodosum [48] (EN) is the most representative example of a septal panniculitis. This is an ischemic and necrotizing process of fat lobules tributaries of a thrombosed artery. Analysis of the artery responsible for the process, the "*erythema nodosum arteritis*," has been already undertaken (p. 103).

In order to perform a satisfactory microscopic study in a case of EN, a deep punch biopsy of the lesion is required (Fig. 5.79). This may allow the microscopist to find the pathognomonic combination of EN, that is, an intense panniculitis with a damaged and frequently thrombosed midsized artery, which along with the pertinent clinical information leads to the conclusive diagnosis of the lesion.

Erythema nodosum leprosum [49] or Lucio phenomenon is a type III hypersensitivity reaction bound to occur in

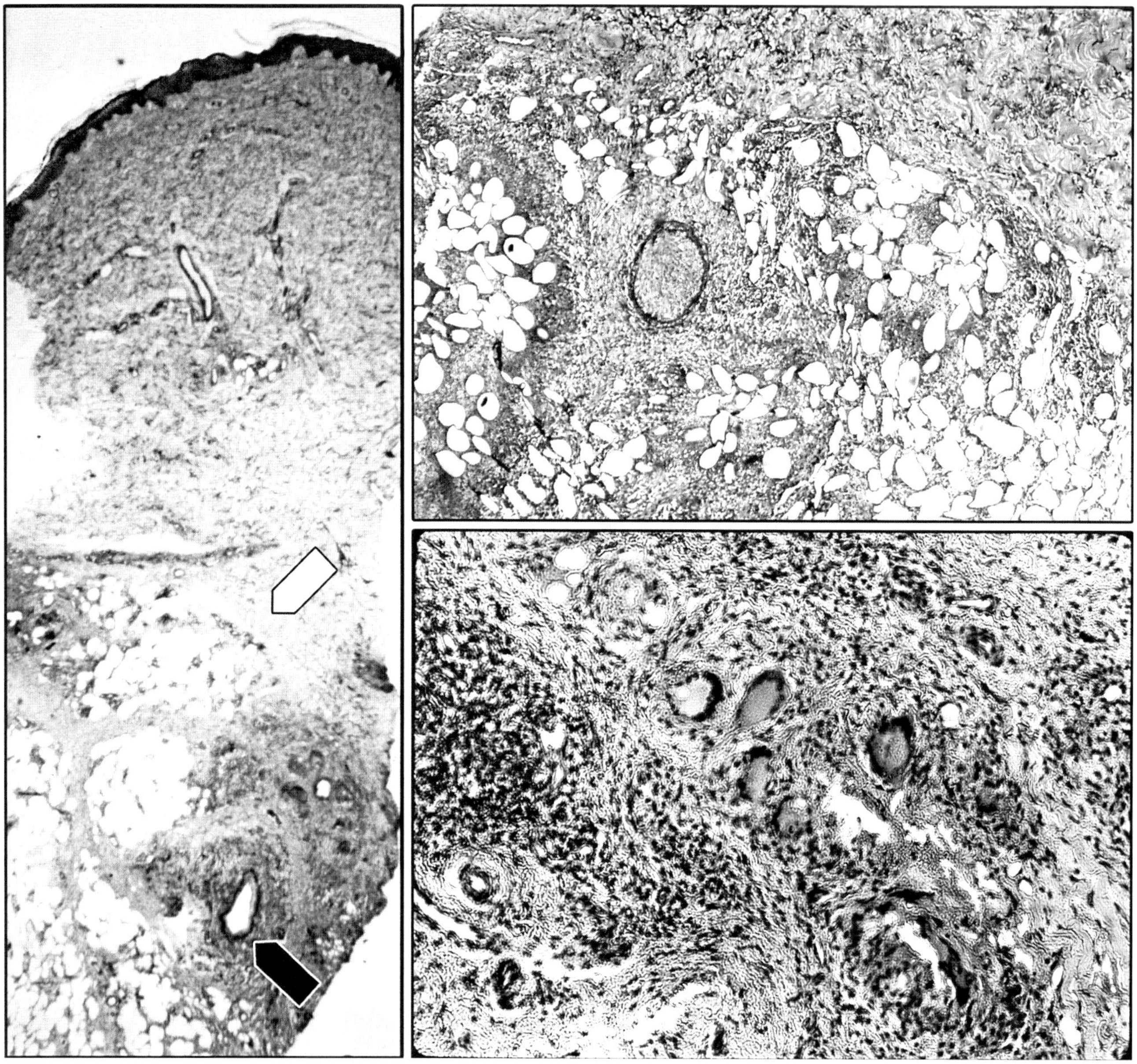

Fig. 5.79 Erythema nodosum. (*Left*) Microscopic examination of a deep punch biopsy demonstrates the simultaneous presence in the section examined of a heavy panniculitis (*white arrow*) and a heavily damaged midsized artery (*black arrow*). At higher magnification (*right above*), the picture reveals, in another case of EN, a thrombosed artery surrounded by an aseptic panniculitis. Late stage of an erythema nodosum lesion (*right below*), containing fibrosis and abundant multinucleated giant cells. Remnants of the destroyed vessel are present at the right lower corner of figure. H&E ×20; ×100; ×100 o m

lepromatous patients with high levels of circulating Abs. Under chemotherapy, a sudden liberation of dead bacilli occurs, which combine with the circulating Abs, forming ICs. The deposition of these ICs on arterial walls is followed by extensive tissue damage.

Lucio phenomenon should not be mistaken with the disfavorable reaction occasionally experienced by lepromatous patients on chemotherapy. This other reaction underlies the massive destruction of *M. leprae* and the liberation of toxic products and must be regarded as closely similar to the already discussed Jarisch-Herxheimer reaction which occurs in syphilitic patients in treatment with penicillin (p. 99).

Lesions of Predominantly Adnexal Localization

The inflammatory lesions of the adnexae may be subclassified as of follicular, sebaceous, tubuloglandular, and ungual localization. Arbitrarily, a fifth Subclass of lesions of cartilaginous nature was added to these (Fig. 5.80).

Lesions of the Hair Follicle

Folliculitis constitutes the most frequent and conspicuous Subclass of adnexal lesions. As indicated in Fig. 5.80, they may be separated into two Groups: infectious and aseptic.

Infectious Folliculitis

The group of infectious folliculitis is the most numerous and variegated, responding to three main pathogenic organisms, viral, bacterial, or fungal [50].

Subclasses	Groups	Subgroups
Of the hair follicle	Infectious	Viral
		Bacterial
		Fungal
	Aseptic	
Of the sebaceous gland		
Of tubular glands	Apocrine	
	Eccrine	
Of the nail		
Of the cartilage		

Fig. 5.80 Evolutive inflammatory lesions of predominantly adnexal localization: Subclasses, Groups, and Subgroups

Folliculitis, Viral

Herpetic folliculitis of the bearded region is the most significant lesion in this subgroup. It is caused by herpesvirus infection, which produces damage similar in the follicular infundibulum and in the skin. This consists of a profound destruction of the epidermis, with acantholytic cells, globular and reticular degeneration, multinucleated giant cells, etc. (p. 77). The result of this process is the irreversible destruction of the follicle (Fig. 5.81, left).

Folliculitis, Bacterial

Folliculitis, the common "follicular pyoderma," is caused in most of the cases by *gram-positive* organisms.

Sycosis barbae is a variant of follicular pyoderma. This appears in the beard and neck regions as multiple pustules each centered by a hair featuring gross structures which in the past, for some reason, were compared to figs (*sycon* [G] a fig).

Folliculitis, acute superficial, or Bockhart's impetigo appears under the microscope as a superficial abscess filling the follicular infundibulum and covered by a crust.

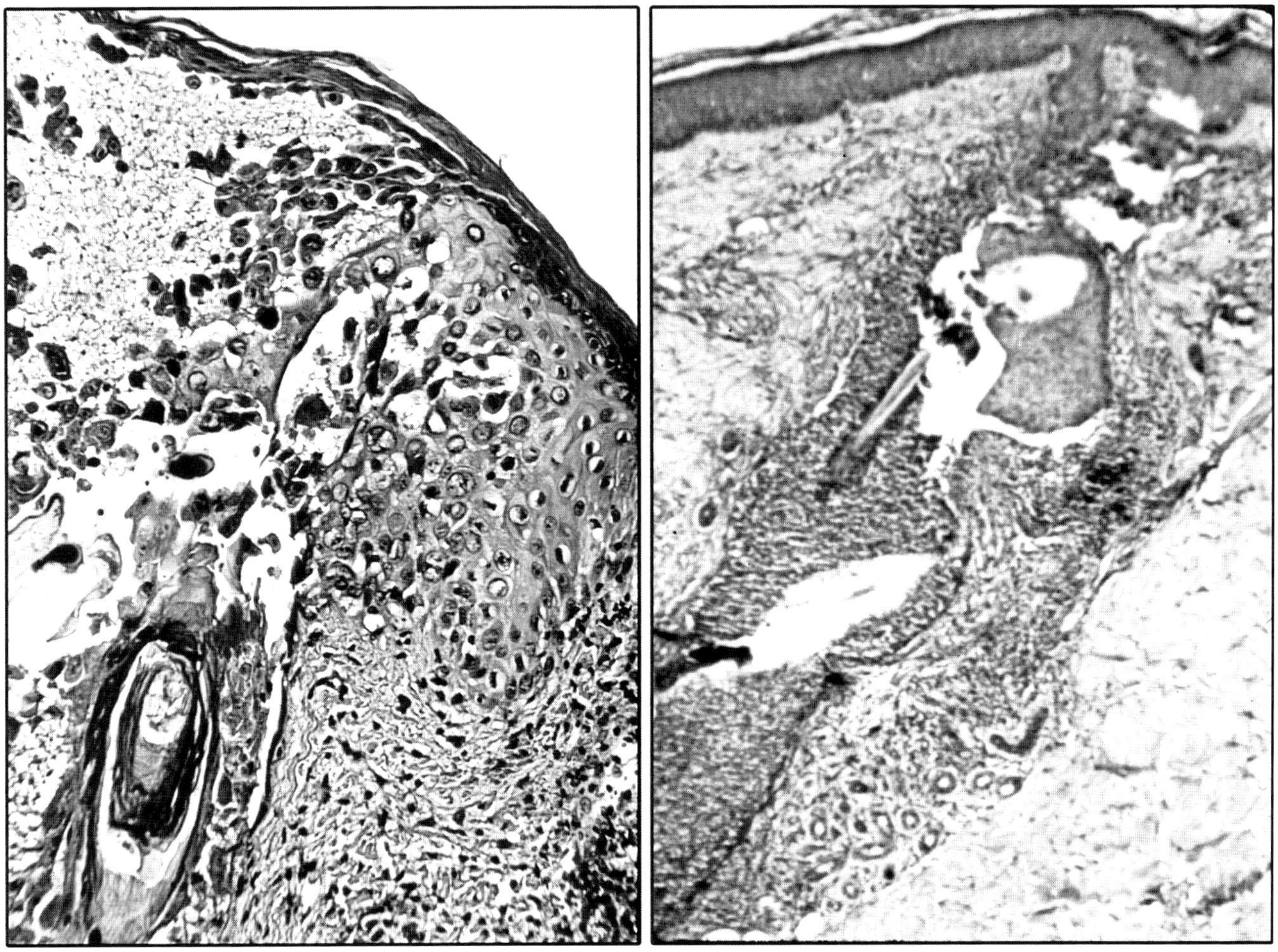

Fig. 5.81 Herpetic folliculitis of the bearded region and furuncle. In the first case (*left*), note heavy damage to the follicular region as described in the text. Observe in the second case (*right*) the presence of purulent material and a fragment of a hair shaft in a slanted infundibulum. H&E ×100; ×40 o m

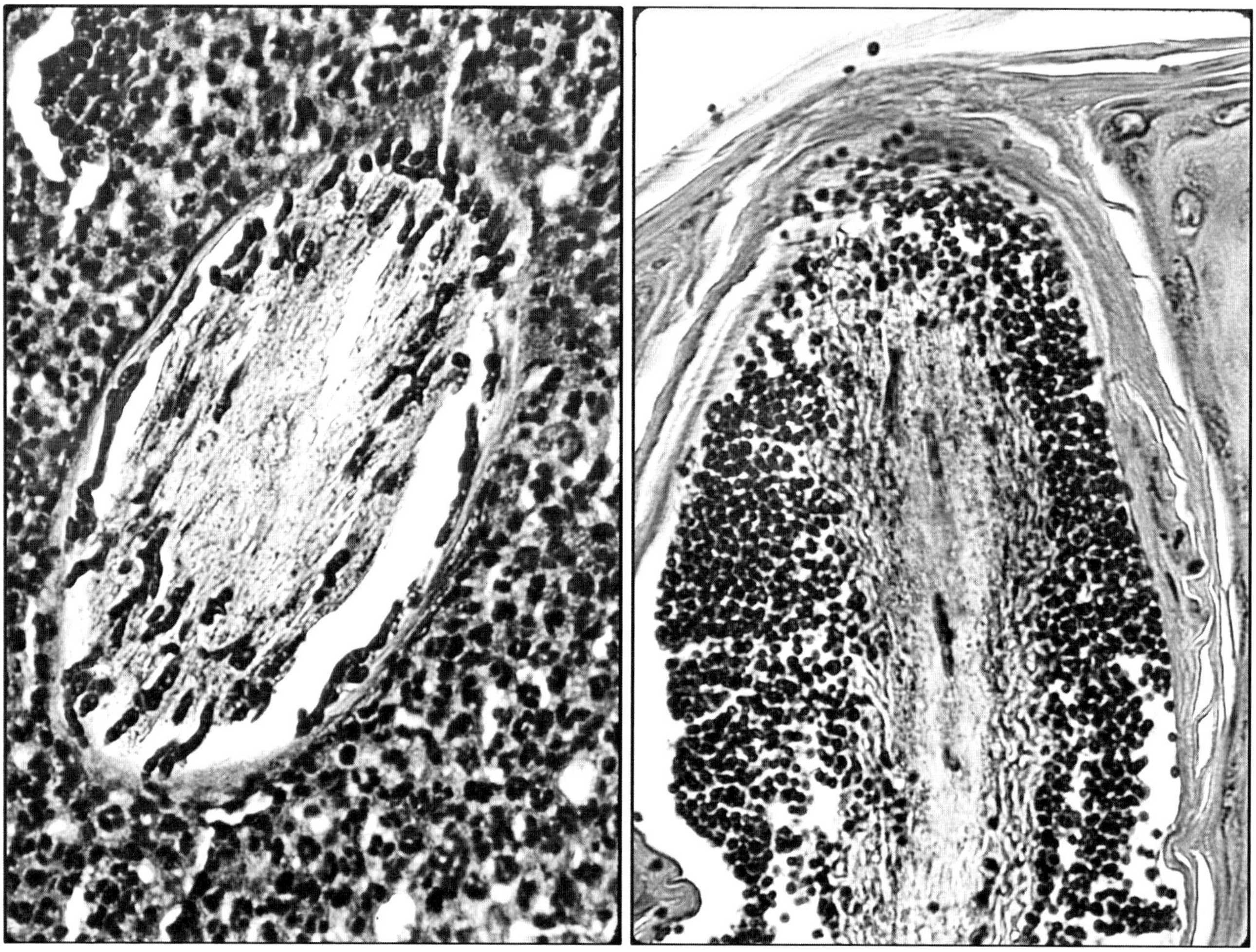

Fig. 5.82 Two infrequent invaders of the hair follicle. *T. violaceum* in a case of Majocchi's granuloma (*left*) and *A. niger* (*right*) an occasional finding in a folliculitis. PAS ×400

Folliculitis, acute deep, the common "furuncle," is a more severe form of folliculitis which appears under the microscope as an irreversibly damaged hair follicle surrounded by an area of purulent necrosis, often featuring a disconnected hair shaft in the center. (Fig. 5.81, right.) Carbuncle is the extreme form of this folliculitis. It is formed by a group of furuncles, with associated cellulitis and necrosis.

Folliculitis balneotermaria is an example of a gram-negative folliculitis caused by *P. aeruginosa*. This lesion is frequent in users of thermal baths where the prolonged contact with warm water favors skin maceration and infection by the *gram-negative* flora of that particular environment. Its microscopic examination fails to reveal significant differences with *gram-positive* folliculitis.

Folliculitis, Fungal

Dermatophytic folliculitis is caused in general by the same agents responsible for the epidermal fungal infections, which belong in their majority to the genera *Microsporum*, *Trichophyton*, and *Epidermophyton*. Nevertheless, less frequently occurring organisms may also be found on occasions (Fig. 5.82).

Although in general dermatophytes are not pyogenic, in some cases, they do produce pus, as in the cases of *kerion* and *favus*. Indeed, the root of both names *keri* [G] and *favus* [L] refers precisely to the same object, that is, a *honeycomb*, making an analogy to the honey (for pus) flowing from the lesions.

Kerion Celsi, associated with the Roman doctor of that name is caused by *M. canis*. This causes a marked purulent reaction on the scalp, where the lesion is located. It has an oozing quality and is often associated to subcutaneous abscesses (Fig. 5.83).

Favus is a lesion endemic in Middle East and the Mediterranean basin and is caused by the fungus *T. schoenleinii*. The lesion, a yellowish crust, is formed by purulent material derived from innumerable infected hair follicles below.

Majocchi's granuloma is a granulomatous and purulent folliculitis generally due to infections by *T. rubrum* or

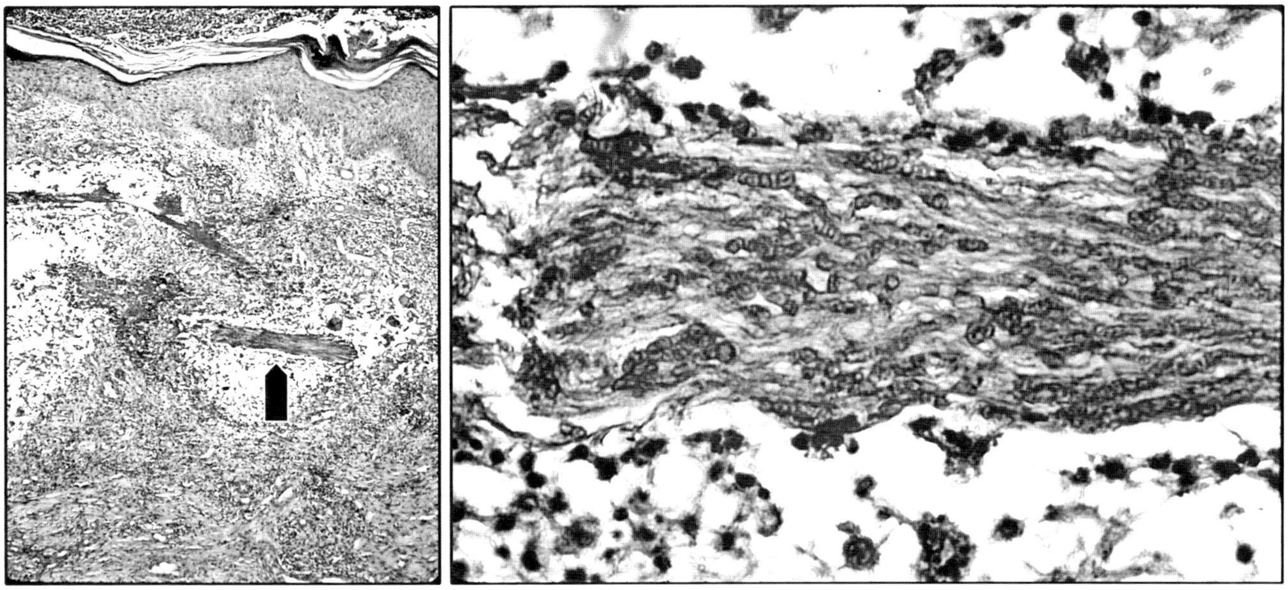

Fig. 5.83 Kerion. Note, at low magnification, the purulent quality of the lesion. It shows up in the center a fragment of hair shaft. Observe at high magnification the presence of hyphae adherent to the external surface of the hair shaft (*arrow*). H&E ×40; ×400 o m

T. violaceum and appearing on the legs of people who have the habit of shaving them. Microscopic examination of the affected area often reveals in the affected follicle the responsible agent wrapped around a hair shaft and surrounded by an intense inflammatory reaction (Fig. 5.82, left). The toxins generated by the infectious process may diffuse into the surrounding tissues and are able to generate acute inflammatory reactions.

Folliculitis, Aseptic

A variegated group of folliculitis exists in which microorganisms are not the etiologic agent. [51] The lesion originally known by the name of "perifolliculitis abscedens and suffodiens" may be more conveniently referred to by its English concise version "dissecting folliculitis." This lesion is a component of the triad of occluded adnexae [52], whose two other members are *acne conglobata* and *hidrosadenitis suppurativa*. These lesions are not due primarily to the aggression of any living organism but rather to the occlusion of the outlet of the adnex involved, caused by a selective hyperkeratosis. This leads to the accumulation of detritus in the occluded follicle and to the formation of sterile abscesses. In the particular case of dissecting folliculitis, confluent follicular abscesses spreading beneath the hairy skin through the subcutaneous tissue may lead to the separation of the scalp from the bone, to which the word "*dissecting*" actually refers (Fig. 5.84).

Among purulent aseptic folliculitis may be included those belonging to cases due to the ingestion of halogens, such as bromoderma and ioderma [53], which are clinically manifested as acneiform eruptions, in cases of intolerance to these elements.

Sebaceous Gland Inflammatory Lesions

Sebaceous gland changes are incidentally involved in the inflammatory changes of the pilosebaceous complex, but there are some conditions under which the sebaceous gland is specifically affected. One of them is chalazion [54] (*chalazion* [G] a pebble). This is a granulomatous inflammation of the sebaceous gland of the eyelid, the Meibomian gland. The most important differential diagnosis in this case is sebaceous gland carcinoma which may be masked by the inflammatory reaction in that area.

Inflammatory Lesions of the Tubular Glands

The term "hordeolum" or "sty" [55] covers indistinctly inflammatory conditions of both tubular glands in the eyelid. Otherwise, the occlusion of the outlet of the tubular glands may be separately considered (Fig. 5.80).

Inflammatory Conditions of the Apocrine Glands

The occlusion of the outlet of the apocrine gland is manifested in the region where these are located, mainly the axilla, nipple, and anogenital region. These appear as tiny cutaneous nodules, a condition called "miliaria" (*milium* [L] millet). Since this term was originally applied to a condition of the *eccrine* gland (see below), in the present case, the lesion is called "apocrine miliaria" in order to distinguish it from the former. Fox-Fordyce's disease is a disseminated apocrine miliaria.

Hidradenitis suppurativa, another member of the beforementioned adnexal occlusion triad is associated to the

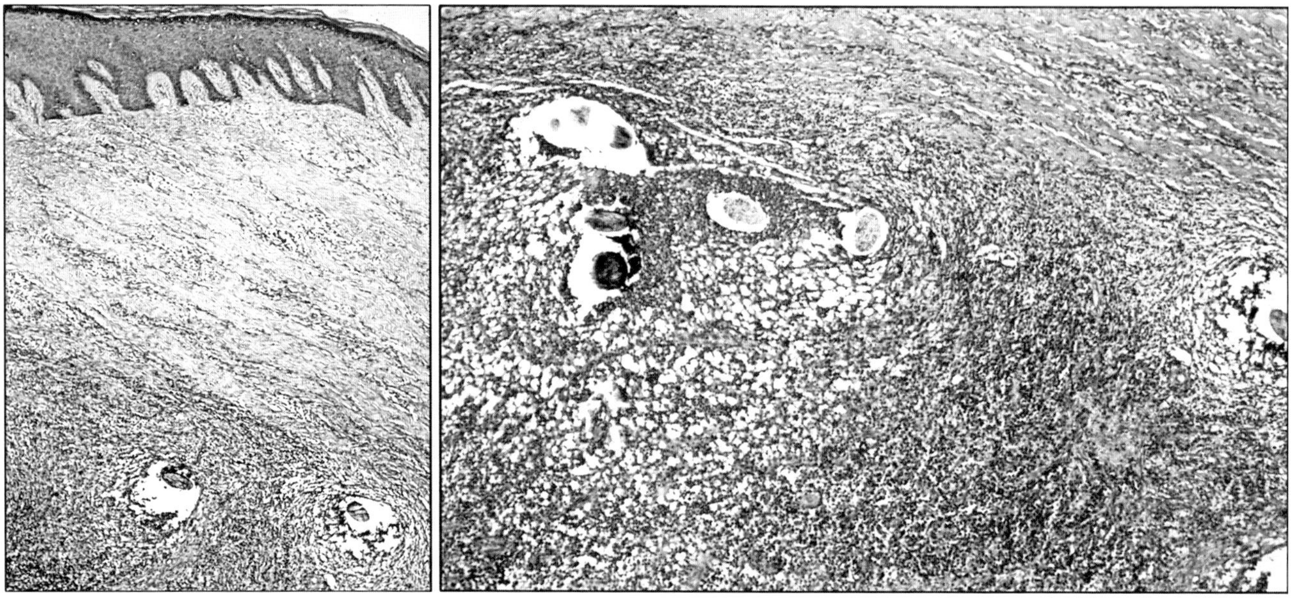

Fig. 5.84 Dissecting folliculitis. (*Left*) Note the area of diffuse inflammatory infiltration below the epidermis, as well as remnants of hair follicles in the lower part of the figure. (*Right*) The lesion is shown at higher magnification. H&E ×40; ×100 o m

occlusion of the apocrine gland. This process appears predominantly in women, in the axilla and anogenital region. Abscess formation frequently occurs and is associated to extensive cellulitis, often with a superimposed septic component, resulting ultimately in the destruction of the glandular elements.

Inflammatory Conditions of the Eccrine Glands

Among these lesions, two types are recognized. One, miliaria crystalina or sudamina, occurs as dew-like drops on the skin of babies shortly after birth: they are due, presumably, to an excess of sweat which causes dilatation of the sweat gland excretory duct. The other, miliaria rubra, occurs in adults and are associated to heat and intense muscular exercise. Contrary to the former type, the lesions in miliaria rubra occur as reddish patches, which regress shortly after relief of the conditions producing the stress. A retention cyst pertaining to a case of miliaria rubra is illustrated in Fig. 5.85.

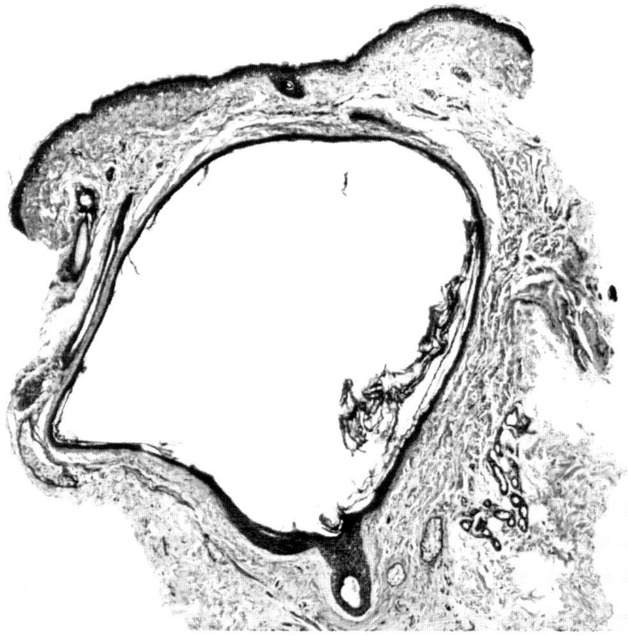

Fig. 5.85 Retention cyst originated in an eccrine gland. The lesion does not contain keratin scales but is filled with inspissated sweat. Note the end of the eccrine duct at the bottom of the cyst. H&E ×40, o m

Inflammatory Conditions of the Nail

The anatomy of the nail has been previously reviewed, and the reader is referred to that section for the present discussion (p. 17, Fig. 1.19). Although the nail and periungual tissue (p. 17) may be affected, as follicles are, by viral, bacterial, and fungal agents, the present discussion shall be limited to infections by the latter agents. The discussion will be focused on the dermatophytic infections, such as the ones caused by *T. rubrum* and *T. mentagrophyte*. These infections are designated as "onychomycosis" or "tinea unguium." The speciation of these organisms is carried via cultures. If they turned positive the general term "tinea unguium" may be replaced by the name of the infectious organism.

Dermatophytes are found on ungual folds and periungual tissue. These are also found between the grooves of the nail bed and the longitudinal ridges of the nail. They are passively dragged to that position by the nail plate in its distal progression from the nail matrix. The nail matrix is indeed, the most favorable environment for dermatophyte proliferation. Whereas these organisms may be relatively easily removed from their external location, it is very difficult to eradicate them from the nail matrix, requiring for this purpose the avulsion of the nail plate, the administration of systemic antifungal agents, or the combined use of both measures.

Cartilaginous Inflammatory Conditions

This section refers specifically to the process affecting the ear rim and the underlying cartilage. The before-mentioned pathogenic combination of cold and external trauma – not necessarily heavy but sustained (p. 104) – affects the very thin skin, from which the nutrition of the underlying tip of the cartilage depends. Therefore, damage on the skin is reflected in the latter, which undergoes localized ischemic necrosis. This process, called "chondrodermatitis nodularis helicis," requires the presence of necrotic cartilage for its microscopic diagnosis (Fig. 5.86). Otherwise, only a suspicion of this condition can be expressed, and this, solely after having ruled out the presence of a squamous cell carcinoma. The latter is the most important differential diagnosis in this case.

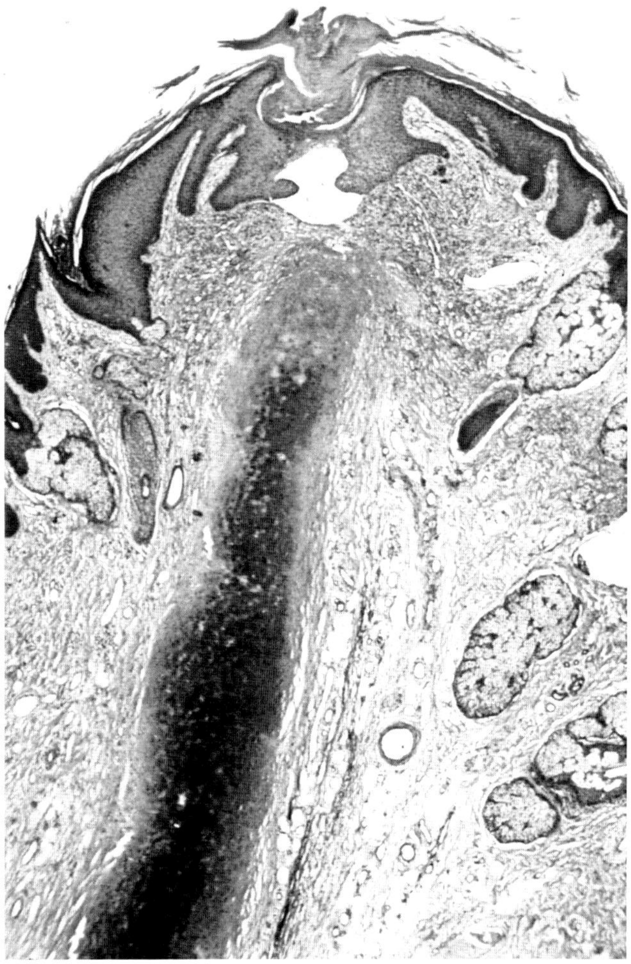

Fig. 5.86 Chondrodermatitis nodularis helicis. Cross section of the ear helix showing the ulcerated skin and the cartilage underneath. Note the inflammatory reaction around the tip of the cartilage which shows necrotic changes. H&E ×40

Postevolutive Inflammatory Lesions

The alterations suffered during inflammatory processes deeply alter the architecture of the skin, erasing the hallmarks on which the classification of the acute inflammatory lesions was based. Therefore, a simplified system of three Classes of post-inflammatory lesions was devised, separating them into dystrophic lesions, atrophic lesions, and scars based on the *anatomic alterations*, the *loss of function*, and the *scarring* the various cutaneous parts presented after the acute inflammatory process subsides.

Table 5.12 Scarring alopecias

Trauma
Burns
Discoid lupus erythematosus
Lichen planopilaris
Morphea "*coup de sabre*"

Dystrophic Lesions

The term "dystrophy" applies particularly to the pilosebaceous and ungual complexes. These feature, after the acute inflammatory phase, a distorted although still recognizable structure, but they are only able to deliver their products – hair and nail – of a defective quality.

Scarring alopecia is the most appropriated example of dystrophic lesion to be mentioned. As already stated, alopecias may be distinguished as either "scarring" or "nonscarring." The first ones, pertinent to this section, are to be discussed in continuation; the study of the second shall be postponed to the next chapter.

Scarring Alopecias

Scarring alopecias to the contrary of nonscarring ones – which may eventually regress – are *irreversible*. Table 5.12 presents several agents involved in the production of scarring alopecias.

The two first-mentioned agents are of a violent physical nature, leading to a sudden change in the affected skin. The three following agents (Fig. 5.87) are associated to disorders in which the alopecia sets progressively along inflammatory processes. Among scarring alopecias, morphea alopecia is included because if its pathogenesis is actually not inflammatory, this condition causes an irreversible alopecia, in the area of the scalp it affects (p. 180).

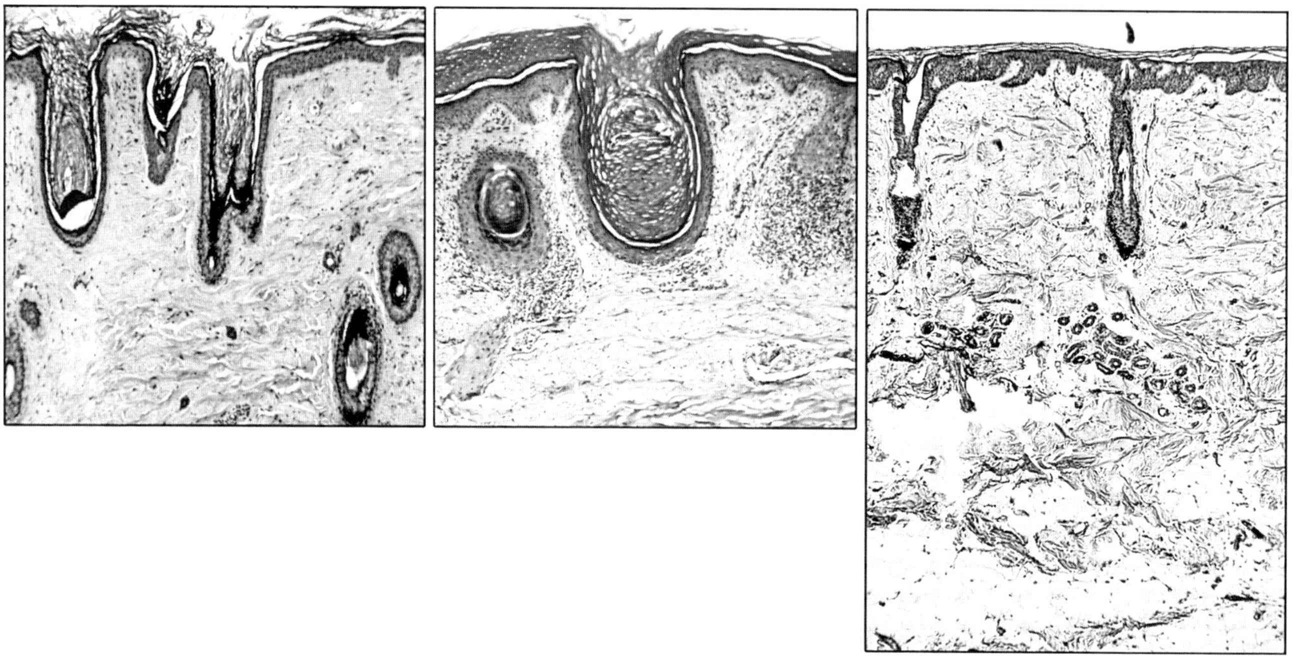

Fig. 5.87 Scarring alopecia. Note in the three cases presented, discoid lupus erythematous (*left*), lichen planopilaris (*center*), and morphea (*right*), a similar, profuse scarring and the presence of atrophic hair follicles. H&E ×40 o m

Atrophic Lesions

Because of its accomplished atrophic features, senile atrophic skin is to be mentioned as the first condition in this Class, even if it does not actually represent a post-inflammatory condition but rather the result of a normal wear. The epidermis appears thinned and frequently scaly, lying flat on the dermis because of the absence of its normal ridges. The lack of a functional dermoepidermal barrier allows the migration of melanin granules into the dermis, where they are often engulfed in macrophages. This feature is called **secondary incontinentia pigmenti**, in order to differentiate it from the previously mentioned *primary incontinentia pigmenti*. In the post-inflammatory conditions of the skin, the presence of scattered chronic inflammatory elements may provide a clue, allowing the differentiation of a post-inflammatory from a plain senile atrophy.

Poikiloderma atrophicans vasculare may be the result of a previous inflammatory process. It leaves a flat epidermis with mild liquefaction degeneration of the dermoepidermal junction and a dash of mononuclear elements with dilated vascular elements in the superficial dermis with secondary incontinentia pigmenti. A similar microscopic picture, however, may represent, alternatively, the initial form of a cutaneous lymphoproliferative process.

Scars

The reparative process subsequent to an aggression of the skin is followed by a mesenchymal reparative response. This is usually a self-limited process, which, after collagen deposition and vascular neoformation, ends up with a dense mass of collagenous tissue overlaid by a thinned epidermis. This is called a "scar." If the scarring process continues beyond the reparative scope but with an autolimited end, the resulting lesion is referred to as a hypertrophic scar. It is very important not to mistake a hypertrophic scar for a keloid. Keloid, a condition delivered from a faulty controlled collagen synthesis (p. 179), contrary to a hypertrophic scar, is not autolimited, but grows indefinitely, reaching considerable volume (p. 180).

A lesion closely related to a hypertrophic scar can occasionally occur following an exaggerated mesenchymal proliferation after an inflammatory process in the subcutaneous tissue. This process ends up as a bulky mass which masks the underlying atrophy of the adipose tissue, reason for which it is called "proliferating atrophy" or "Wucheratrophie" in the German language.

Special forms of scars worth mentioning are Morton neuroma and amputation neuroma. Contrary to what their names indicate, these *are not* neoplastic lesions but rather *reactive fibroproliferations* akin to scars. Morton neuroma develops in the foot, characteristically between the first and second metatarsal bones, while amputation neuroma grows around a nerve in an amputation stump. Amputation neuroma is characteristically a painful lesion and is also included in the acronym SLANG, which groups five painful tumors of the skin.

For the sake of completion of this section, "comedo tunnel" may be finally mentioned. This lesion consists of a fistulous epithelized tracts connecting affected hair follicles in acne cases (Fig. 5.88).

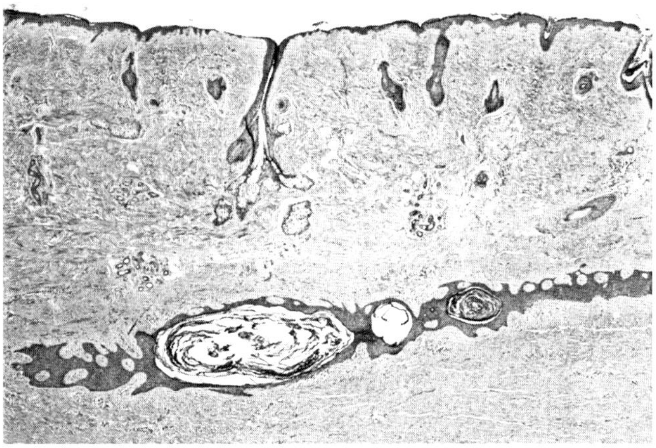

Fig. 5.88 Comedo tunnel in scarred skin. H&E ×40 o m

Table 5.13 Transitional inflammatory lesions

Histiocytic
Rosai-Dorfman disease
Histiocytic cytophagic panniculitis
Malignant histiocytosis
Of Langerhans cells
Langerhans cell histiocytosis
Hand-Schuller-Christian disease
Of T cells
Lymphomatoid papulosis
Lymphomatoid granulomatosis
Midline facial granuloma

Transitional Inflammatory Lesions

Among post-inflammatory lesions, there are a few which do not totally fit into the category of "postevolutive," since after the postevolutive phase, they may undergo a reactivation. Since the quality of these lesions has still not been totally clarified, it is convenient to provisionally regard them as "transitional." According to their nature, these lesions may be grouped as histiocytic, of Langerhans or of T cells (Table 5.13).

Histiocytic Lesions

The group of the histiocytic lesions has been reduced after various of its members were recognized as Langerhans cell proliferations or as cutaneous T_{cell} lymphomas. On the other hand, upon recognition of its histiocytic nature, Rosai-Dorfman disease was incorporated in this group.

Langerhans Cell Lesions

The recognition of the histiocytic nature of the lesions which used to be known by the mysterious name "histiocytoses X," allowed the replacement of this name with the straightforward label of "Langerhans cell histiocytosis." Hand-Schuller-Christian disease and eosinophilic granuloma were also recognized as being of Langerhans progeny, although their actual nosologic character has still not been settled.

T Cell Lesions

In the third group of Table 5.13, there are three conditions whose outcome into malignancy may be eventually contemplated: lymphomatous papulosis or Macaulay disease, lymphomatoid granulomatosis, and midline facial granuloma.

References

1. Schwarz T. In: Bolognia JL, Jorizzo JL, Rapini RP, et al., editors. Dermatology. Edinburgh: Mosby; 2004. p. 65–79.
2. Roitt J, Brostoff J, Male D. Immunology. St. Louis: C.V. Mosby Company; 1985. p. 19.1–19.17.
3. Martin AG, Kobayashi GH. In: Freedberg IM, et al., editors. Fitzpatrik dermatologia en medicina general, 5th ed. Buenos Aires: Editorial Medica Panamericana; 2001. p. 2477.
4. Braun-Falco O, Plewig G, Wolff HH, Burgdorf WHC. Dermatology. 2nd ed. Berlin: Springer; 2000. p. 613.
5. Mehregan AH, Hashimoto K, editors. Pinkus' guide to dermatohistopathology. 5th ed. Norwalk: Appleton & Lange; 1991. p. 194–7.
6. Roberts KB. In: Florey HW, editors. General pathology, 4th ed. Philadelphia: W.B. Saunders Co.; 1970. p. 370–5.
7. Lever WF, Schaumburg-Lever G. Histopathology of the skin. 7th ed. Philadelphia: J.B. Lippincott Company; 1990. p. 104–5.
8. Dorland's illustrated medical dictionary, 28th ed. Philadelphia: WH Saunders; 1994. p. 816.
9. Mehregan AH, Hashimoto K, editors. Pinkus' guide to dermatohistopathology. 5th ed. Norwalk: Appleton & Lange; 1991. p. 187–8.
10. Mehregan AH, Hashimoto K, editors. Pinkus' guide to dermatohistopathology. 5th ed. Norwalk: Appleton & Lange; 1991. p. 241–6.
11. Lever WF, Schaumburg-Lever G. Histopathology of the skin. 7th ed. Philadelphia: J.B. Lipppincott Company; 1990. p. 319–20.
12. James WD, Berger TG, Elston MD, editors. Andrews' diseases of the skin. 10th ed. Pennsylvania: W.B. Saunders; 2000. p. 143–4.
13. Braun-Falco O, Plewig G, Wolff HH, Burgdorf WHC. Dermatology. 2nd ed. Berlin: Springer; 2000. p. 579–82.
14. Lever WF, Schaumburg-Lever G. Histopathology of the skin. 7th ed. Philadelphia: J.B. Lippincott Company; 1990. p. 320.
15. Mehregan AH, Hashimoto K, editors. Pinkus' guide to dermatohistopathology. 5th ed. Norwalk: Appleton & Lange; 1991. p. 194.
16. Mehregan AH, Hashimoto K, editors. Pinkus' guide to dermatohistopathology. 5th ed. Norwalk: Appleton & Lange; 1991. p. 290.
17. Mehregan AH, Hashimoto K, editors. Pinkus' guide to dermatohistopathology. 5th ed. Norwalk: Appleton & Lange; 1991. p. 115.
18. Lever WF, Schaumburg-Lever G. Histopathology of the skin. 7th ed. Philadelphia: J.B. Lipppincott Company; 1990. p. 158.
19. Lever WF, Schaumburg-Lever G. Histopathology of the skin. 7th ed. Philadelphia: J.B. Lippincott Company; 1990. p. 400.
20. James WD, Berger TG, Elston MD, editors. Andrews' diseases of the skin. 10th ed. Pennsylvania: W.B. Saunders; 2000. p. 379.
21. James WD, Berger TG, Elston MD, editors. Andrews' diseases of the skin. 10th ed. Pennsylvania: W.B. Saunders; 2000. p. 478.
22. Braun-Falco O, Plewig G, Wolff HH, Burgdorf WHC. Dermatology. 2nd ed. Berlin: Springer; 2000. p. 663–75.

23. Mehregan AH, Hashimoto K, editors. Pinkus' guide to dermatohistopathology. 5th ed. Norwalk: Appleton & Lange; 1991. p. 159.
24. Braun-Falco O, Plewig G, Wolff HH, Burgdorf WHC. Dermatology. 2nd ed. Berlin: Springer; 2000. p. 670–2.
25. Beutner EH, Chorzelski TP, Bean SB. Immunopathology of the skin. 2nd ed. New York: John Wiley & Sons; 1979. p. 183–224.
26. Lever WF, Schaumburg-Lever G. Histopathology of the skin. 7th ed. Philadelphia: J.B. Lippincott; 1990. p. 125–30.
27. Lever WF, Schaumburg-Lever G. Histopathology of the skin. 7th ed. Philadelphia: J.B. Lippincott; 1990. p. 131.
28. James WD, Berger TG, Elston MD, editors. Andrews' diseases of the skin. 10th ed. Pennsylvania: W.B. Saunders; 2000. p. 476–47.
29. Braun-Falco O, Plewig G, Wolff HH, Burgdorf WHC. Dermatology. 2nd ed. Berlin: Springer; 2000. p. 687–9.
30. Lever WF, Schaumburg-Lever G. Histopathology of the skin. 7th ed. Philadelphia: J.B. Lippincott; 1990. p. 79.
31. James WD, Berger TG, Elston MD, editors. Andrews' diseases of the skin. 10th ed. Pennsylvania: W.B. Saunders; 2000. p. 153–5.
32. Florey HW. In: Florey HW, editors. General pathology, 4th ed. Philadelphia: W.B. Saunders Co.; 1970. p. 370–5.
33. Cochrane CG. In: Cohen S, Ward PA, McCluskey RT, editors. Mechanisms of immunopathology. New York: Wiley; 1979. p. 29.
34. Bisno AL. In: Goldman L, Ausiello D, editors. Cecil textbook of medicine, 22nd ed. Philadelphia: Saunders; 2004. p. 1788.
35. Mehregan AH, Hashimoto K, editors. Pinkus' guide to dermatohistopathology. 5th ed. Norwalk: Appleton & Lange; 1991. p. 149.
36. Mehregan AH, Hashimoto K, editors. Pinkus' guide to dermatohistopathology. 5th ed. Norwalk: Appleton & Lange; 1991. p. 138.
37. Mehregan AH, Hashimoto K, editors. Pinkus' guide to dermatohistopathology. 5th ed. Norwalk: Appleton & Lange; 1991. p. 139.
38. James WD, Berger TG, Elston MD, editors. Andrews' diseases of the skin. 10th ed. Pennsylvania: W.B. Saunders; 2000. p. 688–90.
39. Lever WF, Schaumburg-Lever G. Histopathology of the skin. 7th ed. Philadelphia: J.B. Lippincott; 1990. p. 192–293.
40. Braverman IM. Skin signs of systemic diseases. 3rd ed. Philadelphia: W.B. Saunders Company; 1998. p. 373–81.
41. Braun-Falco O, Plewig G, Wolff HH, Burgdorf WHC. Dermatology. 2nd ed. Berlin: Springer; 2000. p. 221–9.
42. Hinshaw M, Longley BJ. In: Elder DH, et al., editors. Lever's histopathology of the skin, 9th ed. Philadelphia: Lippincott Williams Wilkins; 2005. p. 603–14.
43. Lever WF, Schaumburg-Lever G. Histopathology of the skin. 7th ed. Philadelphia: J.B. Lippincott; 1990. p. 387.
44. Lever WF, Schaumburg-Lever G. Histopathology of the skin. 7th ed. Philadelphia: J.B. Lippincott; 1990. p. 270–2.
45. Lever WF, Schaumburg-Lever G. Histopathology of the skin. 7th ed. Philadelphia: J.B. Lippincott; 1990. p. 201–92.
46. James WD, Berger TG, Elston MD, editors. Andrews' diseases of the skin. 10th ed. Pennsylvania: W.B. Saunders; 2000. p. 630.
47. Braun-Falco O, Plewig G, Wolff HH, Burgdorf WHC. Dermatology. 2nd ed. Berlin: Springer; 2000. p. 872–3.
48. James WD, Berger TG, Elston MD, editors. Andrews' diseases of the skin. 10th ed. Pennsylvania: W.B. Saunders; 2000. p. 487–9.
49. Braun-Falco O, Plewig G, Wolff HH, Burgdorf WHC. Dermatology. 2nd ed. Berlin: Springer; 2000. p. 227.
50. Braun-Falco O, Plewig G, Wolff HH, Burgdorf WHC. Dermatology. 2nd ed. Berlin: Springer; 2000. p. 142–54.
51. Braun-Falco O, Plewig G, Wolff HH, Burgdorf WHC. Dermatology. 2nd ed. Berlin: Springer; 2000. p. 147–54.
52. Lever WF, Schaumburg-Lever G. Histopathology of the skin. 7th ed. Philadelphia: J.B. Lippincott; 1990. p. 322.
53. Braun-Falco O, Plewig G, Wolff HH, Burgdorf WHC. Dermatology. 2nd ed. Berlin: Springer; 2000. p. 1971.
54. Braun-Falco O, Plewig G, Wolff HH, Burgdorf WHC. Dermatology. 2nd ed. Berlin: Springer; 2000. p. 156.
55. Braun-Falco O, Plewig G, Wolff HH, Burgdorf WHC. Dermatology. 2nd ed. Berlin: Springer; 2000. p. 155.

6 Proliferative Cutaneous Lesions

The integrants of the Division of proliferative cutaneous lesions may be distributed into two Subdivisions following their primary *reactive* or *neoplastic* nature (Fig. 6.1).

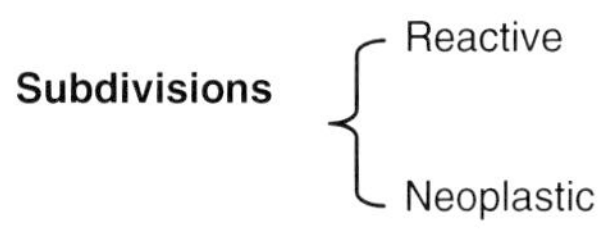

Fig. 6.1 Cutaneous proliferations

Reactive Cutaneous Proliferations

According to the tissues involved in the process, the reactive cutaneous proliferations may be classified as epidermal, dermoepidermal, adnexal, and mesenchymal (Fig. 6.2).

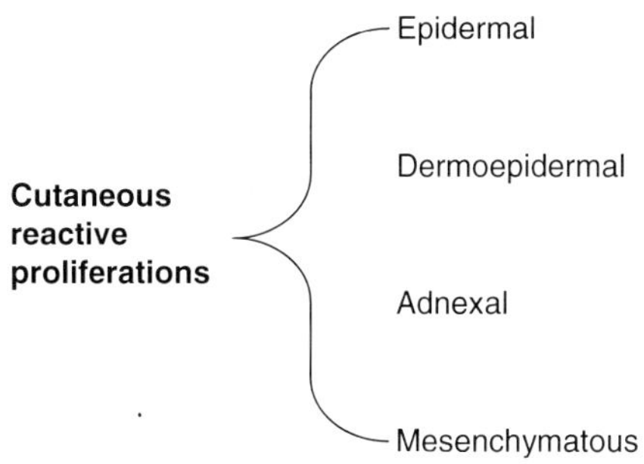

Fig. 6.2 Reactive cutaneous proliferations: classes

Reactive Epidermal Proliferations

The reactive epidermal proliferations are formed by keratinocytes which, in response to a determined stimulus, grow or spread over the skin surface although without trespassing the limits set by the BM. These lesions may be subclassified according to the origin of their proliferative stimulus as *exogenous* and *endogenous*.

Reactive Epidermal Proliferations: Exogenous

The most important example of an externally mediated epidermal reactive proliferation is solar or actinic keratosis (AK). The *reactive* character of this lesion is evidenced by the close relationship it keeps with its specific stimulus, that is, solar radiation. Indeed, AK consistently appears on areas of the body, particularly the scalp, face, and dorsum of the hands, most frequently exposed to sunlight. Females, whose lower limbs are usually less protected against actinic radiation than those in males, may present AK lesions on the anterior aspect of the lower legs. In both sexes, the inferior lip is also a frequent site of presentation for AK, being called in this case "actinic keilitis" (*cheil* + *itis* [G] lip + inflammation).

The dependency of AK on solar light is confirmed by the fact that, by protecting affected areas of the body, it is possible to stop its progression, or even cause it to regress.

When AK is examined under LM (Fig. 6.3), a band of moderate dysplasia is found, mainly restricted to the lower level of the epidermis. The keratinocytes of the germinal layer appear bulky and in disarray, featuring pyknotic nuclei, although no significant increase in mitotic activity. The stratum spinosum appears thinned and deteriorated, whereas the granular layer looks diminished, irregular, and covered by a thick layer of keratin and parakeratin scales.

The superficial expansion of AK may be limited by the barrier consisting of surrounding normal tissues: the repeated folding of the germinal layer, however, creates buds, whose surfaces offer additional room for the expansion of the lesion (Fig. 6.4, left). These buds, highly characteristic of the lesion of AK, are outlined by the BM, meaning that they are still *within* the epidermis. This does not exclude the possibility that upon malignant transformation these buds trespass the BM and actively invade the underlying tissues in the fashion of a squamous cell carcinoma (Fig. 6.4, right). This possibility shall be discussed below.

E. Zappi, E.A. Zappi, *Dermatopathology*,
DOI 10.1007/978-1-4471-2894-6_6, © Springer-Verlag London 2013

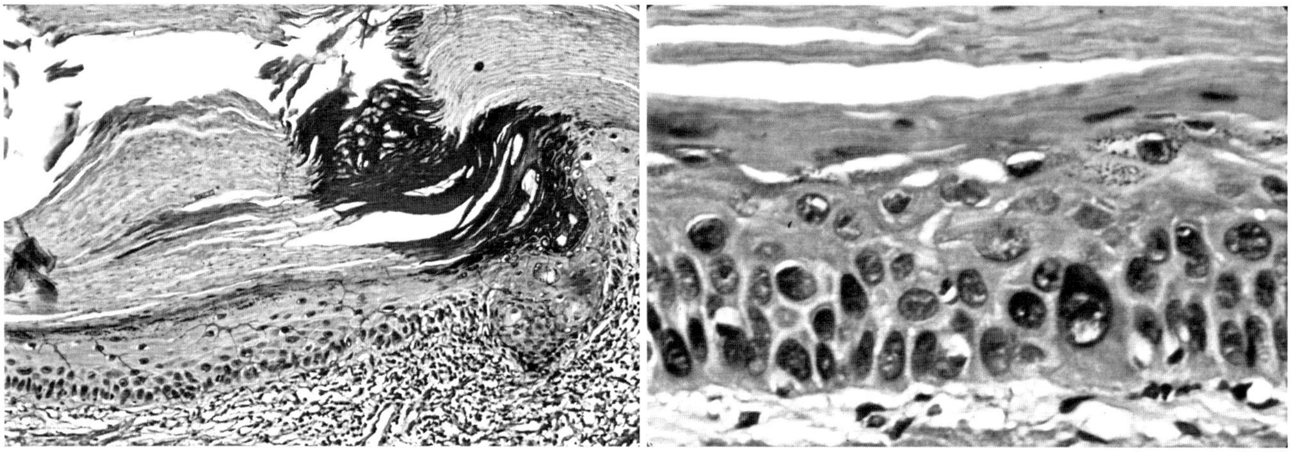

Fig. 6.3 Actinic keratosis. (*Left*) Lesion at low magnification. (*Right*) Detail of the germinal layer. See details in the text. H&E ×40; ×400, o m

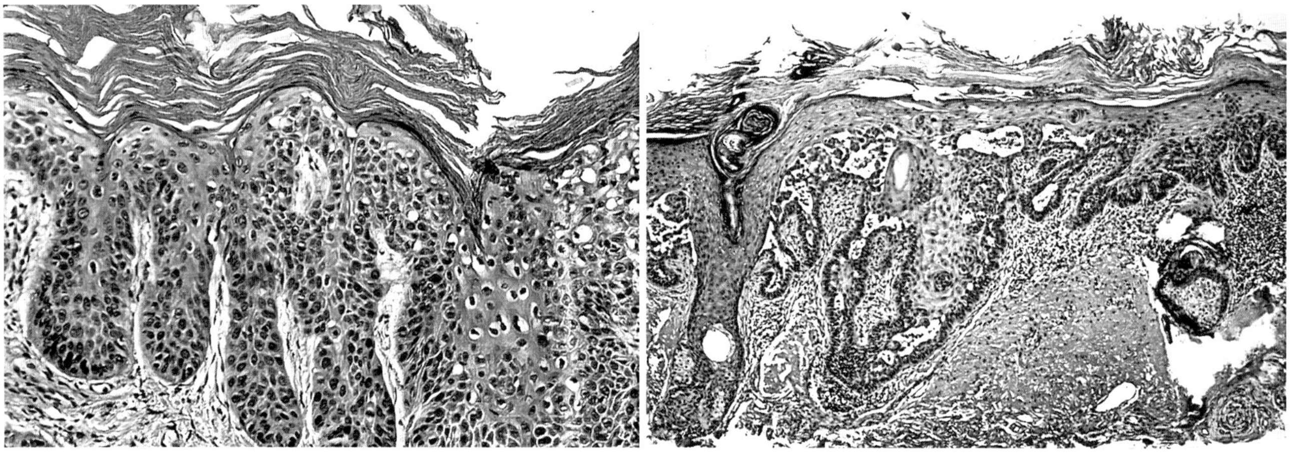

Fig. 6.4 Actinic keratosis. (*Left*) Buds of actinic keratosis dropping down from the epidermis but still contained by the BM. (*Right*) An invasive squamous cell carcinoma originated in these buds is freely invading the underlying dermis. H&E ×100; ×40, o m

Whereas under LM an eosinophylic hue predominates in the epidermis in H&E-stained sections of AK, the dermis of these lesions often shows a steel gray discoloration as a consequence of the degeneration of the elastic network, whose fibers are thickened and agglomerated into amorphous masses (Fig. 6.5).

The damage of the BM and the germinal layer may lead to the development of suprabasal acantholysis, configurating the so-called Darier's type of AK. Alternatively, the confluence of inflammatory round cells into a band-like infiltrate transforms the lesion into a "lichen planus type" of AK. (Fig. 6.6).

The *proliferative* character of AK is not as obvious as its *reactive* character. Indeed, although there are hypertrophic forms of AK which may even feature bulky cutaneous horns, AK usually appears in the atrophic form.

Cutaneous horn, incidentally, is a *clinical entity* whose name appropriately describes its external aspect, but not its histopathologic nature (Fig. 6.7). This latter aspect can only be determined through the microscopic examination of its base, in which several entities may be found. Among the most frequent, AK, verruca vulgaris, squamous cell carcinoma, and seborrheic keratosis should be mentioned. Accordingly, the correct diagnostic formulation of a cutaneous horn would be, for instance, "actinic keratosis (or any other condition) featuring a cutaneous horn."

The cutaneous adnexae are closely related to AK by two characteristic microscopic details: the first is the presence of inverted cones of normal epithelium around the outlets of their adnexae. This detail was brought to the general attention by H. Pinkus [1], who considered these repositories of healthy epithelium engaged in a constant "ebb and flow" process, with the dysplastic one, analogous to that noted between the dysplastic mucosal epithelium of the cervix uteri and normal epithelium emerging from the cervical glands [2] (Fig. 6.8, left and center). The second characteristic histologic detail of AK is the presence of basophilic cell columns surrounding excretory eccrine ducts, comparable in shape to chimneys, which traverse the entire thickness of the epidermis (Fig. 6.8, right).

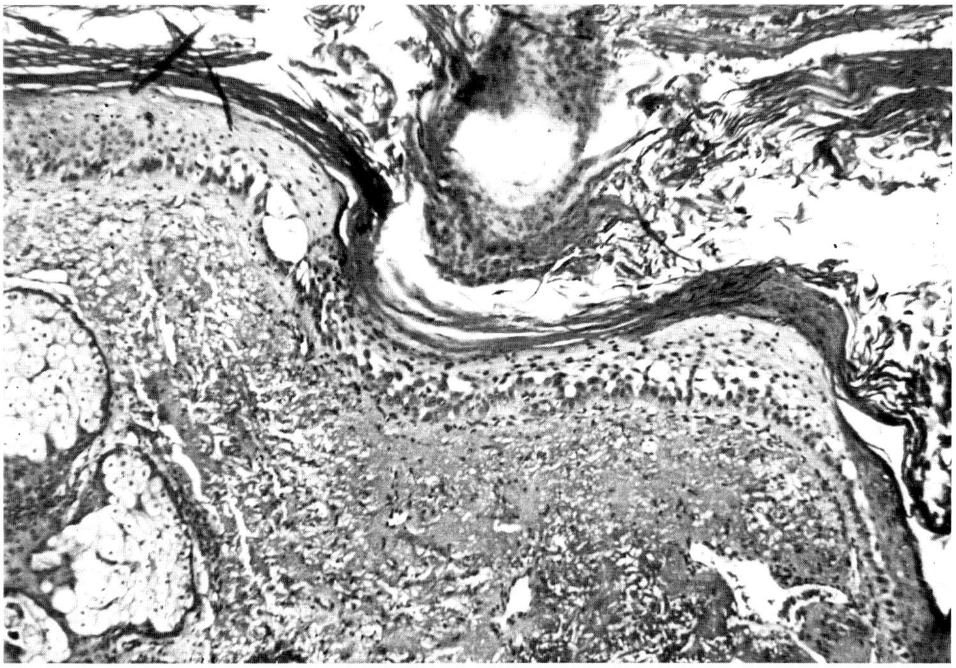

Fig. 6.5 Actinic keratosis. The dermis of the specimen has been transformed into an amorphous, basophilic mass as a consequence of the actinic degeneration of the elastic fibers. Note also the marked atrophy of the epidermis which appears covered by parakeratin scales and the hydropic degeneration of the basement membrane underneath. H&E ×100, o m

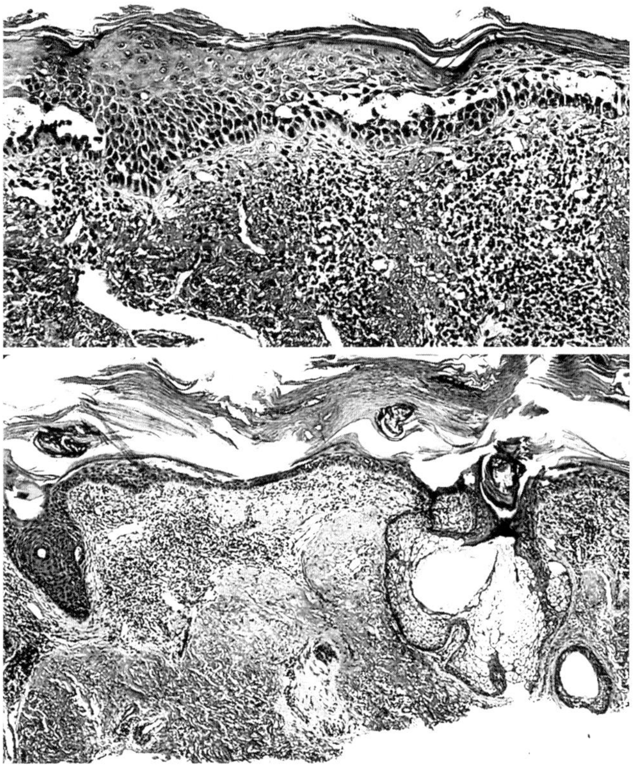

Fig. 6.6 Actinic keratosis "Darier's" and "lichen planus type." Note in the first picture (*top*) the suprabasal acantholysis with cleft formation, similar to the one in Darier's disease, and in the second picture (*bottom*), the band-like infiltrate comparable to the one seen in lichen planus. H&E ×40, o m

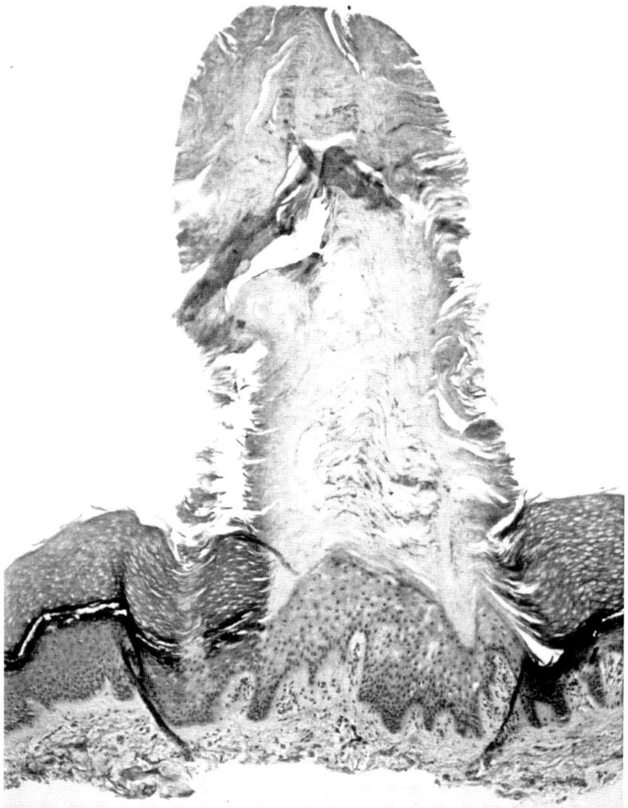

Fig. 6.7 Actinic keratosis featuring a cutaneous horn. Note the histologic changes corresponding to AK at the base of the lesion. H&E ×40, o m

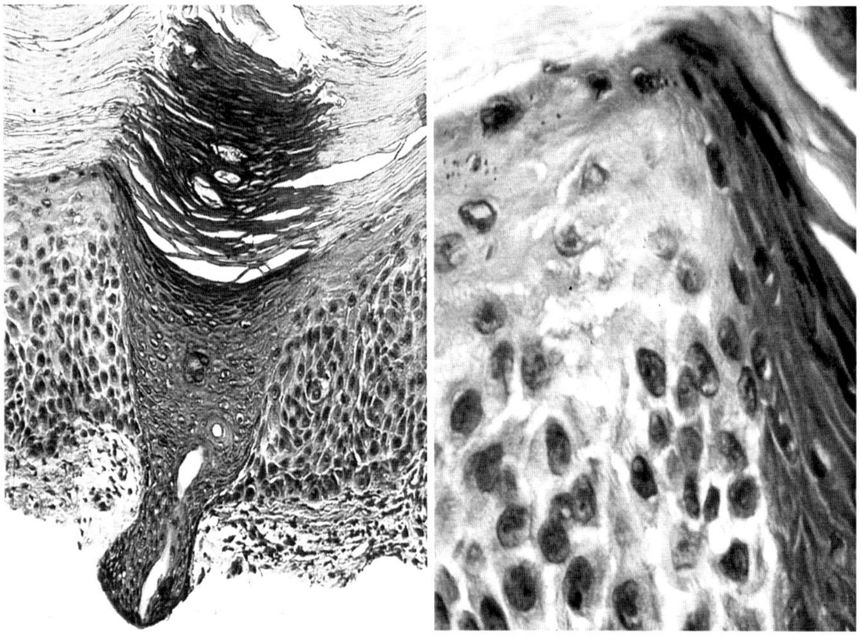

Fig. 6.8 Actinic keratosis. (*Left*) Inverted cone of normal cells surrounding an eccrine excretory duct. (*Center*) Transition of the normal epithelium into the dysplastic one. (*Right*) "Chimneys" of basophilic cells traversing the epidermis. H&E ×100; ×400; ×40, o m

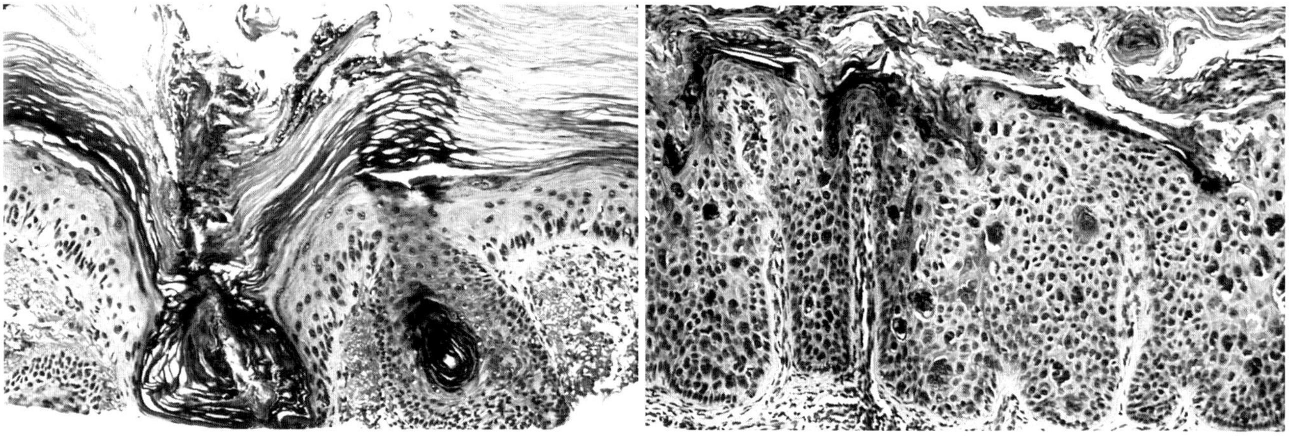

Fig. 6.9 Comparative microscopic study of AK and BD. In AK (*left*), the epidermis appears thinned, featuring moderate dysplasia at its lowermost level. In BD (*right*), the epidermis appears significantly thickened, with severe dysplastic changes involving the entire thickness. Note in BD the dysplastic keratinocytes with pyknotic nuclei. The absence of adnexae is characteristic of the lesion and contrasts with AK, in which adnexae are present. H&E ×40, o m

The taxonomic position that AK occupies in this classification among the *reactive* proliferations helps to distinguish it from Bowen disease, with which it is frequently mistaken. Bowen disease (BD), even though **in situ**, is a true *neoplastic* proliferation, as explained below (p. 130).

The histopathologic differences between AK and BD are apparent as a result of their comparative microscopic study (Fig. 6.9).

These differences are summarily listed in Table 6.1.

An important clinical point to remember in the differential diagnosis between AK and BD is *the site* from which the lesion has been removed. Since AK is restricted in its incidence to sun-exposed areas, the diagnosis of a lesion removed from a sun-protected area would be tilted toward BD, since this condition may appear both on sun-exposed and sun-protected areas.

In the diagnostic workout of AK, actinic reticuloid may be introduced as a differential possibility. This consideration may be easily dismissed, however, because in spite of the analogies insinuated by their names, actinic reticuloid is an entity totally different from AK. That first condition represents a poorly understood form of allergic cutaneous reaction against solar radiation but lacks any of the dysplastic features of AK.

Table 6.1 Comparison of the microscopic features of actinic keratosis and Bowen disease

Histopathologic feature	Actinic keratosis	Bowen disease
Predominant staining on H&E	Eosinophilic	Basophilic
Intercellular bridges	Present	Diminished
Parakeratin scales	Abundant	Scanty
"Chimneys"	Present	Absent
Cutaneous adnexae	Present	Absent
Epidermal buds	Present	Absent
Mitotic activity	Low	High
Atypic mitotic figures	Absent	Present
Epidermal dysplasia	Lower level	Massive
Degree of dysplasia	Low	High
Epidermal polarity	Preserved	Lost

Table 6.2 Agents of endogenous reactive epidermal hyperplasia

Halogenodermas
Acne keloidalis nuchae
Deep fungal infections
Lupus vulgaris
Osteomyelitis
Fibrohistiocytoma
Granular cell tumor

Minor, persistent, and localized mechanical traumas on the skin may lead to the production of masses of solid keratin which, if they are exophytic, carry the designation of "tyloma" (*tyloma* [G] a callosity), the common "callus," whereas if endophytic, they are designated as "clavus." Mild external irritation of mucosal surfaces, such as those produced by ill-adjusted protheses or by cigarette smoke, cause the normally nonkeratizing mucosal epithelium, to keratinize. The area where this occurs, characterized by a whitish appearance, is known as leucokeratosis.

The counterpart of leucokeratosis is "leucoplasia" (*leuco+plasia* [G] white+development). The latter is a mucosal lesion of external aspect similar to the previous one but which, upon microscopic examination, shows dysplastic changes, reason for which it is considered of premalignant nature.

Reactive Epidermal Proliferations: Endogenous

It may be speculated that agents such as those listed in Table 6.2 may in some way inhibit the regulatory activity that the BM exerts over the epidermis, and that when the latter enters a phase of uncontrolled proliferation, it can breach the epidermal boundary and invade the underlying tissues in the form of angulated cords of keratinocytes of marked likeness with a well-differentiated squamous cell carcinoma. This process is exemplified by pseudocarcinomatous or pseudoepitheliomatous hyperplasia (Fig. 6.10).

Reactive Dermoepidermal Proliferations

Contrary to what occurs in the previous Class, in which the proliferative activity is restricted to the epidermis, in the reactive dermoepidermal proliferations (RDEP), a synergistic growth of both layers is noted. This results in epidermal formations supported by a framework of mesenchymal tissue, reason for which they often protrude over the external level of the skin. The importance of viral agents in the pathogenesis of these lesions justifies the division of this class of lesions into two Subclasses: that in which the reactive proliferation is caused by viral infections and the other in which the lesions do not respond to these agents. Table 6.3 exposes a series of RDEP belonging to both subclasses.

Reactive Dermoepidermal Proliferations: Viral

The RDEP of viral origin develops soon after the time of infection by the responsible agents. These are in their great majority DNA viruses of the papova and parapox families.

The individualization of the papovaviruses accounting for viral papillomas, the "human papilloma viruses" (HPV), offers difficulties, first of all, because new strains of these organisms are continuously being reported and, second, because it is not infrequent to find several types of HPVs in a same lesion. For these reasons, discrepancies arise among different authors regarding the identity of the agents responsible for the pathogenesis of these lesions. Table 6.4 shows the essential concordance of five authors regarding the identity of the HPV strain responsible for four of the most common types of these lesions.

It must be emphasized that the production of any particular type of viral papilloma is strongly dependent on the keratinizing capacity of the epithelium on which that lesion is developing. Therefore, verruca vulgaris, regardless of by which HPV it is caused, is only found on strongly keratinizing epithelium, such as that of palms and soles, and by the opposite token, condyloma acuminatum and verruca plana, develop on mucosal surfaces, or on the weakly keratinizing surfaces of adults such as the face, or on infants, irrespective of their pathogenic agent.

Verruca vulgaris (VV) (Fig. 6.11, left), the most frequent of all the lesions caused by HPV, shows an exophytic and clearly circumscribed contour with a strongly keratinizing epidermis when observed under LM. This is located over a framework of thickened and elongated dermal papillae, evidently participating in the proliferative process.

Verruca palmoplantaris. This lesion features a papillomatous contour comparable to the one of VV. However, instead of presenting an exophytic disposition, the lesion appears in an endophytic setting, encased in the dermis and covered by a thick keratin layer. A somewhat simplistic explanation for this difference is offered in Fig. 6.11, right. It postulates that the light external pressure exerted by the environment on the external surface of the body allows the exophytic development

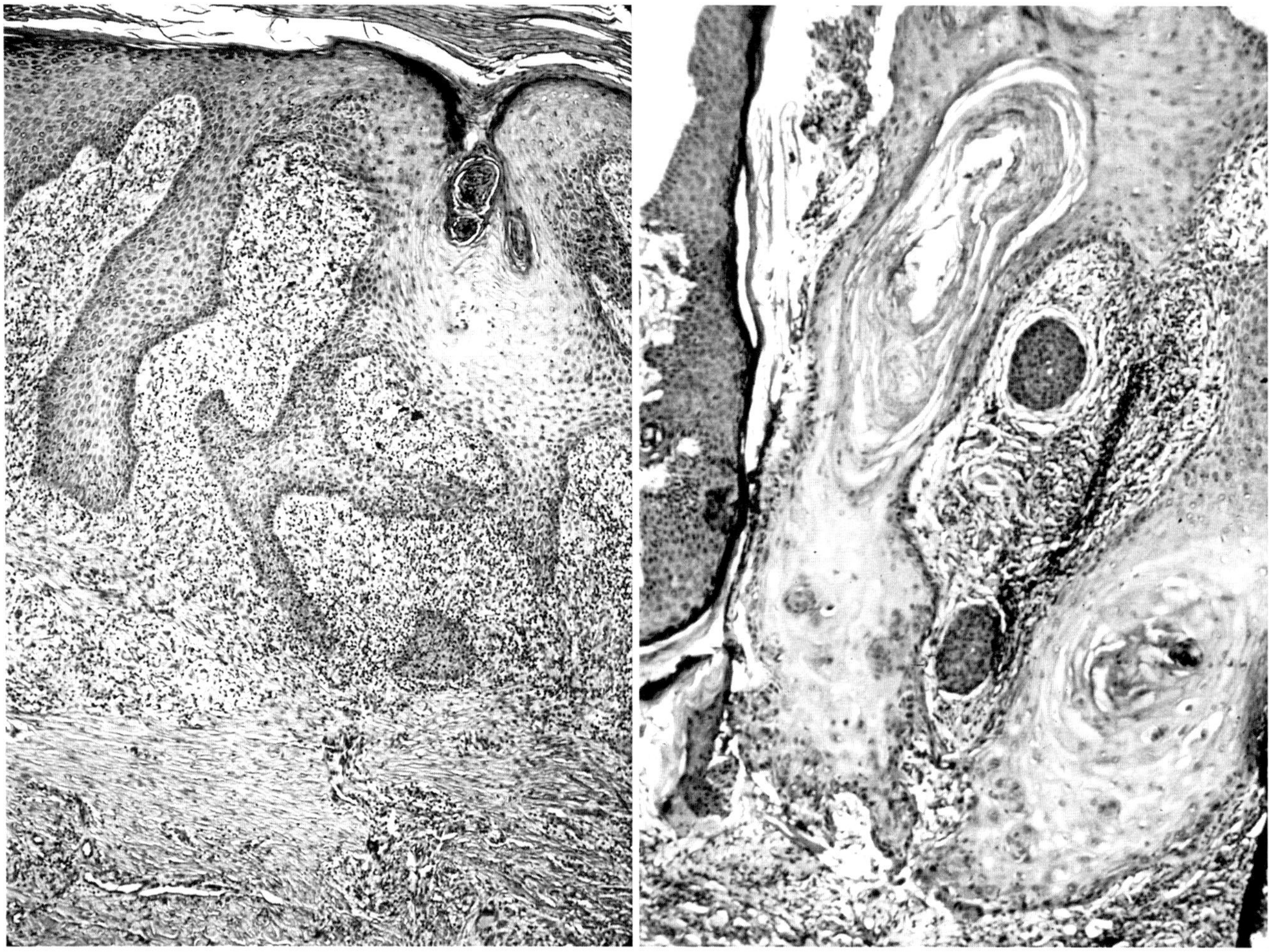

Fig. 6.10 Pseudocarcinomatous hyperplasia. The lesion corresponds to an acne keloidalis nuchae. (*Left*) Note the irregular cellular cords projected into the deep dermis. (*Right*) Examination at higher magnification fails to reveal keratin pearls, mitotic figures, or other elements of squamous cell carcinoma. H&E ×40; ×100, o m

Table 6.3 Reactive dermoepidermal proliferations: Subclasses

Viral
Verruca vulgaris
Condyloma acuminatum
Molluscum contagiosum
Milker's nodule
Keratoacanthoma
Nonviral
Picker's nodule
Nummular eczema
Fixed drug eruption
Lichen simplex chronicus
Acariosis

of VV (left), whereas the high external mechanic pressure sustained particularly on palms and soles forces verruca palmoplantaris to grow downward in these two areas.

One of the most prominent features of both lesions, but more evident in verruca palmoplantaris, is the tendency of the elongated dermal papillae to curve inside to almost meet at the center of the base (Fig. 6.12, left). At low magnification, the epidermis of the verruca presents a thick granular layer dotted by large empty cells, the koilocytes or "empty cells" (*koilo* + *cyto* [G] empty + cell). At higher magnification, these cells show punctiform nuclei surrounded by clear halos and solid, irregular masses of basophilic keratohyaline, both in intra- and extracellular positions (Fig. 6.12, right).

Table 6.4 Concordance of five authors [3–7] regarding the identity of the HPV involved in the pathogenesis of four papillomatous lesions

Lesion	Verruca vulgaris	Verruca plana	Verruca palmoplantaris	Condyloma acuminatum
Responsible HPV	1, 2	3, 10	1	6, 11

Contrary to VV, verruca plana presents an extended, spiky external surface with tiny papillomatous projections. The presence in the lesion of a granular layer studded with koilocytes stands as evidence for its relation with VV and is a necessary feature for positive LM diagnosis of the lesion (Fig. 6.13, left and right).

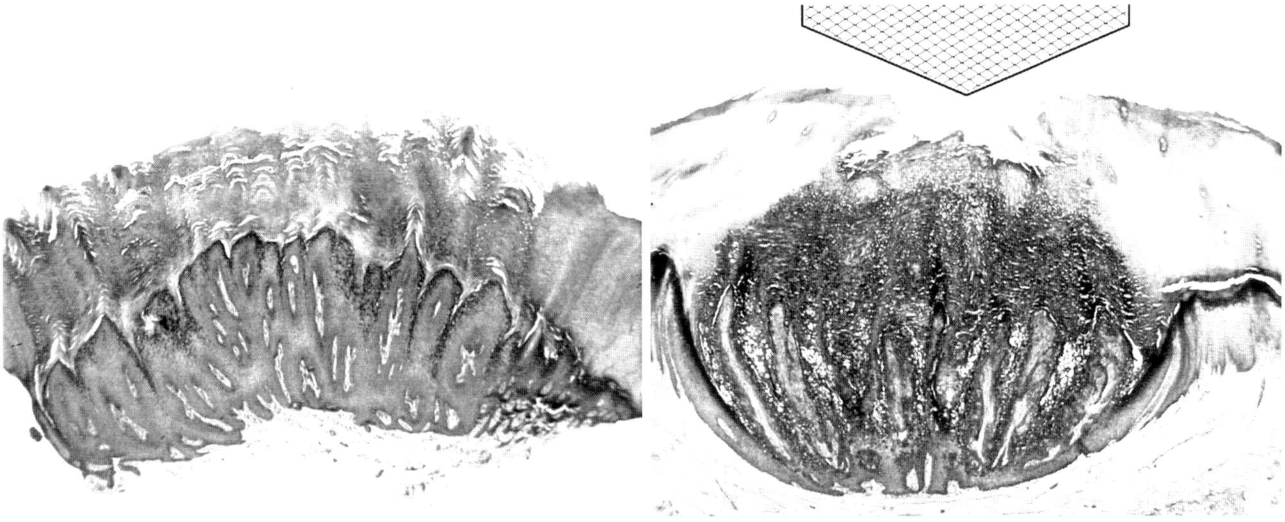

Fig. 6.11 Verruca vulgaris and verruca palmoplantaris. Verruca vulgaris. (*Left*) Note the exophytic and strongly keratinizing character of the lesion. Verruca palmoplantaris. (*Right*) Observe the endophytic character of the lesion, which has been displaced downward by the heavy external pressure sustained in palms and soles, symbolized by the cross hatched (*arrow*). H&E ×40, o m

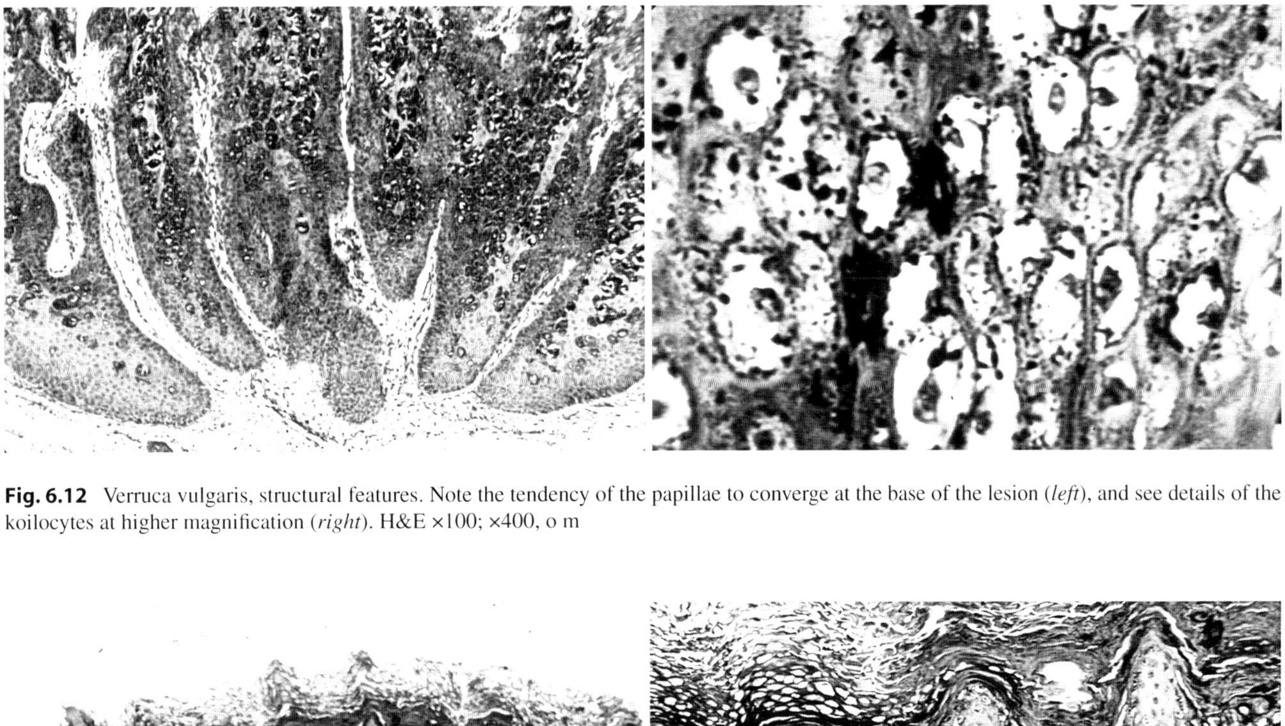

Fig. 6.12 Verruca vulgaris, structural features. Note the tendency of the papillae to converge at the base of the lesion (*left*), and see details of the koilocytes at higher magnification (*right*). H&E ×100; ×400, o m

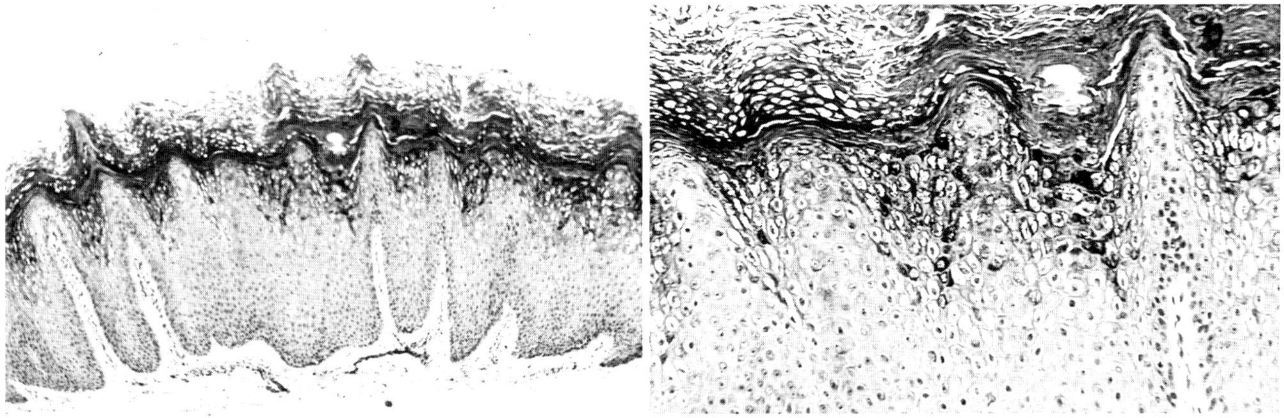

Fig. 6.13 Verruca plana. See details in the text. H&E ×40; ×100, o m

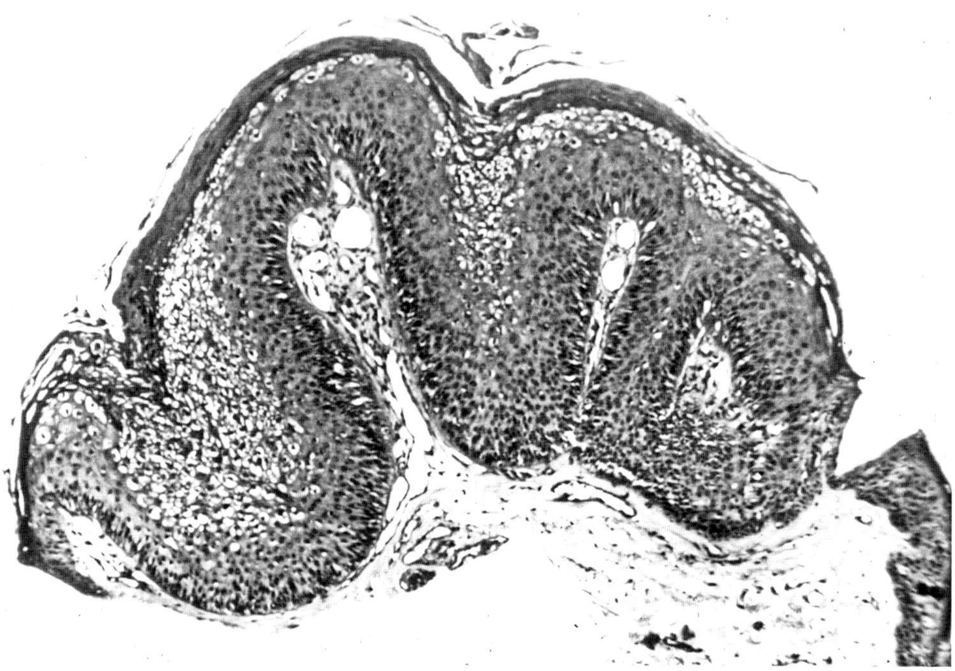

Fig. 6.14 Condyloma acuminatum. Note the exophytic profile of the lesion and the scant amounts of koilocytes located predominantly in its upper levels. H&E ×40, o m

Condyloma acuminatum (*condylus* + *acuminatus* [L] knuckle + pointed) is a lesion closely related to the just mentioned ones, although modified by the fact that it arises on mucosal epithelium. For this reason, the granular layer is very thin, and koilocytes are also very scant. Again, however, koilocytes are indispensable for positive LM diagnosis of "condyloma acuminatum" (Fig. 6.14).

Although classically, condyloma acuminatum is located on the genital mucosa, this lesion may also appear on the oral or other mucosal surfaces. Therefore, "genital wart," as these lesions are frequently referred to in general terms, induces confusion and should rather not be used.

Bowenoid papulosis of the genitalia is a lesion which appears on the genitalia in the form of pinhead-sized nodules. It receives its name from the histopathologic resemblance it bears to Bowen disease, a neoplastic condition. However, this designation imparts on bowenoid papulosis an undeserved suggestion of malignancy since this lesion tends to regress spontaneously [8]. For this reason, it is convenient to replace that frightening name with the term "viral keratosis" [9] which does not give it an unnecessary malignant connotation.

Epidermodysplasia verruciforme, in contrast to the previous lesion, is a complex entity. Besides HPV-5 and a few other HPVs which have been implicated in its pathogenesis, half of the cases of this condition appear to be inherited in an autosomal recessive fashion. Initially, the lesion resembles verruca plana both grossly and microscopically. However, as it evolves, this condition differs significantly from the latter by the persistent nature of its papules. It also differs from verruca plana in that it shows a tendency to grow and to undergo malignant degeneration, capable of ending up as squamous cell carcinomas, either in situ or invasive [10].

Molluscum contagiosum is the most common example of a parapox virus-related RDEH. Its lesions appear as solitary or multiple, raised, and umbilicated nodules from which a cheesy material may be extruded. Low-power examination of its meridian section reveals a sharply delimited basophilic half-moon surrounding a core of soft and deeply altered keratinocytes. These are enlarged and enclose viral masses agglutinated into a basophilic matrix, "inclusion bodies of molluscum contagiosum" (Fig. 6.15).

Other RDEPs caused by the parapox virus are ecthyma contagiosa, also known by the dialectal term "orf" and "milker's nodule" contracted upon handling infected sheep or cows, respectively. These two lesions present an autolimited, although complex vital cycle lasting several months. This cycle starts with an inflammatory phase, later transformed into a proliferative/necrotizing one, before finally involuting (Fig. 6.16).

Keratoacanthoma (KA) may be mentioned now as a lesion of quite probable viral etiology, although its causal agent has not been substantiated. The autolimited life cycle of KA favors that assumption and is further supported by its tendency to involute spontaneously rather than pursuing an aggressive course. For this reason, KA was nicknamed "self-healing squamous cell carcinoma." KA usually begins as a keratinous papule bearing some morphologic resemblances with VV. After an abrupt growth during a few months, the lesion may reach a maximal size of a pea, involuting and disappearing spontaneously afterward.

A meridian section of the lesion at its point of maximal development (Fig. 6.17) reveals a crater delimited on each side by an epidermal formation, the so-called "lips" of the keratoacanthoma. These are two projections thrown from the

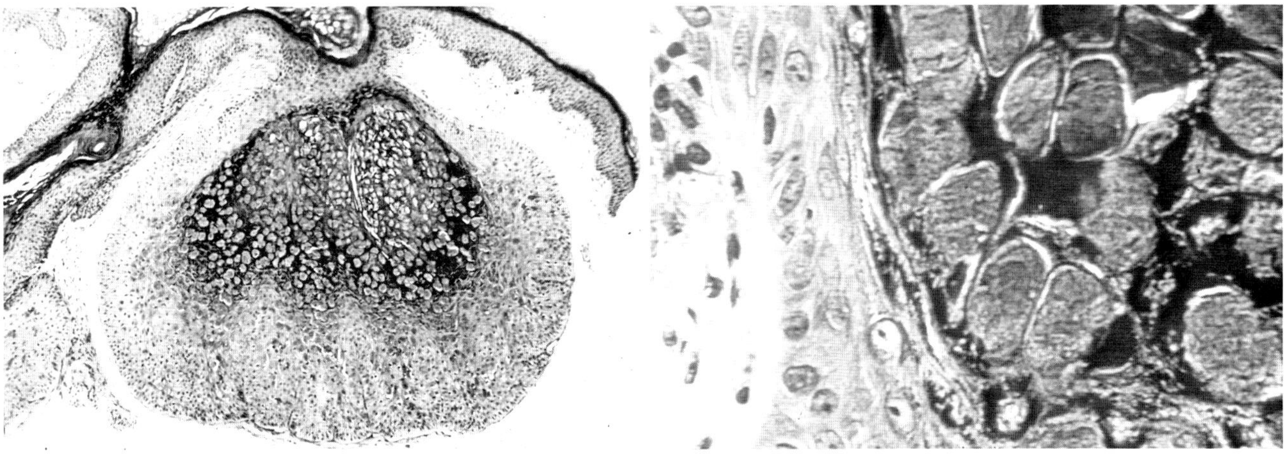

Fig. 6.15 Molluscum contagiosum. Meridian section of the lesion (*left*) and detail of the inclusion bodies (*right*). See details in the text. H&E ×40; ×400, o m

Fig. 6.16 Milker's nodule. The epidermis of the lesion in the early phase of development is hypertrophic but devitalized, as evidenced by its paleness, vacuolization, and disappearance of the granular layer. H&E ×100, o m

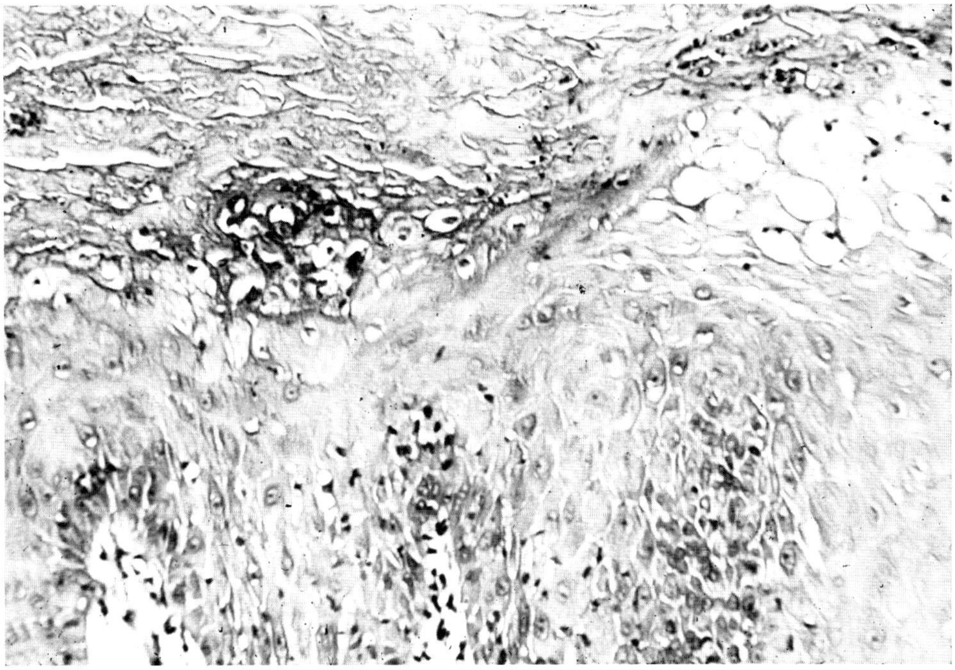

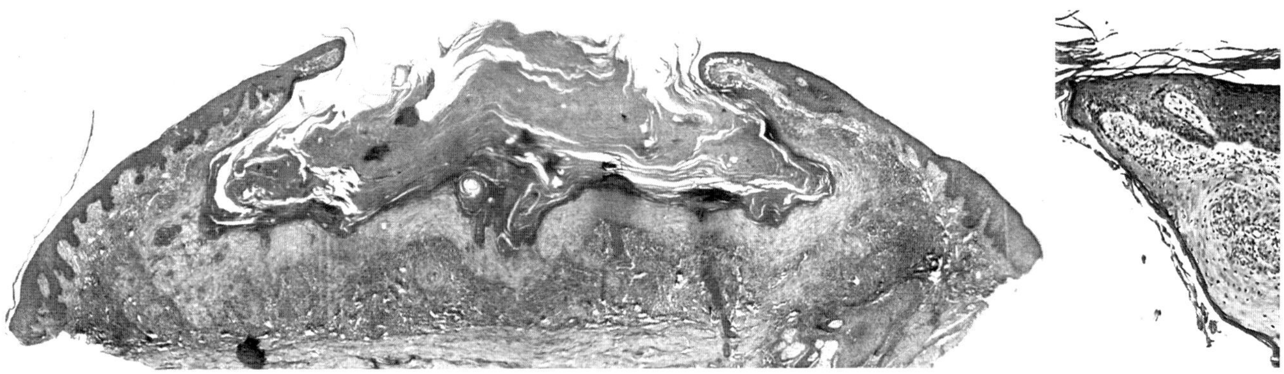

Fig. 6.17 Keratoacanthoma. (*Left*) Meridian section of the lesion. Note the "lips" of the lesion and see further details in the text. (*Right*) The higher magnification picture illustrates the sudden change of the covering epithelium from normal to highly dysplastic, as it is reflected to the inside of the lesion. H&E ×20; ×100, o m

surrounding epidermis into the center of the lesion, although failing to meet there. The epithelial covering the external surface of the "lips" appears unremarkable, but as soon as it is reflected to the inside, it suddenly transforms its character and becomes highly dysplastic. The base of the lesion is formed by a layer of highly dysplastic keratinocytes, which spread out aggressively into the dermis, forming a lesion which could not be distinguished from a well-differentiated squamous cell carcinoma, were it not for "*the lips*," its recognized microscopic hallmark.

Seborrheic keratosis (SK) is probably the most frequent cutaneous lesion in both sexes after 40 years of age. The denomination "*seborrheic*," although incorrect, reflects its external aspect accurately. Due to its indolent character devoid of complications, SK should be considered a proliferative lesion of *reactive* rather than of *neoplastic* character. The viral etiology attributed to it [11] – which, as in the case of KA, is far from proven, could tentatively be accepted. Nevertheless, such an assumption is weakened by the fact that in the already mentioned hereditary Leser-Trélat syndrome, SK is associated with internal malignancies.

SK is formed by small and uniform basophilic cells with scant cytoplasm, which does not show any mitotic activity. The lesion presents countless morphologic variations between two basic forms, the solid or acanthotic and the reticular or adenomatoid (Fig. 6.18).

In the acanthotic or solid type of SK, the proliferative activity is manifested by the buildup of cellular masses. In typical cases, such as the one illustrated in Fig. 6.18, left, these masses are clearly raised above the external surface of the skin. The irregular growth of the lesions leads to the formation of recesses or pseudocysts in which keratin scales accumulate.

In the reticular type of SK on the contrary, the growth of the lesion occurs in the form of cellular cords which spread out and anastomose in the dermis, giving rise to a plexiform structure totally different from the previous one (Fig. 6.18, right).

Minor external traumas cause crusting, congestion, and other general changes, resulting in the nonspecific picture of inflammed seborrheic keratosis. This type should be recognized and distinguished from the irritated form of SK. Irritated seborrheic keratosis has a dysplastic outlook accentuated by the presence of its characteristic elements, the "squamous eddies" (Fig. 6.19). These are masses of whorled keratinocytes of fully benign nature which, nevertheless, simulate the *keratin pearls* of squamous cell carcinoma (see p. 131).

There are two other lesions which may be regarded as forms of irritated SK: clear cell acanthoma and the clonal type of SK.

Clear cell acanthoma, described as a particular entity by R. Degos, may in fact be considered a form of SK because it lacks distinctive clinical features which may help to distinguish it from that entity. In this condition, an external irritative stimulus leads to the storage of abundant glycogen in the keratinocytes. After H&E staining, these appear as masses of clear cells, outlined by basophilic rims (Fig. 6.20, left). These masses yield a strongly positive reaction to PAS, featuring a vivid purple color after that staining procedure has been applied.

Clonal type of seborrheic keratosis is another variant of irritated SB. In it, well-circumscribed intraepidermal masses of keratinocytes are found (Fig. 6.20, right), resembling Jadassohn intraepithelial squamous cell carcinoma (p. 173). However, careful examination fails to reveal in it dysplastic changes or mitotic activity, reason for which this lesion may be considered of benign nature.

Two further lesions worth mentioning in the context of SK are melanoacanthoma and fibroepithelial papilloma. Melanoacanthoma is similar to SK but for some reason has a high melanin content.

These cells account for the increased content of melanocytes in this lesion and for its dark pigmentation, which nevertheless does not imply a malignant tendency.

Fibroepithelial papilloma also known by names such as "acrochordon," "molluscum fibrosum," and "fibroma pendulum," a lesion not very different from SK, is also of high incidence in the clinic and the laboratory. As the latter, it is also formed by an acanthotic epidermis on a supportive mesenchymal framework. Contrary to SK though, fibroepithelial papilloma has a pendulous rather than a sessile contour. In further contrast with SK, it is prone to appear in both young and old individuals.

Prior to pursuing the topic of lesions in the last two Classes of reactive cutaneous proliferations posted in Fig. 6.2, it is convenient to digress on another issue, that is, the pathogenic characteristics of epidermotrophic viruses mentioned in the previous chapter and the current one.

Infections of the skin by *epidermotrophic* viruses, in fact, lead to a wide spectrum of histopathologic manifestations. These cover a range which includes inflammatory lesions on one end and proliferative lesions on the other, with intermediary forms due to *nonepidermotrophic* organisms, which are the cause of morbiliform exanthems (Fig. 6.21).

Reactive Dermoepidermal Proliferations: Nonviral

In addition to the viral conditions, Table 6.3 also mentions nonviral RDEPs. Picker's nodule is the result of the tendency of an obsessive patient to pick on a small area of his or her own skin – frequently out of visual control, such as the nape of neck or the popliteal fossa. Nummular eczema (*nummularis* [L] a little coin), in reference to the rounded shape of the lesion, and fixed drug eruption, two other forms of RDEP, are characterized by their tendency to appear and to persist – for unknown reasons – on the same location of the body.

The terms "lichen simplex chronicus" (LSC) and "lichenified skin" are general, nonspecific designations which cover all the conditions mentioned in the previous paragraph, as well as other itchy conditions associated to a

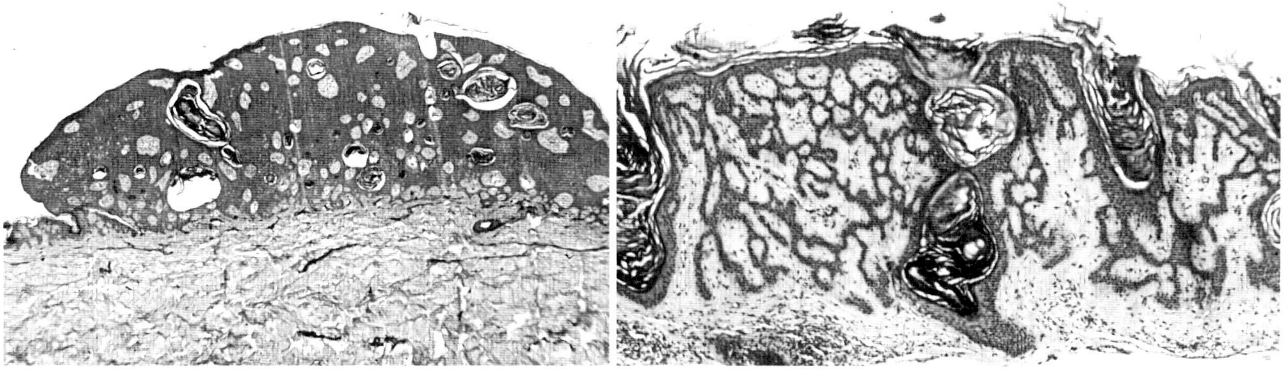

Fig. 6.18 Seborrheic keratosis. The two basic forms are shown: the solid (*left*) and the reticular (*right*). See details in the text. H&E ×40, o m.

Fig. 6.19 Irritated seborrheic keratosis. Note the dysplastic aspect of the lesion and the squamous eddies (*arrows*). H&E ×100, o m

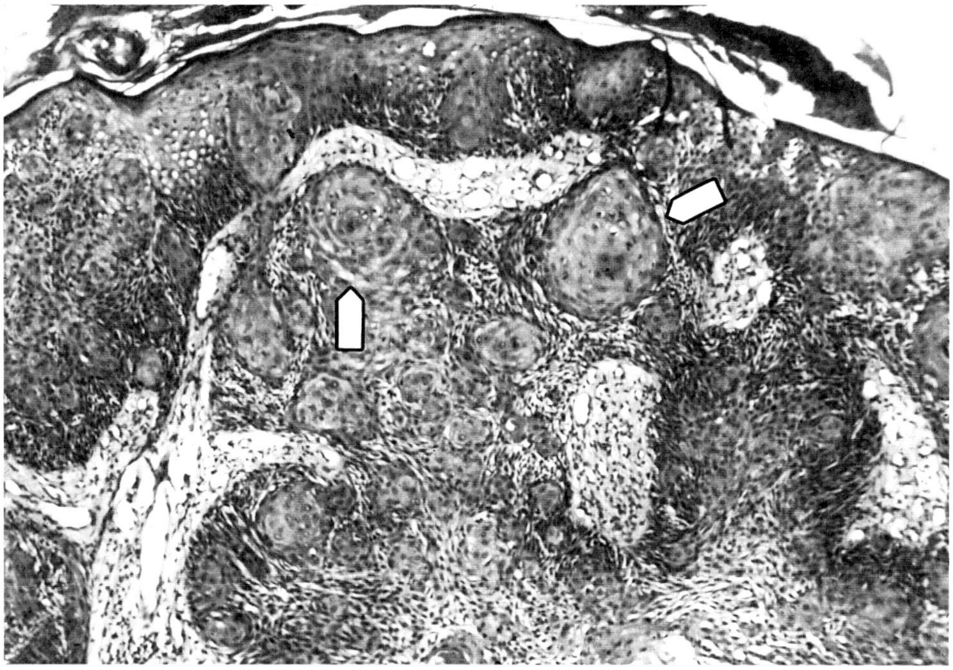

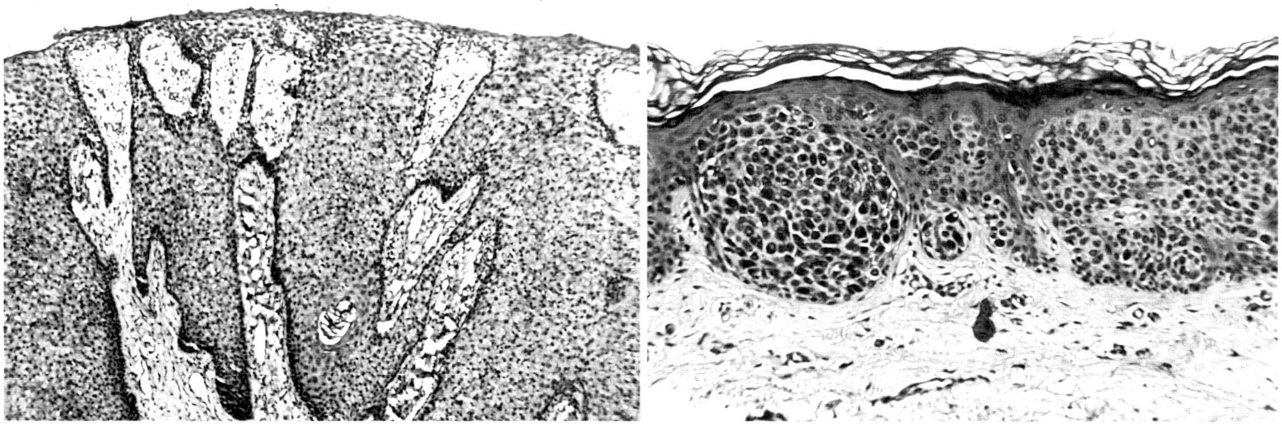

Fig. 6.20 Clear cell acanthoma (*left*) and clonal type of seborrheic keratosis (*right*). See details in the text. H&E ×100, o m

I	II
Herpes virus	Herpes simplex
Varicella zoster virus	Varicella zoster
Poxvirus	Pox
Poxvirus	Vaccinia
Picorna virus	Hand-foot-and mouth dis.
?	Mucha-Habermann disease.
Herpes virus?	Pityriasis rosea
?	Grover disease
?	Juliusberg disease
Epstein–Barr virus	Infectious mononucleosis
Paramixo virus	Measles
Toga virus	Rubella
Parvovirus	Fifth disease
Parvovirus	Sixth disease
?	Seborrheic keratosis
Papova virus	Epidermodysplasia verrucif.
Parapox virus	Milker's nodule
Parapox virus	Orf
Papova virus	Condyloma acuminatum
Parapox virus	Molluscum contagiosum
Papova virus	Verruca plana
Papova virus	Verruca vulgaris
Human papiloma virus?	Keratoacanthoma

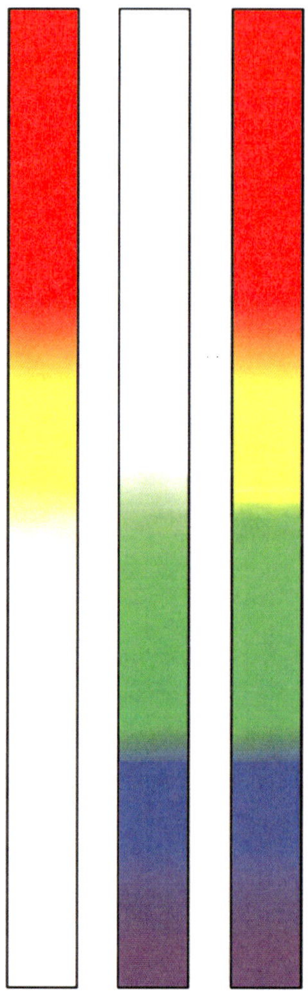

Fig. 6.21 Viral disorders arranged according to the histopathologic character of their lesions. The known or suspected viral agents for 23 cutaneous conditions are posted in column I, on the left hand side of the table. They are arranged from top to bottom according to their decreasing inflammatory character and, conversely, from the bottom to the top of the column according to their diminishing proliferative activity. The clinical conditions corresponding to the mentioned viral agents are exposed in column II. The cutaneous lesions associated to these conditions are separately evaluated for their inflammatory and proliferative activity in columns III and IV, respectively. The inflammatory character in column III goes from bright red for the more acute lesions to orange for the lesser ones. The following *yellow color* indicates that the lesions in that range have a dermal rather than an epidermal component. In column IV, the *color violet* goes for the most vigorously proliferative lesions at the bottom to blue and green for the lesser ones.

The first four entities at the head of column II, due to pox and herpesvirus infections, are bound to cause the sudden destruction of the epidermis via epidermolysis or necrosis. The intensity of the damage is reflected by the bright red color at the top of column III. The following five disorders in column II are due to picorna and other undetermined virosic agents. They lead to milder manifestations, in the form of necrobiosis and spongiosis: these are codified in column III via the color orange. The five following conditions in that column are caused by a heterogeneous array of nonepidermotrophic but inflammatory agents which includes herpes-, paramyxo-, toga-, and parvovirus: these do not directly affect the epidermis but are clinically manifested by exanthems, mainly underlying edema and perivascular infiltrates.

The last disorders in column II do not have any inflammatory activity, as indicated by the corresponding colorless segment of column III, but starting by milker's nodule, caused by a parapoxvirus, they begin featuring a proliferative activity: this is shown by the color green in column IV.

To the group of the verrucae caused by papovaviruses is assigned the color blue and to the two final integrants of column II, keratoacanthoma and seborrheic keratosis, whose pathogenic agents are still unproven, the color violet is assigned, on account of their clear proliferative character.

Overlapping column III on column IV, the entire gamut of viral pathology on the skin is presented from the epidermolytic and necrotizing to the proliferative ones symbolized by the spectrum of light decomposition. In the center of the spectrum, represented by the color yellow, are those lesions with negligible epidermal changes, caused by an array of not epidermotrophic viruses, which are translated in the clinic by various exanthems thickened and deteriorated skin, whose precise diagnosis cannot be established. This condition presents a striking although nonspecific microscopic picture. This is characterized by an acanthotic and hyperkeratotic skin with a thick, frequently irregular granular layer. The rete ridges are hypertrophic, elongated, and deformed, showing a characteristic tendency to bifurcate. The intervening dermal papillae are tortuous and fibrotic, featuring an abundance of thin nerve fibers and a diffuse infiltrate of mononuclear cells. The total absence of spongiosis allows to tell apart the RDEPs in Fig. 6.22 left from dermatitis chronica. Minor clinicopathologic details may allow the identification of Picker's nodule.

Acariosis may involve extense areas of the skin and can be frequently diagnosed from the exterior by the presence of the responsible parasite Fig. 6.22 right.

Figure 6.23 illustrates a RDEP resulting from a parasitic infestation of, in this case an acariosis or mite infestation, by *S. scabiei*, causing the so-called sarna norvegica.

Reactive Adnexal Proliferations

In the following discussion of reactive adnexal proliferations, those concerning the pilosebaceous apparatus will be the only ones discussed.

A fitting example of these conditions is sebaceous hyperplasia. This is presumably caused by a hormonal imbalance, predominant among aged populations, and occurs in areas of the face, which are normally endowed with abundant sebaceous glands. The orderly disposition of the increased numbers of sebaceous glands around central follicular infundibuli is a feature of importance for the distinction of this condition from sebaceous hamartoma which by definition shows a disorderly distribution of its components (p. 46). An orderly arrangement and absence of atypical figures and mitotic activity as observed by LM are also enough to discard the possibility of malignancy in sebaceous hyperplasia (Fig. 6.24).

Also pertinent to the reactive adnexal proliferations is hirsutism (*hirsutus* [L] hairy), that is, the increase in the number of hairs, which may occur in a localized or generalized way. This condition may respond to hormonal imbalances or to other known or unknown stimuli. In this sense, the hirsutism of the porphyrias (p. 37) is a case in point.

Reactive Mesenchymal Proliferations

Among the mesenchymal proliferations, granulation tissue should be mentioned first. Granulation tissue builds up when the borders of recent wounds have not been properly apposed, or when the re-epithelialization of a flat open surface is delayed. Figure 6.25 illustrates the first situation.

Under the microscope, granulation tissue appears as a vascular mass.

It is formed by capillaries running parallel to each other and perpendicular to the external surface of the lesion enmeshed in abundant stroma, in which abundant acute inflammatory cells are noted. This growth is characteristically *devoid of covering epithelium* (Fig. 6.25c), a detail that contributes to differentiate this lesion from *pyogenic granuloma* (p. 129), a benign vascular neoplasia with which it is frequently mistaken.

Metabolic xanthoma is another type of reactive mesenchymal proliferation, this time of cellular rather than vascular character. These lesions are associated to the dyslipoproteinemias discussed under the category of HMEwCR, from where they obtain the name "hyperlipidemic or metabolic xanthomas" (p. 36), in contrast to the "*normolipidemic xanthomas*," which do not require any exogenous stimulus to growth.

Metabolic xanthomas are frequently multiple. Four types exist: eruptive, tuberosum, planar xanthoma, and xanthelasma, as was already pointed out. Particular types of xanthoma can only be determined clinically because with the exception of xanthelasma, they are indistinguishable under the microscope, since all of them feature lipid-loaded epithelioid histiocytes and multinucleated giant cells. In contrast, xanthelasma presents a tenuous stroma in which large epithelioid cells are distributed, along with punctiform nuclei and a foamy cytoplasm with a "*ground glass*" look. These cells are also loaded with lipids (Fig. 6.26).

Neoplastic Cutaneous Proliferations

In order to commence the study on the Subdivision of neo plastic cutaneous proliferations (Fig. 6.27), it is convenient to define three terms which will frequently appear in related discussions: dysplasia, anaplasia, and neoplasia.

Dysplasia (*dys* [G] defective+*plasia* [G] growth) is a term applied to cells which feature atypical changes in size, volume, and/or organization. Currently, this definition is reinforced by changes detected using modern analytical techniques. The meaning of the word "dysplasia" applied here is therefore different from the one with which it was before, applied in reference to post-inflammatory changes of various adnexae (p. 124).

Anaplasia (*ana* [G] reversion+*plasia* [G] growth) refers to cellular reversion to the primitive stage through loss of the corresponding differentiation process. Anaplastic cells are those devoid of differentiation.

Neoplasia (*neo* [G] new+*plasia* [G] growth). According to Willis [12] and substituting the term "*tumor*" from his original definition by "*a mass of tissue*," "*neoplasia is a mass of tissue whose growth exceeds, and is not coordinated with that of normal tissue, and which persists in the same excessive*

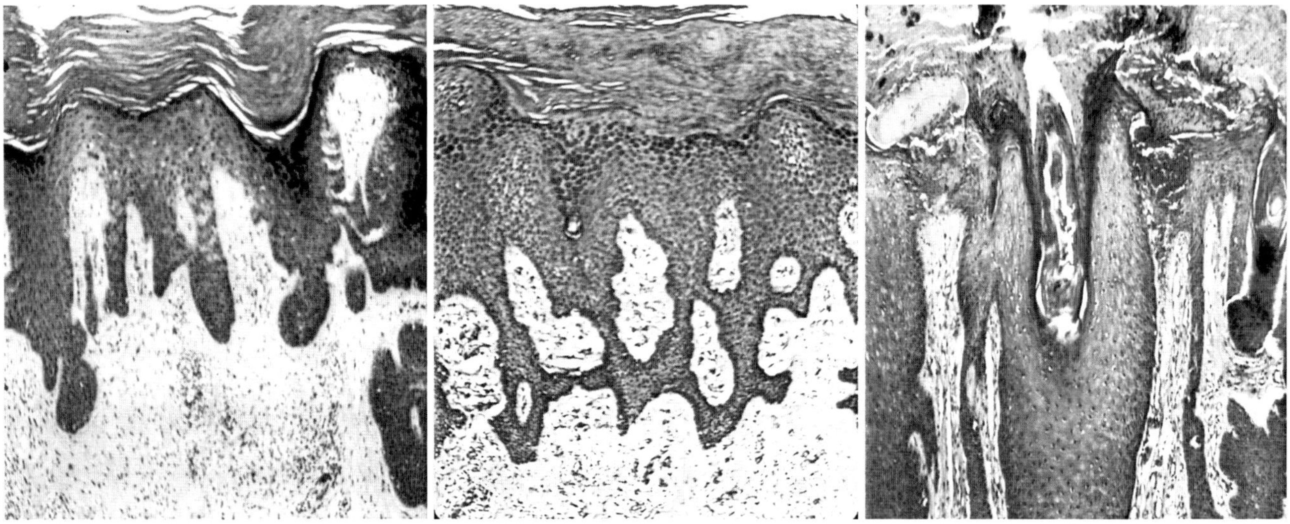

Fig. 6.22 Lichen simplex chronicus and associated lesions. (*Left*) Lichen simplex chronicus: see details in the text. (*Center*) Chronic dermatitis: the presence of spongiosis, even minimal, is the differential feature of the lesion. (*Right*) Picker's nodule presents gross deformation of the architecture and crusting. H&E ×40, o m

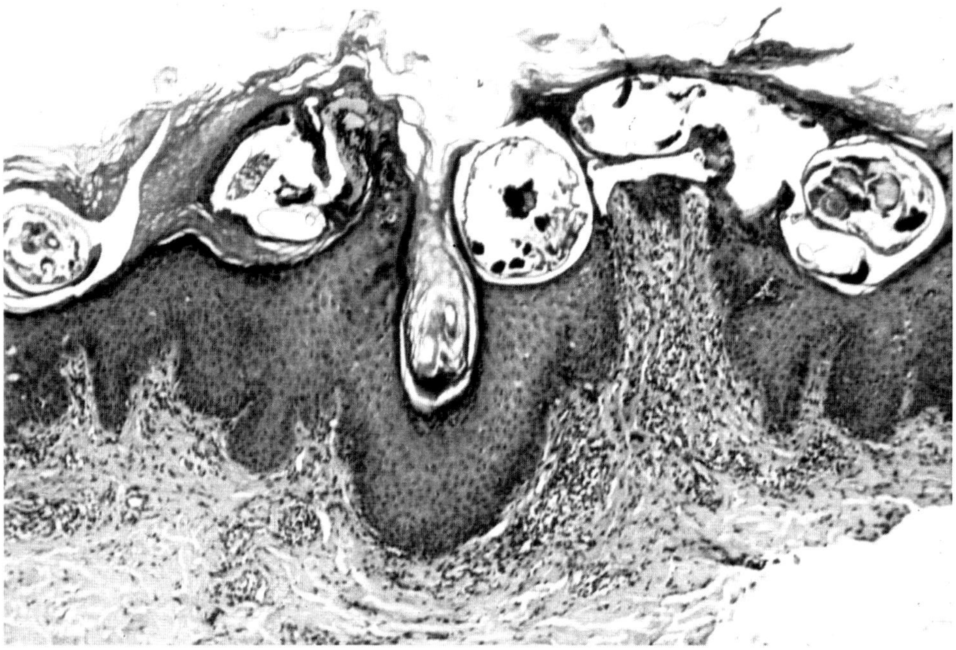

Fig. 6.23 Acariosis (sarna norvegica). Note the hyperplastic and deformed epidermis, the inflammatory infiltrate in the dermis, and the presence of mites underneath the horny layers. H&E ×40 o m

manner even after termination of the stimulus which provoked its growth." Or, said in words used prior to the discovery of cell markers and other elaborated techniques: "*a neoplasia is a mass of tissue exhibiting autarchic and anarchic growth of undefined duration.*"

Following the approach used in systemic pathology, neoplastic growths may be tracked to the organ from where they derive. In such a way, the neoplasias in the lung may be regarded as of bronchial, bronchioalveolar, pleural, or of other components of this organ. Likewise, the neoplasias of the skin may be considered to arise from the epidermis, the adnexae, or its mesenchymatous-lymphohistiocytic component. Accordingly, cutaneous neoplasias may be presented in three Classes: epidermal, adnexal, and mesenchymatous. To these, a fourth Class of neoplasias of extracutaneous origin must be added. The adnexal neoplasias are the so-called "adnexal tumors", and the mesenchymatous, the "soft tissue tumors" (Fig. 6.27).

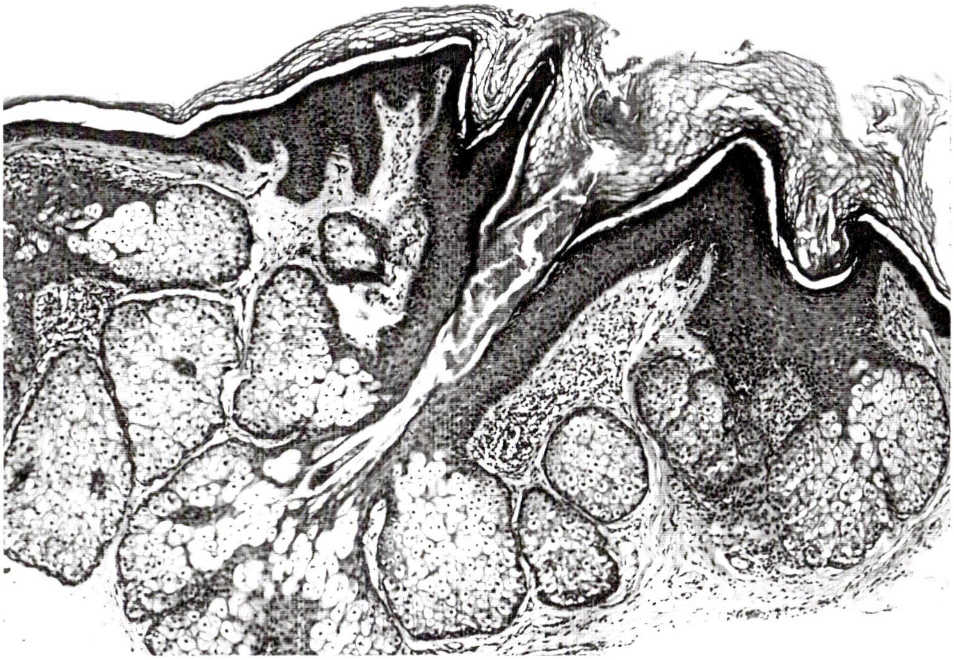

Fig. 6.24 Sebaceous hyperplasia. Note the increased number of sebaceous glands and their orderly disposition around a well-formed follicular infundibulum. H&E ×40 o m

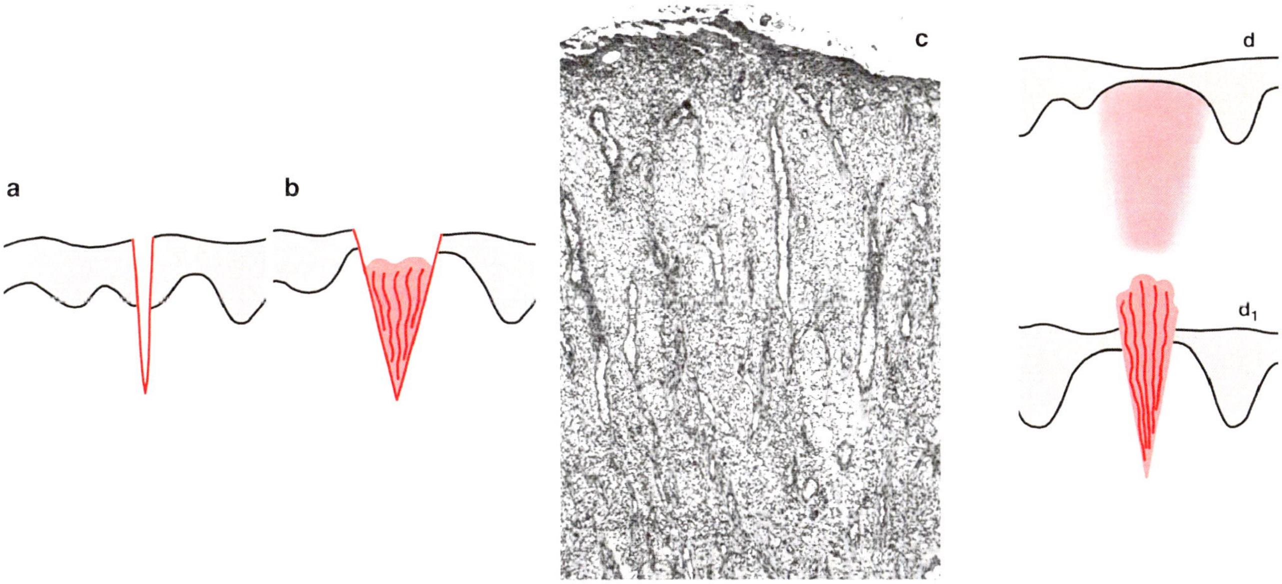

Fig. 6.25 Evolutive cycle of granulation tissue. If the borders of a sharp wound are not properly apposed (**a**), during the first stage of granulation tissue production, active capillary proliferation occurs. The capillaries, growing parallel to each other, tend to occupy the empty space in the wound (**b**). The photomicrograph (**c**) illustrates this situation: note the capillaries running in parallel. When the vascular mass reaches the level of the external surface of the skin, either the epidermis slides over the surface of the wound, closing and healing by "second intention," (**d**) or, if it fails to do so, the proliferating tissue continue growing above the skin surface. In the latter case, it forms a vascular mass, used to be named in the French school a botriomycoma, when it was assumed that it was the result of an infection by a botriomycoma fungus. The lesion is also known colloquially as "proud flesh" ($\mathbf{d}_1$)

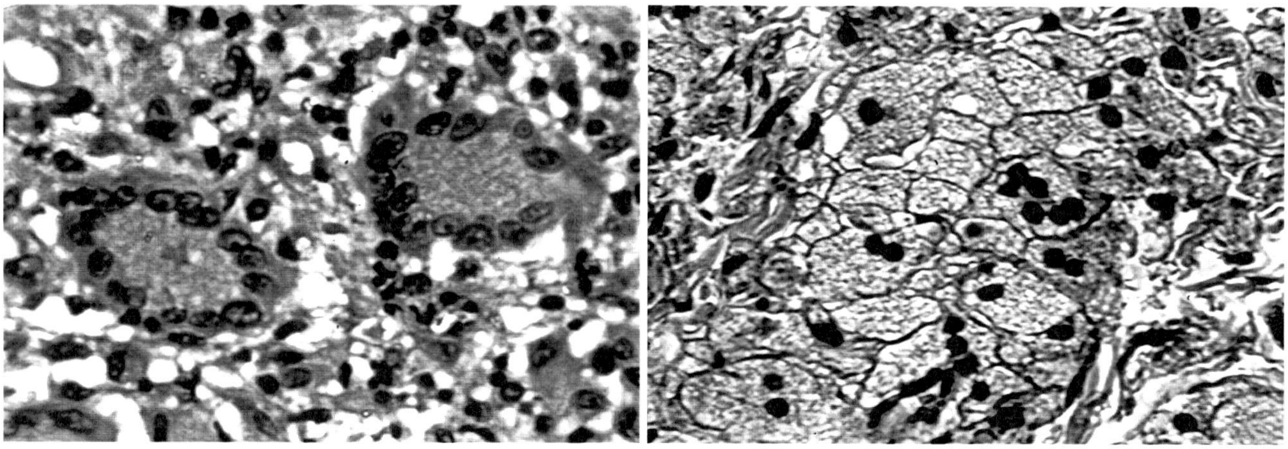

Fig. 6.26 Metabolic xanthomas. (*Left*) General view of a metabolic xanthoma. Note the presence of lipid-loaded histiocytes and multinucleated giant cells. (*Right*) Xanthelasma, with large epithelioid histiocytes, featuring punctiform nuclei and cytoplasms with a "*ground glass*" appearance. H&E ×100 o m

Cutaneous neoplastic proliferations
- Epidermic
- Adnexal (adnexal tumors)
- Mesenchymal (soft tissue tumors)
- Extracutaneous

Fig. 6.27 Neoplastic cutaneous proliferations: Classes

Subclasses
- Keratinocytic
- Melanogenic — **Groups**: Melanocytic; Nevocytic
- Of Merkel cells

Fig. 6.28 Epidermal neoplastic proliferations

Neoplastic Epidermal Proliferations

Three Subclasses can be recognized within the Class of the epidermal neoplastic proliferations: these are the keratinocytic, the ones of melanogenic cells, and the ones of Merkel cells.

The Subclass of melanogenic cells comprises two Groups of neoplasias, melanocytic and nevocytic (Fig. 6.28).

Although both of these melanogenic cells have melanosomes and the capacity for generating melanin, melanocytes *are normal components* of the epidermis, whereas nevocytes *are not*. The pathology of these two elements is quite different, making it necessary to deal with them in two separate Groups.

Langerhans cells are not of cutaneous origin, and their proliferative lesions are not considered at this point.

Neoplastic Keratinocytic Proliferations

Squamous cell carcinoma (SQC) is the general designation for neoplasias of keratinocytes. At the moment it is studied under the microscope, SQC may be found contained within the epidermis or have already spread to invade surrounding tissues: in the first case, the lesion is a "squamous cell carcinoma **in situ**," and in the second, it is an "invasive squamous cell carcinoma" (Table 6.5). In this text, "squamous cell carcinoma" without further qualification means "invasive squamous cell carcinoma."

Table 6.5 Examples of squamous cell carcinoma in situ and invasive

Squamous cell carcinoma in situ
Bowen disease
Erythroplasia of Queyrat
Squamous cell carcinoma invasive
Squamous cell carcinoma, well differentiated
Adenoid carcinoma
Carcinoma cuniculatum
Squamous cell carcinoma, anaplastic

Squamous Cell Carcinoma In Situ

The prototypic squamous cell carcinoma in situ Bowen disease (BD) was described by J.T. Bowen in the first decade of the nineteenth century. This lesion is found in middle-aged and old individuals of both sexes as erythematous plaques, located on sun-exposed, or more frequently, sun-protected regions of the body, such as the trunk and the inguinogenital areas. Under low magnification, the lesion appears as a solid cellular band involving the whole thickness of the epidermis, clearly delimited from the underlying dermis by a preserved BM. Cutaneous adnexae are characteristically *absent* from the lesion and parakeratin scales are barely visible. At higher magnification, the lesion appears formed by large pleomorphic cells, including bizarre elements with hyperchromatic nuclei. The lesion features a high mitotic rate and atypical mitotic figures. The cellular elements appear in profound disarray,

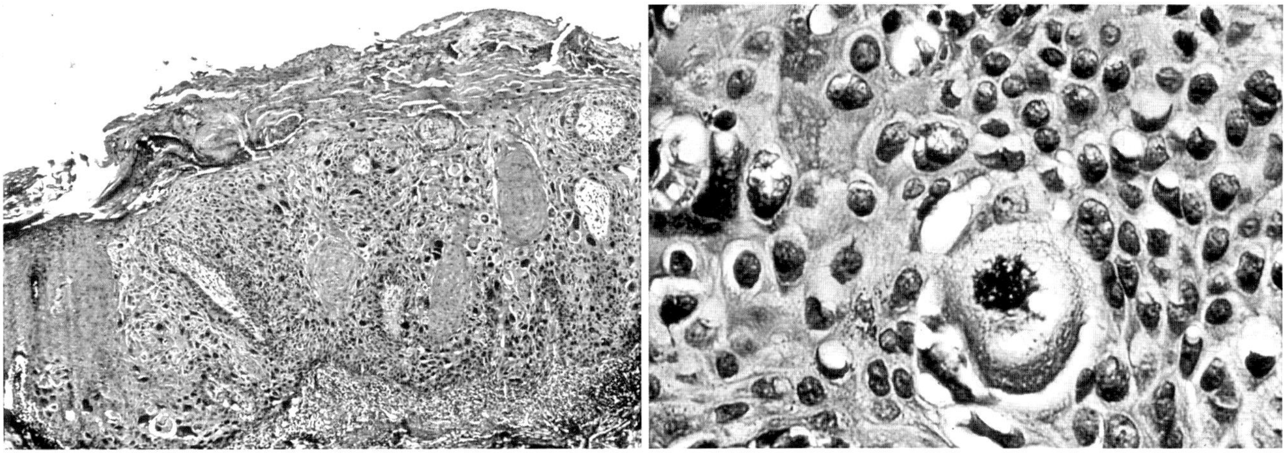

Fig. 6.29 Bowen disease. At low magnification (*left*) the lesion appears as a solid mass occupying the entire thickness of the epidermis, although it does not spread into the dermis. Note at higher magnification (*right*) the profound disorganization of the epidermis and the presence of bizarre cellular elements and the atypical mitotic figures. H&E ×100; ×400 o m

with loss of epidermal polarity. Using a classic comparison, it may be said that the cells in BD appear as "dry leaves which after having been blown around, resettle in a pattern which is totally different from the original" (Fig. 6.29).

BD may acquire invasive properties, being transformed into an anaplastic SQC whose microscopic picture becomes closely similar to that of its in situ counterpart (Fig. 6.30).

From the ongoing discussion, it is obvious that BD is a *neoplastic* lesion, quite different from AK, which is a condition of *reactive* nature (Table 6.1). This fact is emphasized by the important biological difference that separates these lesions, insofar as AK is clearly dependent on actinic radiation for its inception, whereas BD is independent of that agent for its development.

Erythroplasia of Queyrat, reported by A.d. Queyrat in 1910, is another example of an in situ SQC. It is since known by the author's name. This lesion differentiates clinically from BD by the fact that it is selectively found on the genital mucosa. Nevertheless, under microscopic examination, erythroplasia offers a picture alike to that of BD (Fig. 6.31).

As an introduction to the study of the invasive squamous cell carcinoma, it may be said that, based on the assumption that an increasing loss of keratinization of a SQC indicates an increment of its malignancy, A. Broders developed a system known as Broders system for evaluating these lesions [13]. Such system ranges from grades 1 to 4 depending on the increasing loss of keratinization, the least keratinizing being the most malignant. This system does not seem to hold true, however, since keratinizing SQC may prove to be as much aggressive as nonkeratinizing ones. Moreover, the idea that a SQC may change its biological features throughout its life cycle, another fact implied in Broders system, has not been proven either. Rather, a SQC seems to keep invariably its level of keratinization throughout its life cycle. Therefore, many pathologists prefer to classify SQC simply as "well differentiated," "poorly differentiated," or "anaplastic," [14] which is the criterion followed in this text.

Several varieties of SQC may be recognized microscopically, as shown in Table 6.5.

Squamous cell carcinoma, well differentiated, in its most frequent form appears as angulated, irregular, and keratinized cords that spread down from a dysplastic epidermis. The lesion is formed by rather large eosinophylic cells with abundant intercellular bridges and a moderate to high mitotic rate. As they advance downward, the cellular cords may be cut from the main lesion, forming rounded, discrete colonies which frequently enclose "*keratin pearls*" (Fig. 6.32).

Keratin pearls are a pathognomonic feature of the well-differentiated SQC. They are made by laminated scales of keratin concentrically located around a central eosinophylic core. When they are found, the microscopist should devote every effort to confirm their nature and tell them apart from their "*look alikes*," squamous eddies, characteristic of the irritated form of SK (see Fig. 6.19). This will avoid mistaking the latter condition for a SQC (or vice versa).

Acantholytic carcinoma is a special form of keratinizing SQC, which may be regarded as the invasive form of AK (p. 116). Keratinocytes appear intensely eosinophilic in this lesion and devoid of intercellular bridges, forming dehiscent, pseudoglandular structures, from where the original name of the lesion "adenoid carcinoma," given to it by W. Lever [15], derives (Fig. 6.33).

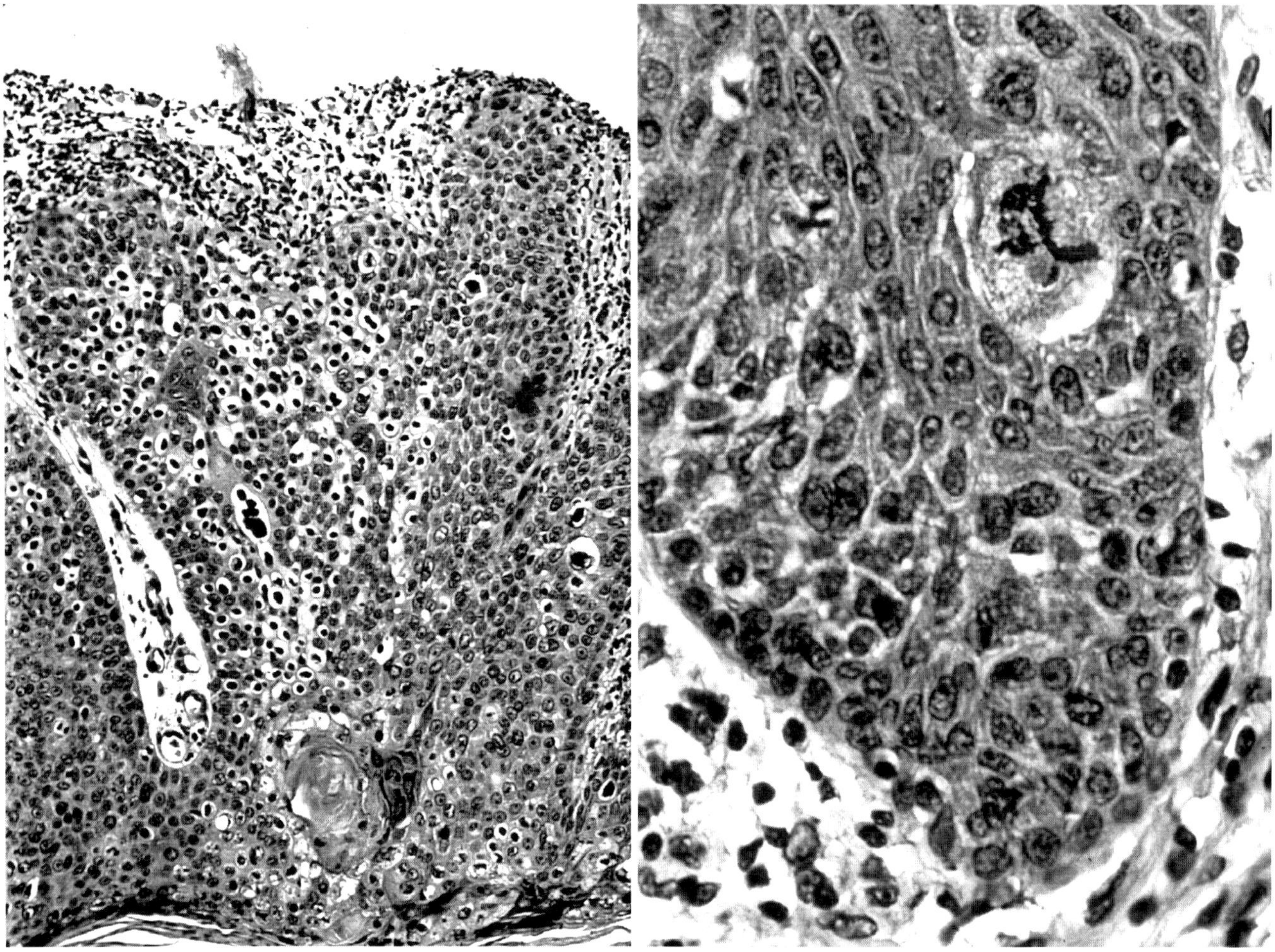

Fig. 6.30 Squamous cell carcinoma originated in Bowen disease. (*Left*) Note the continuity of the severe dysplastic changes in the epidermis, with those noted in the dermis (*right*). H&E ×100; ×400 o.m

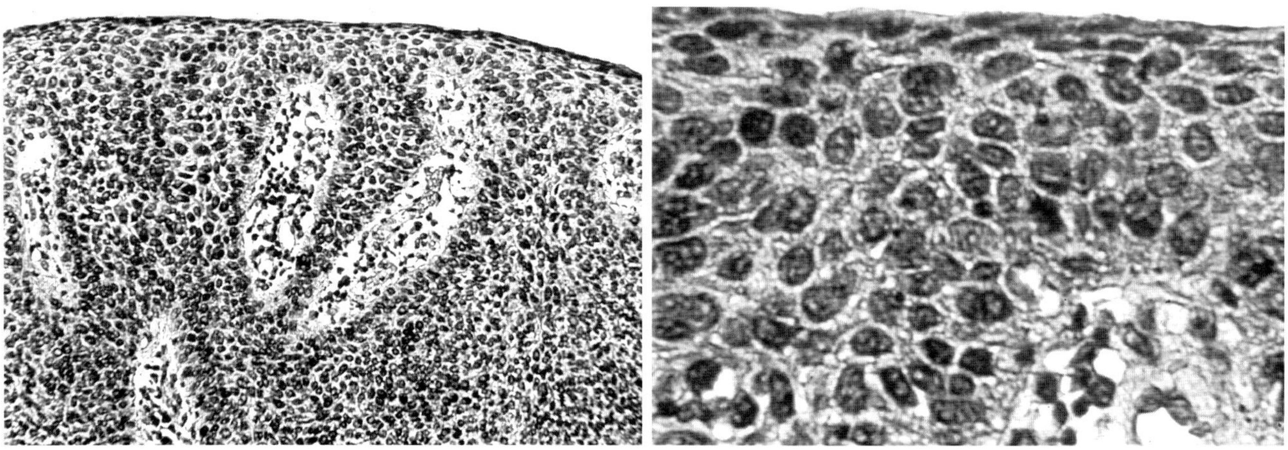

Fig. 6.31 Erythroplasia Queyrat. (*Left*) Note the full-thickness involvement of the epidermis and the disruption of the architecture by bizarre elements (*right*). H&E ×100; ×400 o m

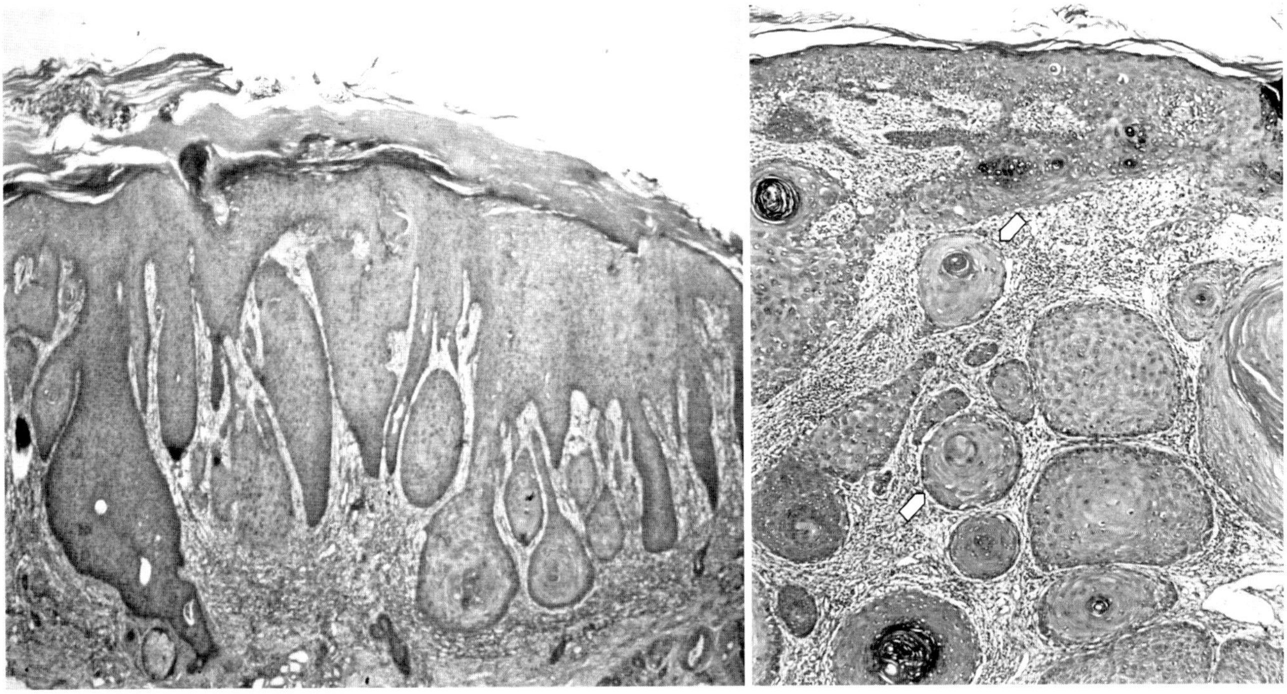

Fig. 6.32 Squamous cell carcinoma: well differentiated. At low magnification (*left*), the lesion appears as a solid eosinophilic mass formed by angulated cords penetrating from a crusted, dysplastic epidermis into the dermis of the specimen. A view of another lesion (*right*) shows rounded colonies of neoplastic cells, disconnected from the main lesion and enclosing keratin pearls (*arrows*). H&E ×40 o m

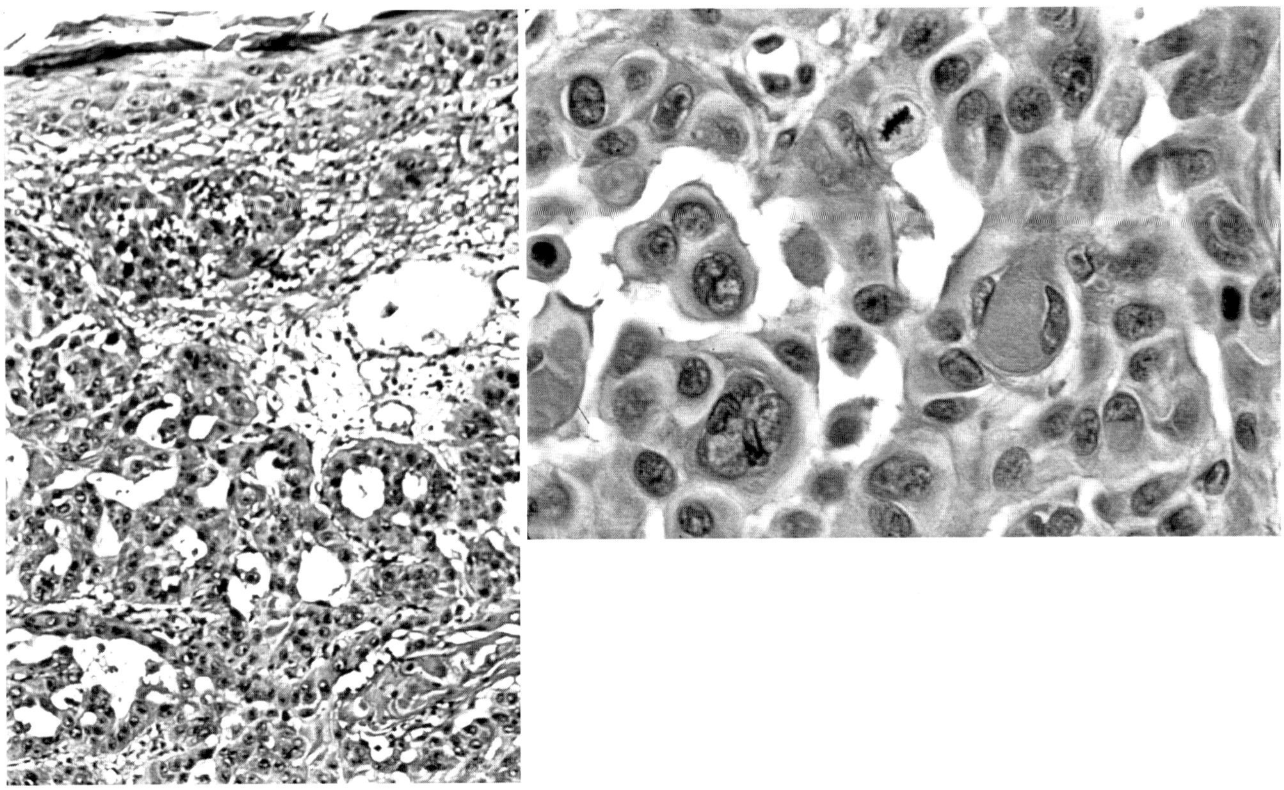

Fig. 6.33 Acantholytic carcinoma. Note the pseudoglandular and invasive character of the lesion (*left*). A higher magnification exposes the acantholytic character and active mitotic rate of the lesion (*right*). H&E ×100; ×400 o m

Squamous cell carcinoma of the oral cavity: In spite of the specific name assigned to it, this lesion is nothing other than an exophytic, well-differentiated SQC, which happens to develop on the mucosa of the oral cavity.

Squamous cell carcinoma featuring a cutaneous horn: An exophytic SQC may also be present at the base of a cutaneous horn, in which case its correct denomination would be "squamous cell carcinoma featuring a cutaneous horn," as explained before.

Giant condyloma of Buschke and Loewenstein has to be included in any discussion on exophytic SQC due to its misleading name. Its denomination may induce a person reading a report that mentions a lesion by this name, to think that he or she is dealing with just an oversized condyloma. However, giant condyloma is a full-fledged exophytic SQC, such as that displayed in Fig. 6.34. For this reason, the name "*giant condyloma*" should be eradicated from the dermatologic lexicon. It should be replaced with the term "squamous cell carcinoma, exophytic" and further qualified as "anaplastic," if it so deserves.

Carcinoma cuniculatum is another variety of SQC found on the sole of the foot [16]. This lesion is not exophytic but features a tendency to grow under the skin, hence resembling rabbit burrows (*cuniculus* [L] a rabbit).

Anaplastic squamous cell carcinoma may appear spontaneously, unrelated to any circumstance. Otherwise, it may represent the invasive form of BD. In both cases, it would display the same level of anaplastic regression, high mitotic rate, irregular mitotic figures, etc., shown in Fig. 6.35, as the most malignant tumors of any other progeny may. In these highly anaplastic lesions, occasional faint desmosomes may hint at their keratinocytic progeny.

It should be noted again that there is an analogy in the process of malignant transformation of AK and BD. In both cases, the invasive form of the lesion offers a microscopic picture quite similar to the lesion in its localized form.

Neoplastic Melanogenic Proliferations

The melanogenic potential of a lesion may be surmised from its pigmented external surface or by melanin granules found during its microscopic examination. In the absence of this finding, the application of cell marker studies may allow the recognition of the melanogenic potential of a lesion. No technique is more conclusive in this regard, however, than EM. Indeed, upon finding melanosomes – the organelles responsible for the production of the pigment (p. 5) – this technique settles without doubt any question on the potential pigment-producing capacity of a lesion.

As already stated, two different cellular elements, melanocytes and nevocytes, are able to generate melanin (p. 8). Therefore, the melanogenic proliferations should be dealt with in two separate Groups, that of the *melanocytic* and the other of the *nevocytic* proliferations (Fig. 6.28). The distinction of the actual progeny of a *melanogenic* lesion has more than taxonomic implications: melanocytic and nevocytic lesions bear significant differences, as it will be evident when they are comparatively studied. Figure 6.48, which the reader is advised to visit during the discussion that follows, illustrates these differences graphically.

Neoplastic Melanocytic Proliferations

In their progression toward malignancy, melanocytes feature a series of three lesions, one benign, another premalignant, and a third overtly malignant. These are *lentigo simplex, lentigo maligna* – or *atypical melanocytic hyperplasia* – and *lentigo malignant melanoma* (see Fig. 6.48). At this point, the reservation should be made that the lentiginous lesions associated to HPDwCP such as Peutz-Jeghers, v. Recklinghausen, and Carney syndrome made of melanocytes of unusual microscopic features should not be included in this discussion.

Lentigo simplex (*lentigo* [L] lentil-shaped) is a simple proliferation of the normal melanocytic population in a restricted area of the skin. It appears in young as in old Caucasian individuals as pigmented spots sitting both on sun-exposed or sun-protected areas of the body. The microscopic examination of these lesions simply shows an increase of melanocytes of normal features disposed as tight rows over the basement membrane, displacing the keratinocytes normally present there. The examination of a mucosal lentigo shows a simplified picture of this lesion, with a tenuous pigmented row made by an increased number of unremarkable melanocytes outlining the epidermis (Fig. 6.36).

Junction nevus is a relic of Unna's obsolete "*Abtropfen Theorie*" proposed in connection with the life cycle of nevocytes over 100 years ago (p. 51). When flat, jet black lesions referred to the laboratory under the presumptive clinical diagnosis of "*junction nevus*" are examined under the microscope, they simply prove to be, in the great majority of cases, lentigines simplex with a heavy load of melanin (Fig. 6.37, left).

Lentigo senilis is still another type of hyperpigmented lesion located on the body of aged people. They are characterized under the microscope by elongated epidermal ridges loaded with melanin (Fig. 6.37, right).

Atypical melanocytic hyperplasia (AMH): Lentigo simplex may increase its size and pigmentation, showing blurred and irregular borders. If, under microscopic examination, this new lesion happens to show atypic, angulated, and vacuolated melanocytes disposed in disarray though *without transgressing the BM limits*, that lesion should be called "atypical melanocytic hyperplasia" (AMH) (Fig. 6.38).

AMH corresponds and is equivalent to the lesion known in the clinic as "lentigo maligna" (LMa). When located on

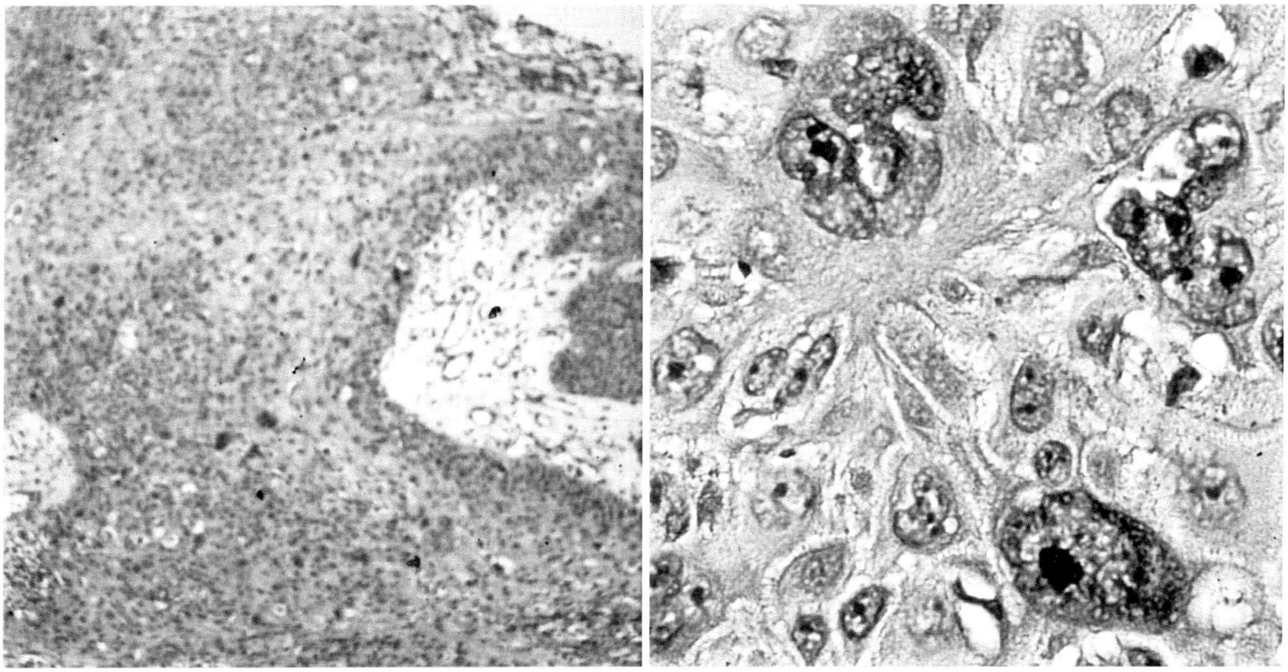

Fig. 6.34 Giant condyloma of Buschke and Loewenstein. Note the profuse growth of the lesion (*left*) and the anaplastic character of its cellular components (*right*). H&E ×40; ×400 o m

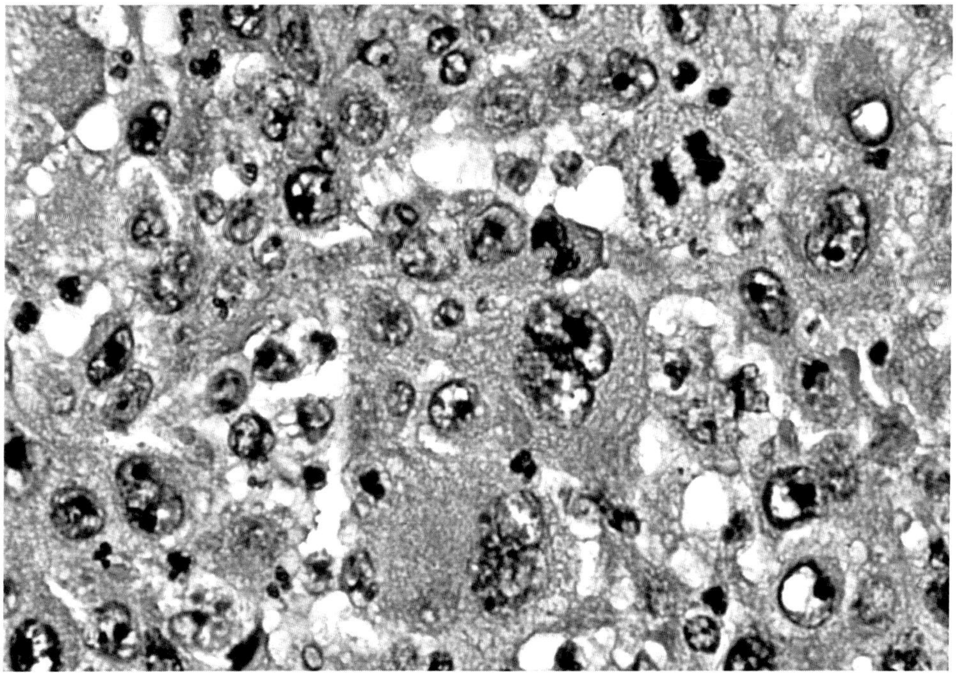

Fig. 6.35 Squamous cell carcinoma: anaplastic. Note the high mitotic rate of the lesion, its irregular mitotic figures, bizarre, often binucleated cellular elements, and monster figures. H&E ×400 o m

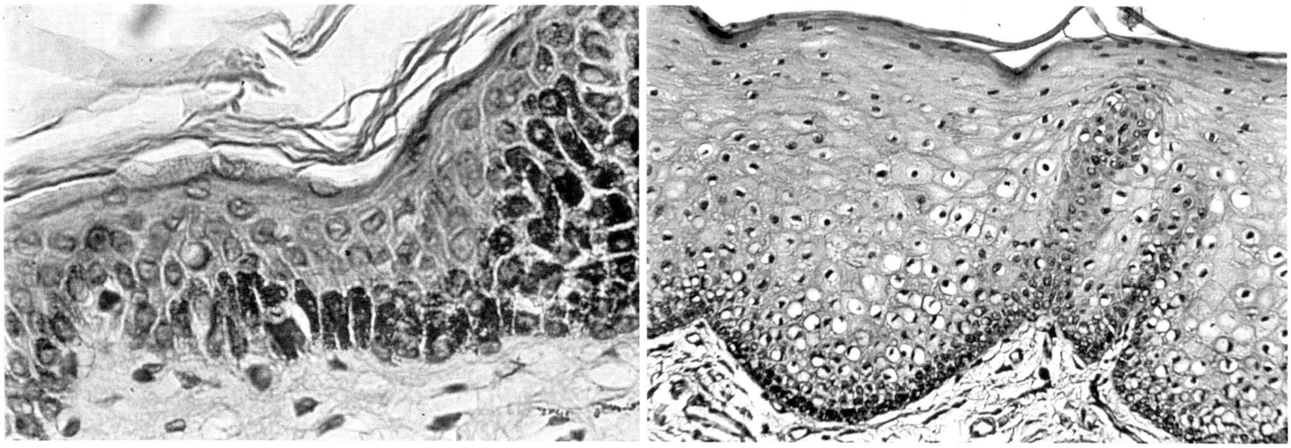

Fig. 6.36 Lentigo simplex and mucosal lentigo. Lentigo simplex (*left*) shows a flat keratinizing epidermis with clusters of unremarkable melanocytes, some of them featuring clear cytoplasms, disposed at the low epidermal level. Mucosal lentigo (*right*) features a subtle layer of melanocytes underlying a nonkeratinizing epithelium. H&E ×100 o m

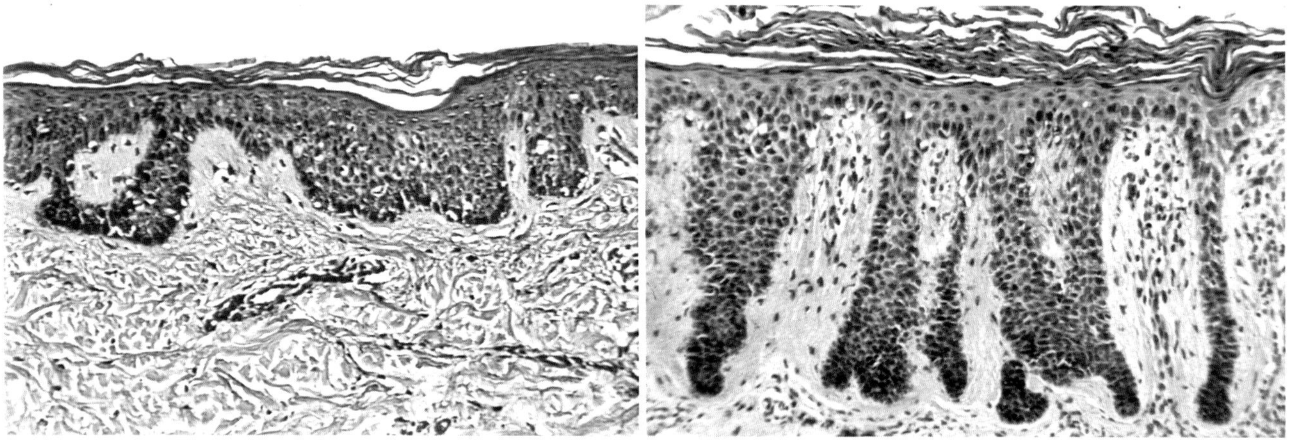

Fig. 6.37 "Junction nevus" and lentigo senilis. Note the similarity of the so-called junction nevus (*left*), with the lentigo simplex presented in Fig. 6.36. A so-called lentigo senilis featuring elongated epidermal ridges is seen at *the right*. H&E ×100 o m

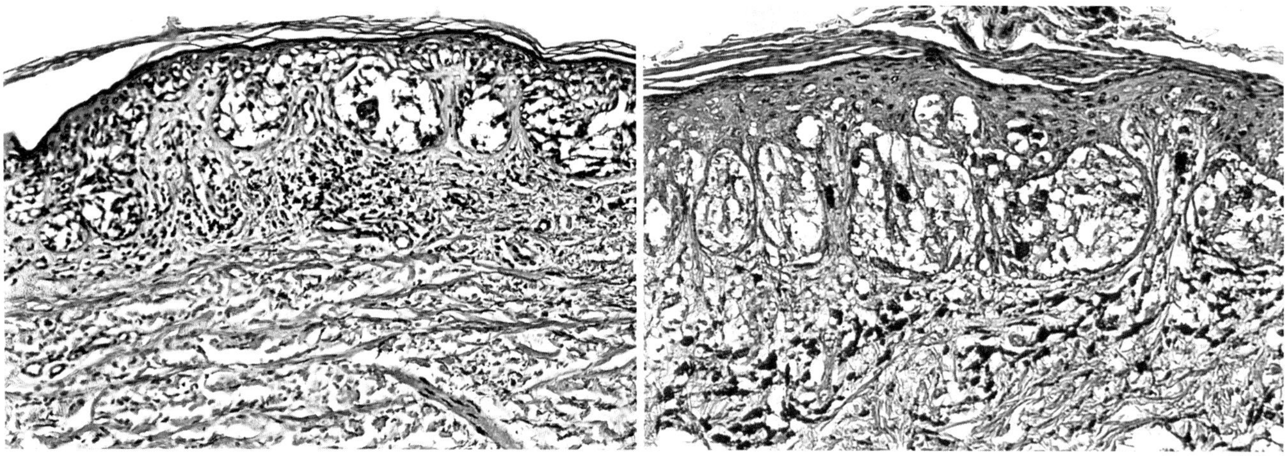

Fig. 6.38 Atypic melanocytic hyperplasia. This figure presents two AMH lesions. The one to *the left* shows globules of spindle-shaped and vacuolated melanocytes attached to the uppermost layers of the epidermis and contained within this layer by a preserved BM. The one to *the right* shows a picture essentially similar to the former but giving the impression that it is about to break out. H&E ×40 o m

the face, LMa is called "melanotic freckle of Hutchinson" or alternatively, "Dubreuilh's melanosis circumscripta blastomatosa." AMH has an indolent evolution which may be prolonged for years without complications. Its malignant transformation, however, cannot be ruled out, reason for which its excision is advised as soon as it is diagnosed.

Lentigo maligna melanoma (LMM): The diagnosis of lentigo maligna melanoma is based on a specific feature, which is *the breakthrough of the BM by an AMH, which invades the underlying dermis* (Fig. 6.39). This change bestows the new lesion, LMM, with a potential for systemic dissemination, justifying the seriousness of its diagnosis.

The retrospective comparison of this Fig. 6.39 with Fig. 6.38 emphasizes the differences between AMH and LMM. In AMH, the lesion is still contoured by a preserved BM, whereas in LMM the lesion, upon breaking through the BM, has invaded the dermis.

Malignant blue nevus: Before closing the discussion of the malignant melanocytic proliferations, *malignant blue nevus* deserves a short comment. This quite uncommon *melanocytic* lesion may either have been of malignant nature from its inception or otherwise, it may be the result of the direct malignant degeneration of a blue nevus (p. 39), but in any case, it appears without any intermediate form, being from the beginning a fully malignant lesion seated in the deep dermis or subcutaneous tissue.

Neoplastic Nevocytic Proliferations

The sequence of transformations ultimately leading to nevocytic malignant melanoma begins very frequently with changes in a *nevocytic nevus* [17] – abbreviated conveniently as IDN. IDN is an abnormal, although most frequently benign lesion of very frequent incidence and widespread distribution on the human skin. Its nature and origin has been previously reviewed.

The dysplastic changes which may transform IDN into a fully malignant lesion are subtle, gradual, and complex and cannot be clenched together in a single description. With didactic intention, these changes may be split into *cytologic* and *structural*.

Among the *cytologic* dysplastic changes IDN may undergo, it should be mentioned a thickening of the cellular membrane of their integrants, the nevocytes. These develop, in addition, a steel gray cytoplasmic discoloration along with nuclear pyknosis and nucleolar prominence. These changes are accompanied by smudgy cellular limits and a tendency of the cells to loosen their attachment to the main lesion and to spread out toward the BM (Fig. 6.40 and 6.48). Since nevocytes are unable to actively mobilize, it may be assumed that their displacement occurs passively, with help of the lymphatic flow or other agents. An important fact that may also contribute to nevocyte mobilization are the changes their external surface may undergo during the course of their dysplastic transformation: those may permit the nevocytes to detach from structures to which they are normally bound and even allow these to pass through the BM in order to invade the epidermis (Fig. 6.40).

Regarding the *structural* dysplastic changes of IDN undergoing malignant degeneration, the most significant are the loss of their nestiform pattern and their transformation into syncytial masses which tend to disgregate. From all the above stated changes, an intermediary entity results, the nevocytic nevus, dysplastic (NND) (Fig. 6.41).

Figure 6.42 captions the ongoing transformation of a dysplastic nevocytic nevus into a malignant melanoma.

Nevocytic malignant melanoma: The accentuation of the above stated cytologic and architectural changes lead to the final stage of transformation of a dysplastic nevocytic nevus into a nevocytic malignant melanoma (NMM) (Fig. 6.43).

The cytology of the malignant melanoma is varied and deceitful.

It is reduced in some cases to sheets of epithelioid or cuboidal elements with a bland aspect, devoid of either mitotic activity or melanin granules (Fig. 6.44, left), whereas in other cases, it is formed by intercrossing bundles of spindle-shaped elements which may cause the observer to think of a soft tissue tumor (Fig. 6.44, right).

Moderate dysplastic microscopic pictures as mustered in Fig. 6.44 are not the rule in NMM, since its cytology may eventually show a spectacular profile, reaching the limits featured by the most anaplastic neoplasias and presenting, in addition, a heavy load of melanin.

The invasion of the epidermis by the MM leads to the so-called phase of radial or horizontal propagation, in a fashion appropriately nicknamed the "*moth-eaten*" or "*buckshot pattern*" in reference to the nests of neoplastic cells, which appear as "holes caused by these insects or by the pellets of a shotgun hitting its target" (Fig. 6.45).

The phase of horizontal dissemination may be followed by another called "vertical propagation" or "propagation in depth," a development which does not always occur as schematically or in that order. Figure 6.46 features a malignant melanoma simultaneously present in the dermis and the epidermis of the specimen.

Nodular malignant melanoma: This lesion, most probably of nevocytic progeny, does not develop from an IDN or any other superficial structure but seems rather to be coming from the depth. If it represents the extension from an underlying local melanoma or if it corresponds to a distant metastasis from an unknown primary, this is a question still to be answered. Its compact texture, its nodular contour, the outward bending or the pilosebaceous complexes at the periphery caused by its expansion, and its characteristic tendency to ulcerate would favor the second possibility (Fig. 6.47).

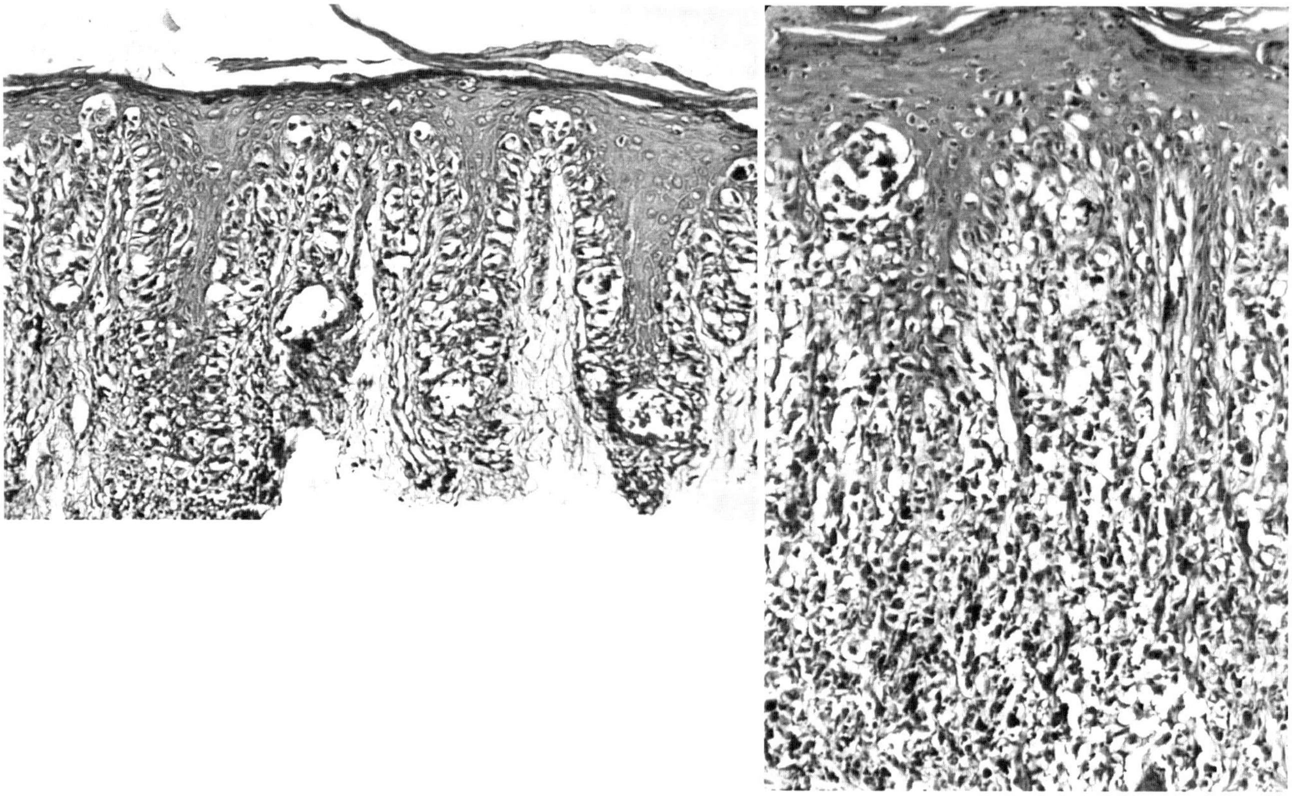

Fig. 6.39 Lentigo malignant melanoma. Note in the lesion to *the left* the incipient invasion of the dermis. Observe in the lesion to *the right* the neoplastic melanocytes "falling as rain drops" from the epidermis and massively infiltrating the dermis and the subcutaneous fat. H&E ×100 o m

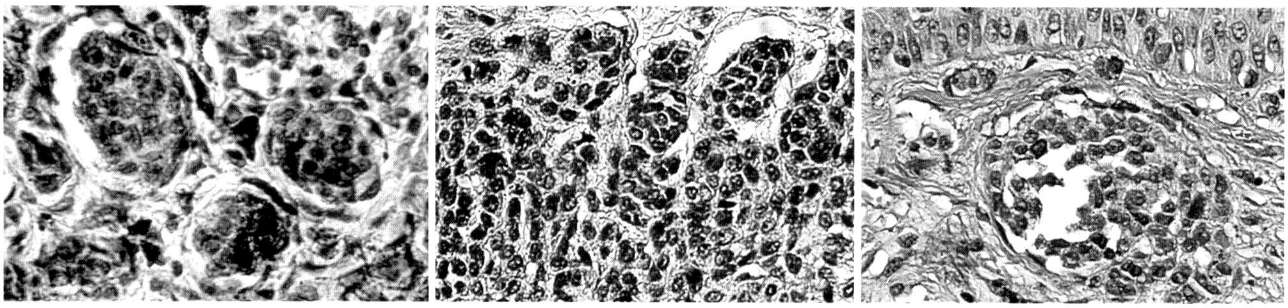

Fig. 6.40 Normal and dysplastic nevocytes. Note the nestiform disposition of the normal nevocytes (*left*), and the loss of this arrangement in the dysplastic ones (*center* and *right*). In the central picture, the nevocytes still show a hint of the nestiform structure, whereas in the figure to *the right*, they are forming a syncytial mass of clearly abnormal aspect, which is approaching the BM. H&E ×100 o m

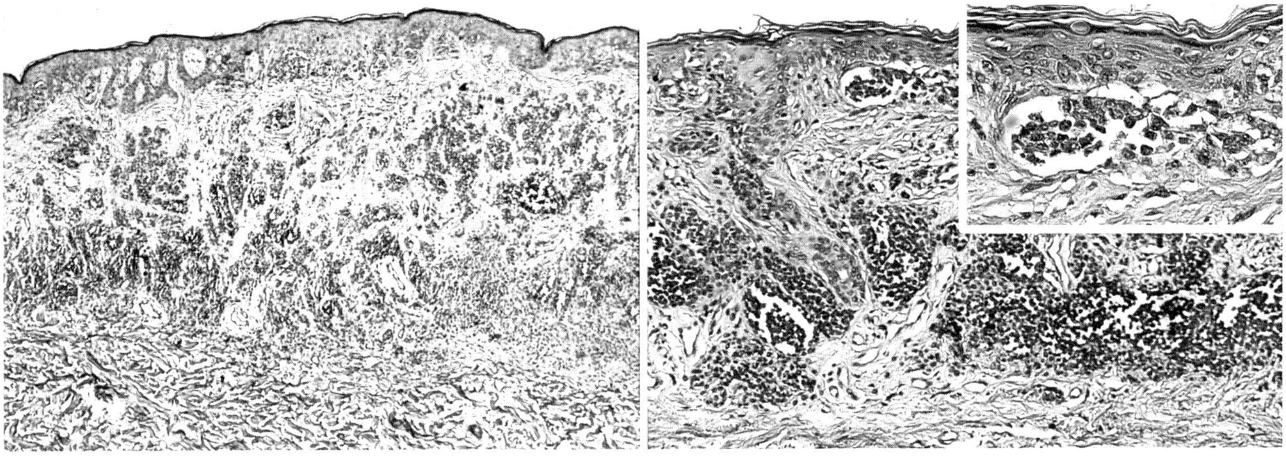

Fig. 6.41 Nevocytic nevi: dysplastic. In the lesion to *the left*, there are remnants of the original IDN in the form of a band of nevocytes in the deep dermis. Above it are scattered isolated or clustered dysplastic nevocytes. In the lesion to *the right*, the malignant transformation has progressed further, and there are groups of dysplastic nevocytes in the process of migration to the BMZ, against which some of these are already impinging (*inset*). H&E ×100; ×400 o m

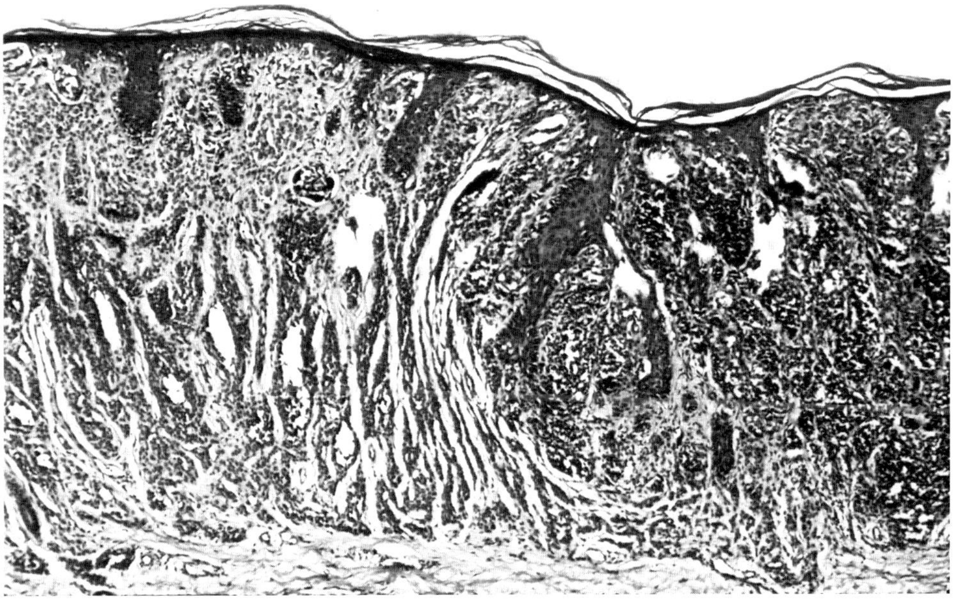

Fig. 6.42 Nevocytic nevus dysplastic undergoing malignant transformation. The left sector of the lesion shows a NND, in which nevocytes are in a cord-like disposition. The right sector of the lesion has lost the organized structure and has been transformed into a solid nevocytic malignant melanoma. H&E ×40 o m

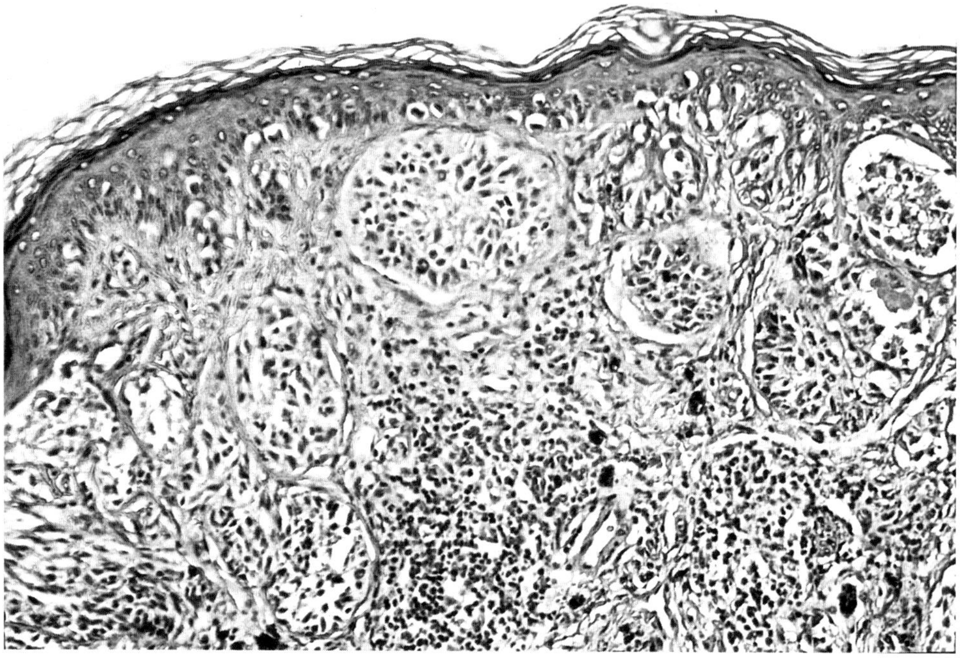

Fig. 6.43 Nevocytic malignant melanoma. The components of the lesion are malignant epithelioid elements, featuring in this particular lesion a low mitotic activity. They are disposed as tightly attached nodules filling the superficial and deep dermis of the specimen. Note that the overlying epidermis appears flat and compressed by the lesion but still uninvolved in the process. H&E ×100 o m

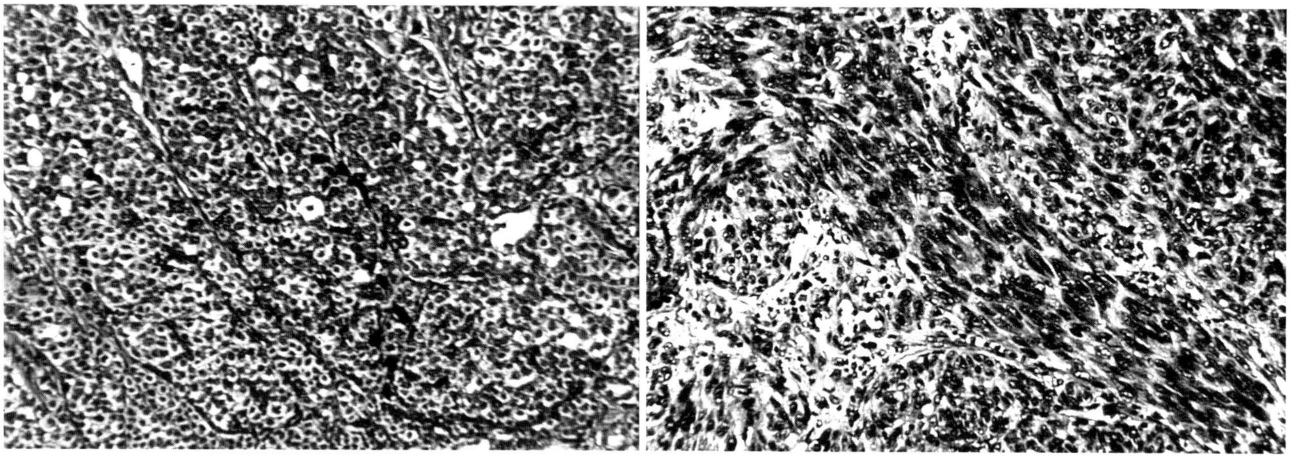

Fig. 6.44 Cytology of the malignant melanoma. The lesion to *the left* is formed by tightly apposed malignant round cells featuring an epithelioid pattern, in which no mitotic activity is noted. The lesion to *the right* is formed by intercrossing bundles of spindle-shaped malignant elements. H&E ×100 o m

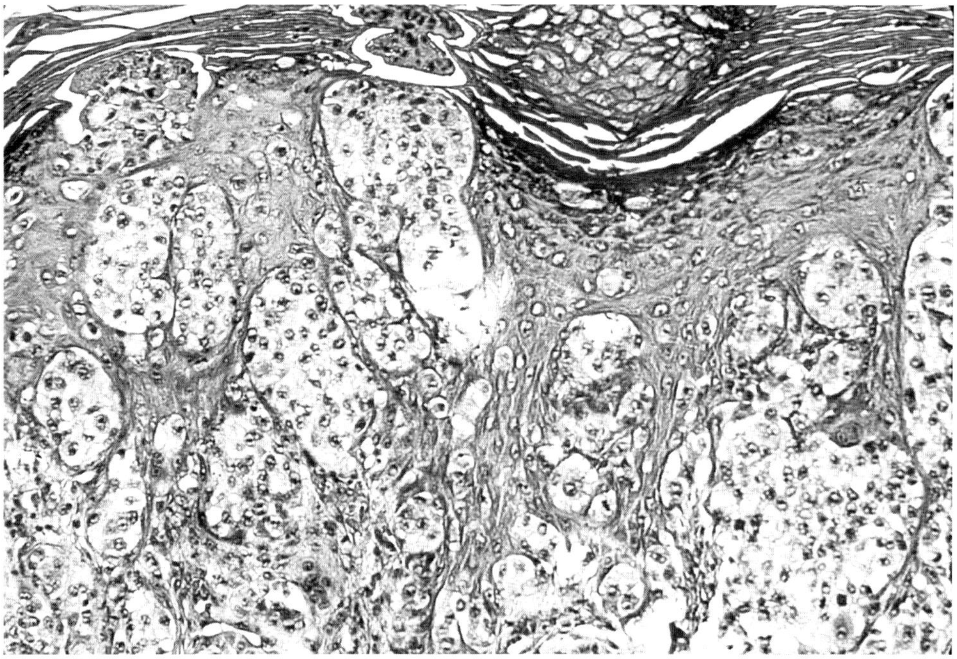

Fig. 6.45 Malignant melanoma in the horizontal phase of propagation. The lesion is present as irregular islets of neoplastic elements spreading within the epidermis in a clear invasive fashion. See further details in the text. H&E ×100 o m

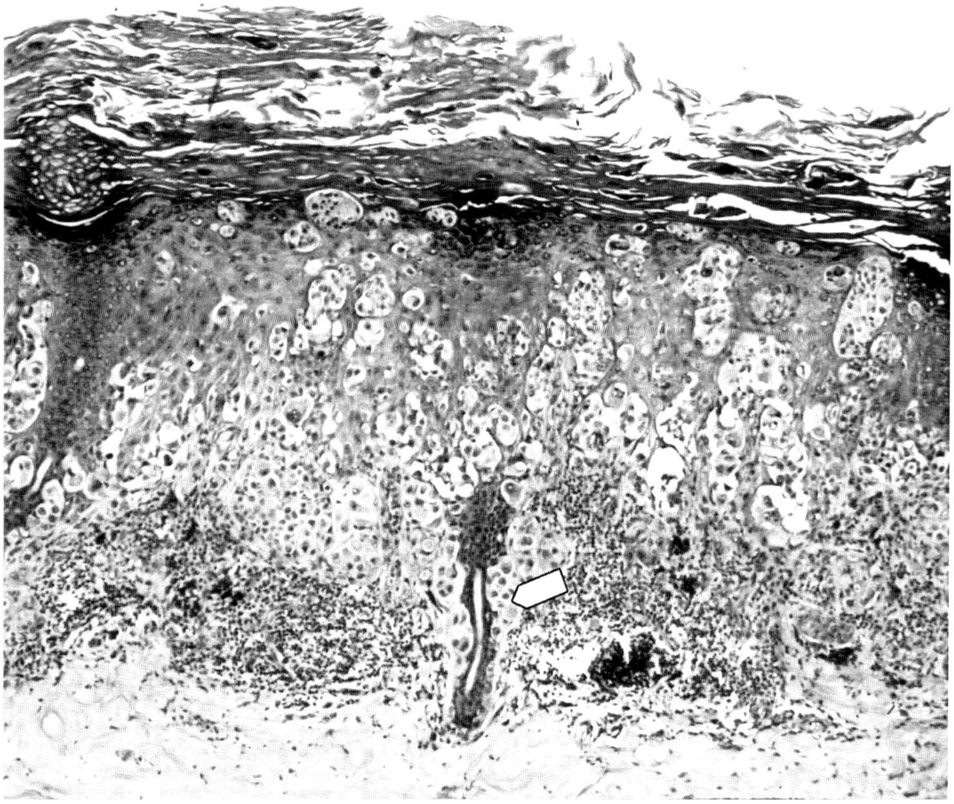

Fig. 6.46 Malignant melanoma presenting simultaneously a clear invasion of the epidermis and a vertical involvement of the deep dermis. The *arrow* points out to a stream of neoplastic cells spreading down along a hair follicle. H&E ×40, o m

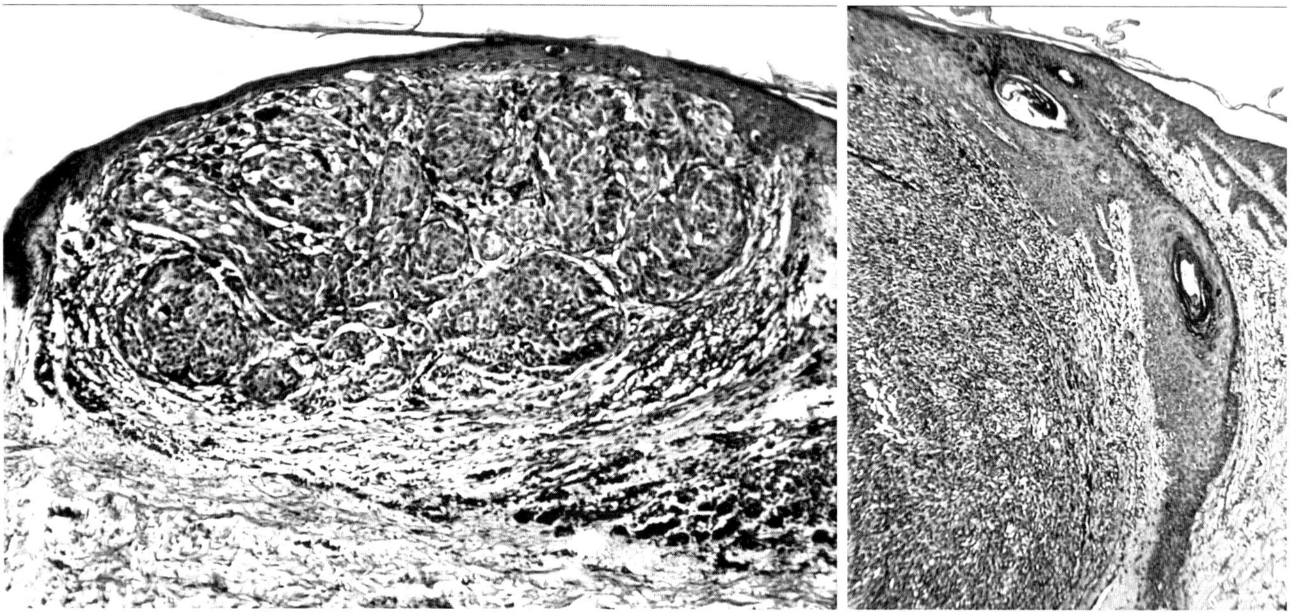

Fig. 6.47 Nodular malignant melanoma. Note at *the left*, the nodular and sharply delimited profile of the lesion. Observe at *the right* the dense cellular population of a larger lesion: this is pushing and bending outward a marginal hair follicle and is simultaneously impinging upon the overlying epidermis, causing its ulceration. H&E ×40, o m.

Comparative Study of Melanocytic and Nevocytic Lesions

The author's ideas regarding the biological cycle of melanocytic and nevocytic lesions exposed below are generally in agreement with those on the dual nature of malignant melanoma, that is, *melanocytic or nevocytic*, initially postulated by Y. Mishima, following the studies of P. Masson (p. 52).

Figure 6.48 is an artistic rendering of the author's conception of the biological cycle of melanocytic and nevocytic lesions. Although largely based on accepted facts in the study of these lesions, and on the observation by the author of a large number of specimens, this conception encloses conjectural elements. Since these cannot be submitted to the rigorous canons of scientific investigation, nor to experimental verification, they confer a speculative character to the conclusions hereby reached which will not escape to the reader.

As shown in the upper rectangle of the figure, upon a benign proliferative process, a group of melanocytes undergo a numeric increase, forming a lesion whose elements are tightly disposed over the BM. This lesion, of totally benign nature, is lentigo simplex. Due to unknown impulses, LS may continue its growth, with production of atypical elements. These, abandoning their linear disposition, tend to heap themselves over the BM, reaching upper epidermal levels. This lesion, still in an intraepidermic position but of a dysplastic character, is the atypic melanocytic hyperplasia or lentigo maligna (LMa). In the last stage of malignant degeneration, the lesion, upon breaking through the BM, penetrates into the superficial dermis and is transformed into a lentigo malignant melanoma (LMM). This landmark is pointed out precisely by the arrow LMM II. In the progress of the invasive process, the lesion increases its "*level of invasion*" from II to V.

The malignant degeneration of the nevocytic lesions (lower rectangle) starts in this drawing with changes on a preexistent benign nevocytic nevus (NN), indicated by the first arrow from the left. These changes lead to a dysplastic lesion, the "nevocytic nevus, dysplastic" (NND), indicated by the second arrow from the left. Through modifications which occur gradually in the period indicated between the arrows NND and MMII, it is transformed into a "nevocytic malignant melanoma level II" (NMM II). As in the case of the melanocytic lesions, the level of invasion of the NMM increases from II to V.

The comparative study of the biological cycle of the melanocytic and nevocytic lesions brings up the differences between them. As already stated, nevertheless, these differences can only be ascertained by the study of early lesions: in advanced lesions, the neoplastic changes obliterate the details which would otherwise have allowed to state the actual melanocytic or nevocytic progeny of the lesion under study.

Summing up, in the author's opinion, *melanocytic lesions originate and develop within the epidermis and only reach a full level of malignancy upon bursting into the dermis through the BM*. Nevocytic lesions, on the other hand, *are generated within the dermis, quite often in IDNs, where they remain*

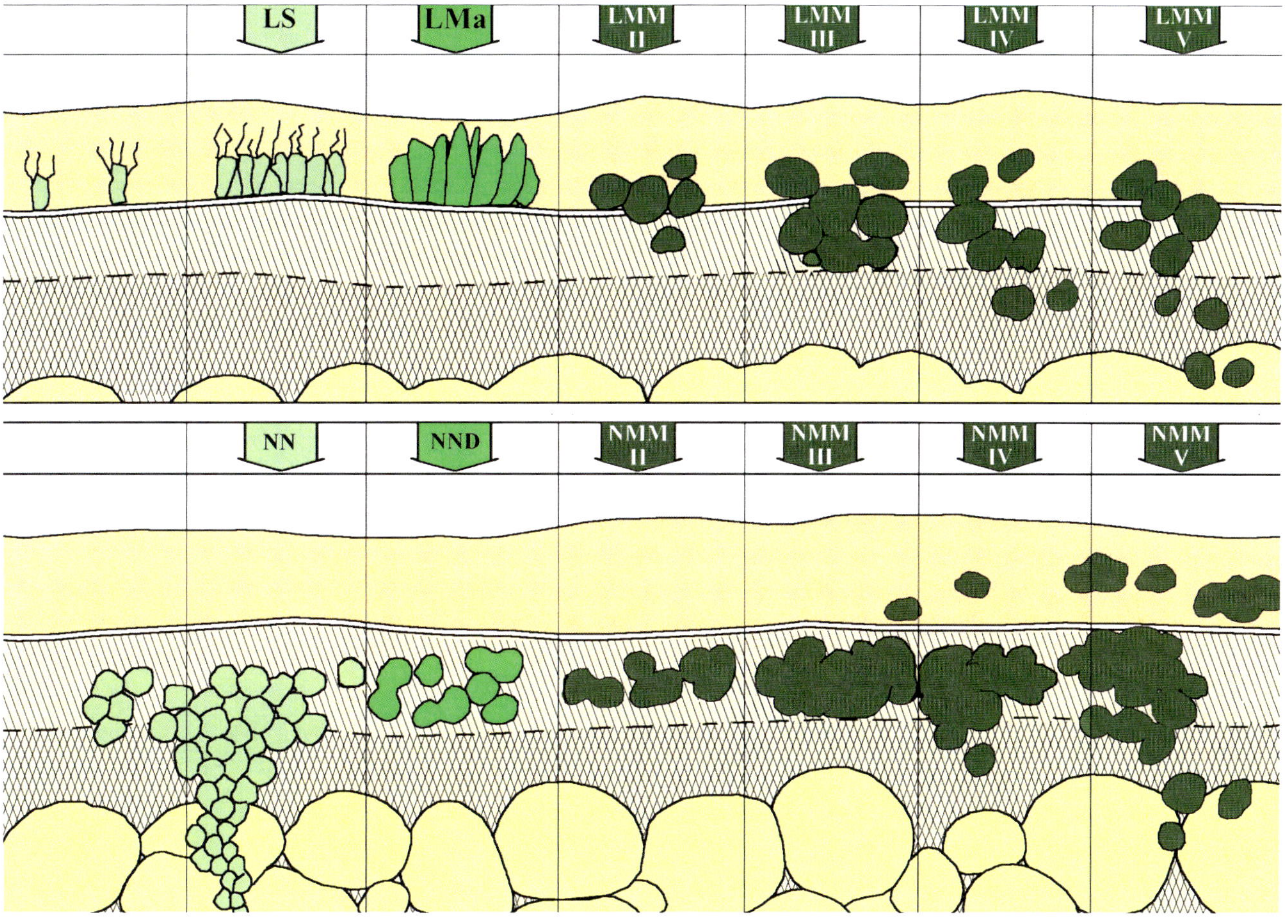

Fig. 6.48 Graphic representation of the author's conception about the development of melanocytic and nevocytic malignant melanoma. In the *upper and lower rectangle* of the figure, a comparable segment of skin is schematically depicted. Same symbols are applicable to the cutaneous elements in both cases: the epidermis is represented as an off-white band and the basement membrane underneath, by a *double line*. The papillary part is depicted hatched in *light pink*, and the reticular part is crosshatched in *darker pink*: they are separated by a *hyphenated line*. Adipose lobules are represented as *light yellow circular* structures. Normal melanocytes and nevocytes are depicted in *light green*; the former, in addition, are showing dendritic projections. The successive change of both types of cells from normal to dysplastic and to full malignancy is indicated by the change in color, from *light to mid green* and then to *dark green*. Additional indications of the progress to malignancy are the loss of the dendritic projections of melanocytes and, for both types of cells, the disappearance of cellular boundaries, with transformation of the cellular masses into solid agglomerates. The initials in the *arrows* in the upper rectangle, LS, LMa, LMM, stand for "lentigo simplex, lentigo maligna, and lentigo maligna melanoma": the Roman numbers underneath indicate the depth of the lesion. The initials in the *arrows* in the lower rectangle, NN, NND, NMM, stand for "nevocytic nevus," "nevocytic nevus dysplastic," and "nevocytic malignant melanoma," whereas the Roman numbers indicate, again, the depth of the lesion

and, through gradual changes, are transformed into fully malignant melanomas. These, secondarily, may or may not invade the overlying epidermis. Accordingly, the diagnosis of LMM relies on a specific detail, that is, *the invasion of a LMa from the epidermis into the dermis*. In the case of the dysplastic nevocytic nevus, its transformation into NMM is simply a matter of gradual intensification of the dysplastic changes, and the diagnosis of the lesion depends on the observer's criteria for evaluating these. Of these changes, the most categoric is the invasion of the epidermis by the malignant cells (Figs. 6.45 and 6.46). This, however, does not happen invariably or as an early event. Therefore, the microscopist must be prepared to formulate a diagnosis of NMM in the absence of epidermal invasion.

Histopathologic Report of Malignant Melanoma

In the case of a lesion such as the one on Fig. 6.39, right, it is licit to use the term "*lentigo maligna melanoma*" for its report, since its histopathologic examination discloses the invasion of the dermis specifically supporting that possibility. Otherwise, in any other case, it is more convenient to report the lesion just as "malignant melanoma," which indicates concisely the primary nature of the lesion, without going into details about its progeny.

Prognosis of Malignant Melanoma

A meaningful prognosis for the melanoma patient can only be issued after careful examination of the excised lesion and a thorough workup of the patient [18]. Nevertheless, the microscopist, based on the examination of the specimen received in the laboratory, may render a preliminary, uncommitted prognosis for the lesion under study based on the two most used parameters for this purpose, that is, the level of cutaneous invasion reached by the lesion at the point of excision, as proposed by W. Clark and/ or the measurement of its maximal thickness as recommended by A. Breslow [19]. The crucial point both methods try to indirectly ascertain is *if the lesion had metastasized before the excision* since that would totally change the patient's prognosis.

Clark proposed five levels of invasion the lesion may have reached at the moment of its microscopic examination: within the epidermis, in the papillary dermis, in the papillary dermis but fully occupying its thickness, in the reticular dermis, and in the subcutaneous fat. Intraepidermal melanomas are appraised as "**in situ**" lesions devoid of metastasizing potential, and melanomas only partially occupying the papillary dermis are also considered devoid of metastasizing potential. For this reason, none of two types of lesion would be expected to affect the patient's postoperative survival. Lesions at the three other level of invasion are considered to display increasing possibility of having metastasized before their excision, curtailing the patient's long-term survival significantly.

Breslow's technique consists of measuring the lesion's thickness directly with a scale attached to the microscope. Lesions measuring up to 0.75 mm stand little chance of having metastasized. Therefore, if they had been totally excised, the surgical intervention should be considered curative. If a lesion measured up to 1.5 mm, it should be regarded in a gray zone, where preoperative metastasis could not be ruled out, whereas if it measured up to 3.0 mm, it must be considered that the patient should already have metastasis at the point of the operation. Finally, if the lesion measures over 3 mm when it is examined, it would be safe to assume that the patient most probably had at that point a metastatic dissemination of the melanoma [20].

Mononuclear Infiltration of the Base of the Lesion

This feature is commonly interpreted as a favorable parameter for the melanoma-operated patient.

Terminology Associated to the Diagnosis of Malignant Melanoma (Alphabetically Ordered)

Acrolentiginous melanoma [21]: This is a clinical term variably interpreted by different authors for melanomas arising peri- or subungually, on the palm or plant, or on other parts of the limbs, provided they show a diffuse blackish discoloration. Acrolentiginous melanoma does not have a histopathologic equivalent.

Atypical melanocytic hyperplasia is a histopathologic term and lentigo maligna is its clinical equivalent.

Dysplastic nevus syndrome: This condition was initially reported by W.H. Clark under the name B-K mole syndrome [22] based on his observation of two unrelated families (B & K), some of whose members presented multiple abnormal nevi with a clear tendency to undergo malignant degeneration. The condition has a clear dysgenetic base which is presently being elucidated. The pigmented lesions in these patients before their transformation into fully malignant ones are called "Clark nevi."

Reed nevus: This lesion is frequently regarded as a pigmented variant of Spitz nevus [23], but since it may display features suggestive of malignant melanoma, it is pertinent to mention it under the differential diagnostic possibilities of that condition.

"Regression phenomenon" is an irregular whitening of the external surface of a melanoma which may lead the observer to believe that the lesion is spontaneously regressing. In fact, the whitening is due to a desmoplastic reaction, and rather than an auspicious sign, it should be considered, if anything, an unfavorable indication for the evolution of the lesion.

Residual nevus is frequently the result of a "*shaving*" excision, which leaves behind the deeper part of the lesion in the dermis. Several months after the operation, a bump may appear on the surface of the operated area, which is frequently regarded as a regrown nevocytic nevus. The microscopic examination of the lesion shows a nevocytic nevus sharply cut horizontally on its upper part, which appears replaced by a scar (Fig. 6.49).

Recurrent nevus is a term used to describe a pigmented spot which appears at the site of the previous excision of a nevocytic nevus. The explanation given to this phenomenon is that melanocytes, dragged toward the center of the lesion during the re-epithelialization process, generate the melanin responsible for the repigmentation of the area (Fig. 6.49, right). The explanation appears valid and can be verified under the microscope, but the caveat must be attached to this interpretation that a closely similar picture may be caused by the subepidermal propagation of a malignant melanoma in the area as shown in Fig. 6.50.

"Satellite malignant melanoma" and "in transit malignant melanoma" are terms which denote melanomas separated from the border of the primary one by less or more than 20 mm, respectively.

Merkel Cell Tumor

The third Subclass of epidermal neoplasias (Fig. 6.28) is formed exclusively by the carcinoma of Merkel cells [24].

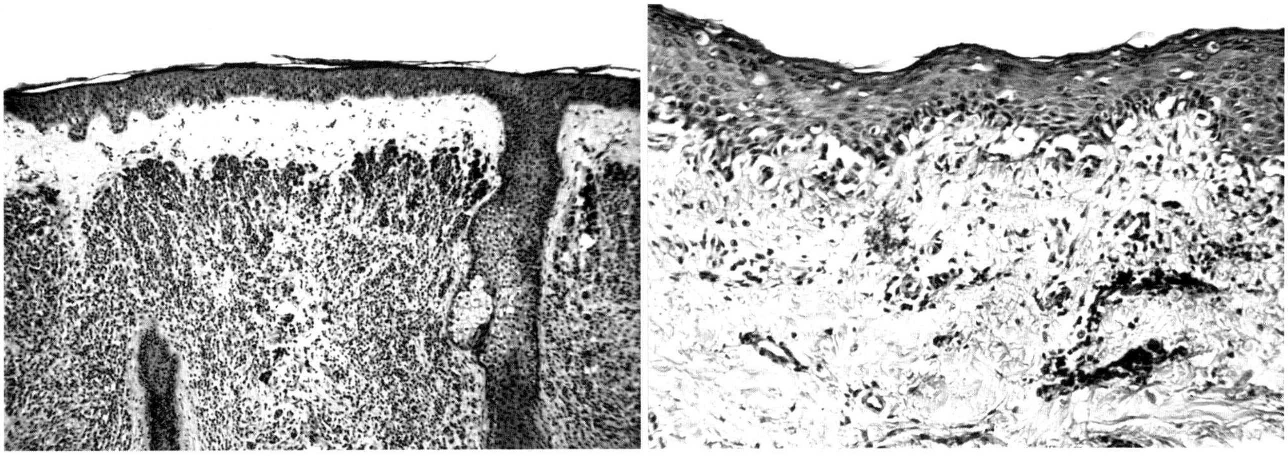

Fig. 6.49 Nevocytic nevus: residual and recurrent. In the residual nevocytic nevus (*left*), a sharp horizontally cut nevocytic nevus is seen, overlaid by a scar covered by a flat epidermis. In the recurrent nevus (*right*), clusters of irregular melanocytes attached to the inside of the epidermis are found in the process of being dragged toward the center of the lesion. H&E ×40; ×100 o m

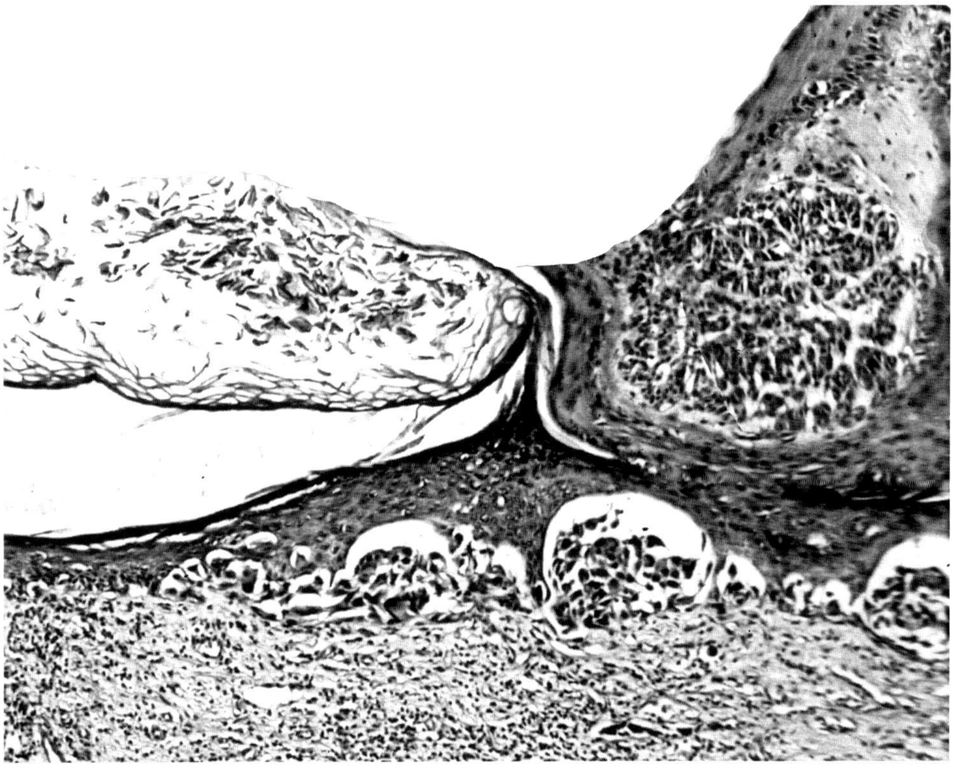

Fig. 6.50 Subepidermal propagation of a malignant melanoma. Note toward *the right* of the figure an exophytic malignant melanoma from which nests of malignant cells are spreading out beneath the epidermis. H&E ×100 o.m

This lesion originates by the proliferation of these elements considered of neuroendocrine nature, reason for which Merkel cell tumor is also known as "cutaneous neuroendocrine carcinoma." Under the microscope, Merkel cell tumor appears formed by cords of cuboidal basophilic cells with blurred contours (Fig. 6.51), being also known as "reticular carcinoma." Merkel cell carcinoma is considered as lesion of aggressivity comparable, at least, to that of malignant melanoma.

Neoplastic Adnexal Proliferations

Neoplastic adnexal proliferations, the so-called adnexal tumors, constitute the second class of the cutaneous neoplastic proliferations (Fig. 6.27).

The class of the adnexal tumors, the "appendage tumors of the skin" [25], is frequently nicknamed the "tribe of the adnexal tumors" because its variegated and confusing character derived from the habit of unrestrictedly including lesions of

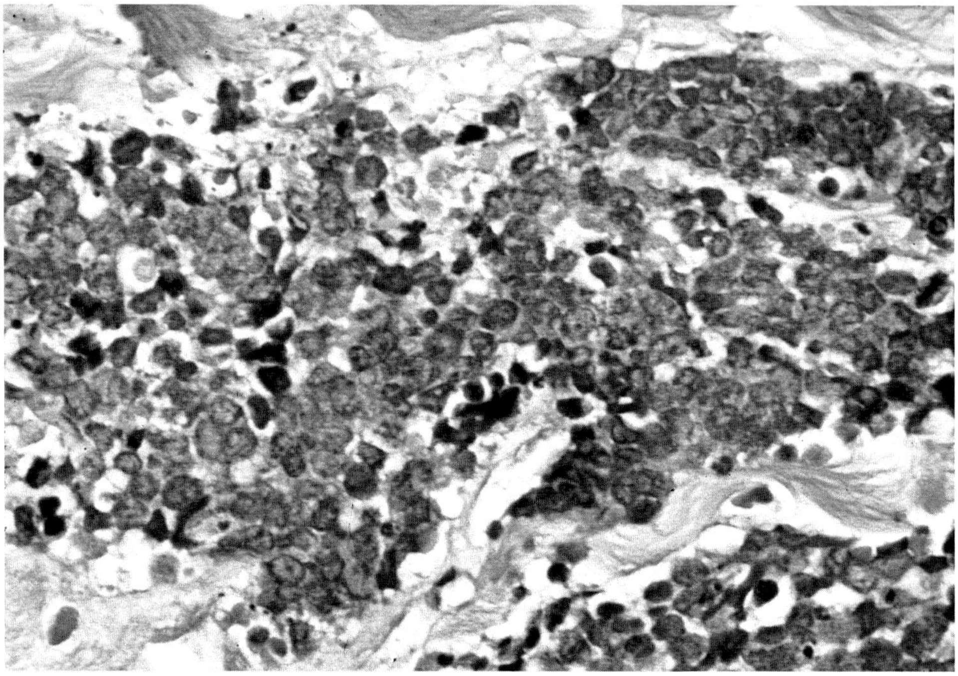

Fig. 6.51 Merkel cell carcinoma. See details in the text. H&E ×400 o m

every sort, such as malformations, reactive proliferations, neoplasias originated outside the cutaneous adnexae, and even inflammatory lesions.

In this text, adnexal tumors are defined as (a) neoplasias, as stated at the beginning of this chapter (p. 127), (b) originated in any of the cutaneous adnexae. These lesions usually present an organoid structure reminiscent of any of these adnexae.

This restrictive definition considerably shrinks the number of integrants of this class of tumors, which may be distributed following the taxonomic approach followed in this text and displayed in Table 6.6.

The Class of the adnexal tumors is separated into two Subclasses, the pilosebaceous on the left half of the table and the tubuloglandular on the right half. The Groups of tumors of each Subclass, follicular and sebaceous and apocrine and eccrine, respectively, are distributed in vertical columns following a tentative topographic approach according to the putative level of the adnexae at which the tumor is supposed to arise. In the Subclass of tubular tumors, below the tubular adenocarcinomas, two lesions are found, cylindroma and spiradenoma, supposedly originated from the secretory coil of either the apocrine or the eccrine gland. Basal cell carcinoma, whose origin is uncertain, is positioned in between the groups of follicular and sebaceous tumors at a midlevel of the two columns.

Insofar as the tumors occupying the niches of Table 6.6, they are prototypic and representative entities of real existence. Adnexal tumors found by the microscopist in the daily practice may be comparatively referred to these for diagnostic purposes, avoiding the copious, redundant, and often misleading nomenclature currently applied to these neoplasias. In fact, it is more important for the pathologist, once he or she has recognized the lesion under study as an adnexal tumor, to assess its malignant potential and its eventual prognosis rather than to find out the name which more accurately fits it

Table 6.6 Class of the adnexal tumors, Subclasses, Groups, and prototypic examples

Adnexal tumors			
Pilosebaceous		Tubuloglandular	
Follicular	Sebaceous	Apocrine	Eccrine
Dilated pore	Cystoma sebaceous	Cystoma apocrine	Eccrine poroma*
Trichoadenoma			Syringomas
Trichilemmoma	Sebaceous adenoma		
Trichilemmoma keratinizing	Sebaceous carcinoma	Apocrine adenoma	Clear cell hidradenoma
Basal cell carcinoma*		Cylindroma*	
Pilomatrixoma			

*The asterisk denotes an eventual hereditary background for the lesion

Figure 6.52 emphasizes structural details of the cutaneous adnexae, which will be of utility in the review that follows.

Pilosebaceous Tumors

The first tumor to be discussed in this context is basal cell carcinoma.

The name basal cell epithelioma was coined at the beginning of the nineteenth century by E. Krompecher [26]. Based on his assumption that this lesion was originated on the *basal*

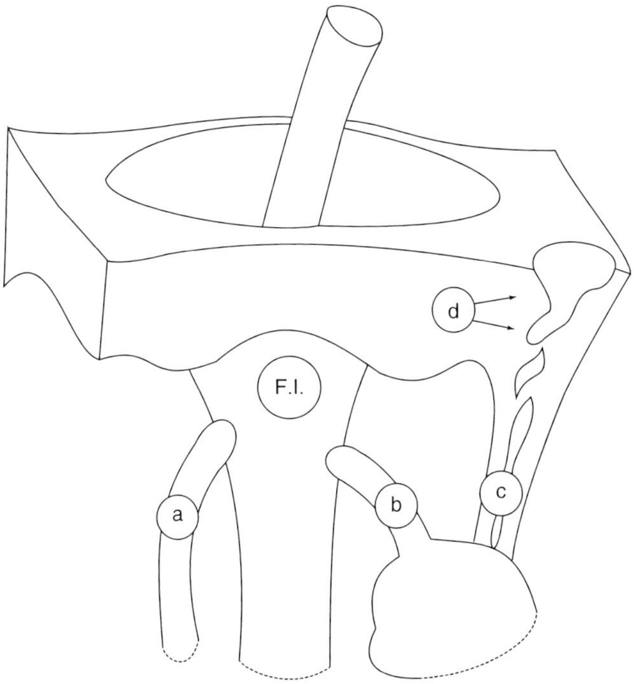

Fig. 6.52 Outlets of the cutaneous adnexae. The excretory duct of the apocrine and sebaceous gland (*a* and *b*) open into the follicular infundibulum (*FI*), whereas the one of the eccrine gland (*c*) does so separately from them, on the external surface of the skin, by means of the acrosyringium (*d*)

cells of the epidermis, which he considered to be different from the upper ones of that layer, he proposed that name. Today it is known that Krompecher's assumption was wrong, but the name he proposed "basal cell epithelioma," or "basal cell carcinoma" (BCC), as it is more frequently called these days, is so deeply ingrained in the literature that no interest exists in replacing it.

BCC, the most common of the adnexal tumors, arises, except in occasional cases, on hair-bearing areas of the skin in males and females, most frequently after 40 years of age. This lesion is formed by small, uniform basophilic elements designated by Pinkus as "basaliomatous cells": these eventually correspond to the cells of the embryonal buds (p. 1). These cells aggregate, forming lesions ranging from isolated, incipient germs attached to the lower aspect of the epidermis to bulky masses visible to the naked eye. The most distinctive microscopic features of BCC are, besides the basaliomatous cells generally devoid of mitotic activity, the presence of cellular palisadings at the periphery of the tumoral masses and clefts outlining them (Fig. 6.53).

The mentioned clefts, although most probably of artifactual nature – due to tissue retraction during processing – are, however, of great usefulness for the LM diagnosis of BCC.

The basaliomatous cells combine with variable amounts of mucin to form a wide morphologic repertoire of solid, cribriform, or pseudoglandular lesions, sometimes with spectacular microscopic features (Fig. 6.54).

The presence of patchy areas of keratinization gives rise to the "basosquamous" or "metatypic" BCC (Fig. 6.55, left), whereas necrotic degeneration of bulky BCC masses causes the central accumulation of debris, lending to these lesions the aspect of comedos, from where the term "comedo-type BCC" obviously derives (Fig. 6.55).

The description of all possible microscopic patterns of BCC does not have an end and nor a practical purpose. There are, however, selected types of this neoplasia which deserve a short comment. In this regard, pigmented basal cell carcinoma should be first mentioned. The LM examination of this lesion discloses melanocytes admixed with the basaliomatous cells: the melanin secreted by the former cells is responsible for the suspicious external pigmentation of the lesion, in which, however, the LM examination may easily rule out the possibility of a melanoma.

Adamantinoid basal cell carcinoma presents angulated basaliomatous cells which make the lesion look like an adamantinoma or ameloblastoma, an odontogenic tumor of the dental enamel, totally unrelated to the cutaneous pathology (Fig. 6.56).

Pinkus premalignant fibroepithelioma [27] is another type of BCC worth of mention since it illustrates the influence of the terrain on the shape BCC may adopt. This lesion, for which the name "Pinkus basal cell carcinoma" is more appropriate since it clearly states its true neoplastic nature, appears on areas of the body, such as the thighs and trunk, particularly the back, furnished with thick skin. Due, perhaps, to the resistance that the fibrotic dermis opposes to the progress of the lesion, this one insinuates as cellular cords crawling between the collagen bundles (Fig. 6.57, left) and expanding whenever tumoral nests find areas of less resistance (Fig. 6.57). A situation comparable to the one in Pinkus BCC occurs in cases of BCC sitting over histiocytomas. Due to the fibrotic consistency of the latter, the neoplasia is unable to penetrate it, becoming deformed to such an extent, that upon LM examination it is sometimes impossible to tell a BCC apart from a rudimentary pilosebaceous complex (see Fig. 6.76).

Sclerosing basal cell carcinoma, a well known variety of BCC, is characterized by threads of neoplastic cells embedded in a fibrous stroma (Fig. 6.58). Because of this fibrotic background, which makes the lesion somehow similar to "morphea" – a condition discussed in Chap. 7 – sclerosing BCC is also called "morphea-type basal cell carcinoma" [28]. This name is, however, misleading, and besides, it does not present any advantage over the term "*sclerosing*," which clearly defines the lesion.

The cords of sclerosing BCC show occasional palisading and peripheral clefts. These, along with the lack of cystic structures, contribute in telling it apart from *desmoplastic trichoepithelioma*. This distinction has important implications

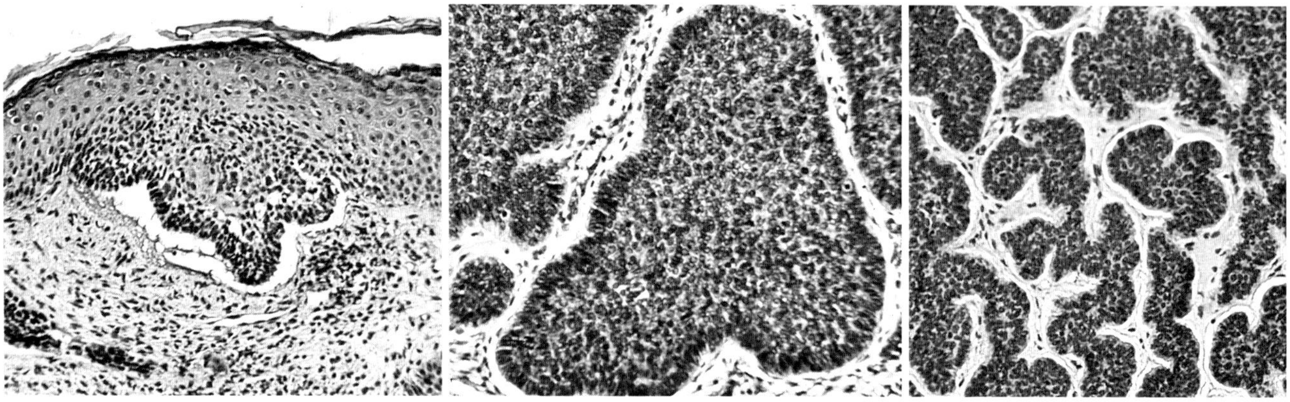

Fig. 6.53 Basal cell carcinoma. Note to *the left* an incipient lesion, in *the center* a solid tumoral mass, and to *the right* a lesion formed by cords of neoplastic basaliomatous cells. The peripheral palisading and the cleft outlining them are visible in the three cases. H&E ×100 o m

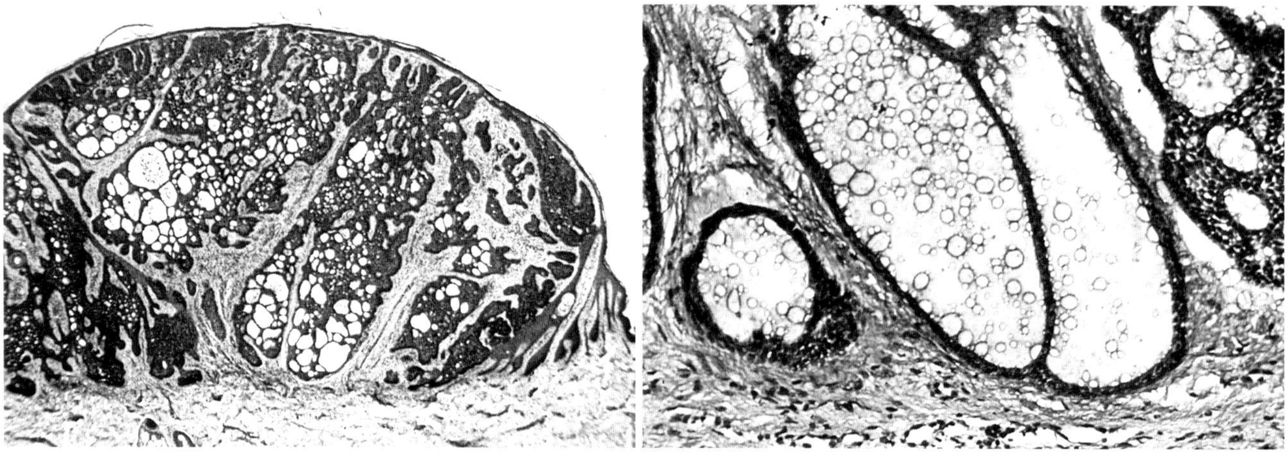

Fig. 6.54 Basal cell carcinoma, cribriform, and pseudoglandular. The resemblance of the lesion to *the left* to a strainer is obvious. The glandular aspect of the lesion to *the right* is provided by layers of BCC surrounding masses of mucin. H&E ×40; ×100 o m

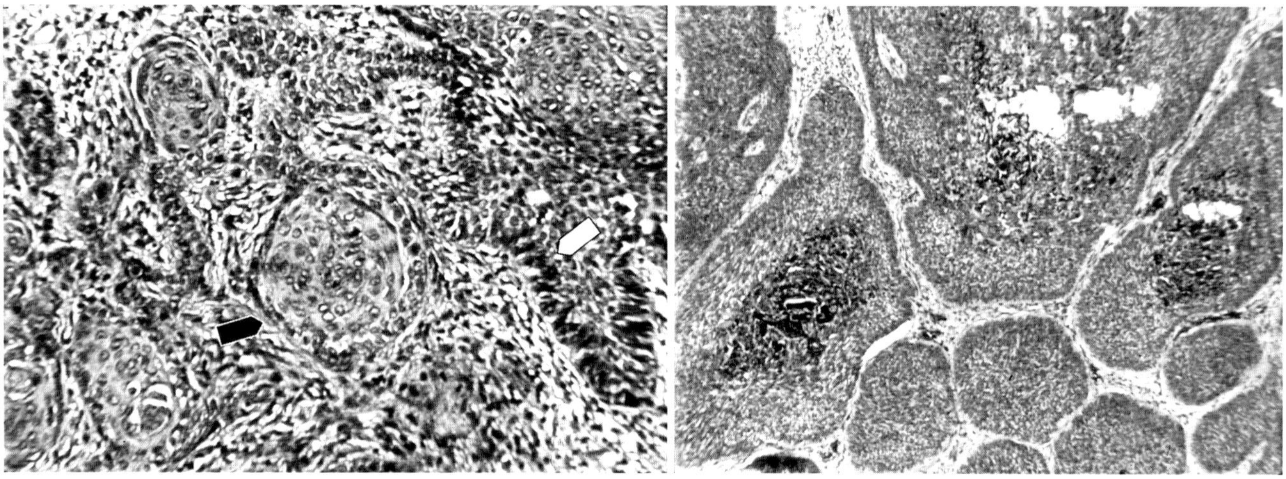

Fig. 6.55 Basosquamous and comedo type of basal cell carcinoma. In the first one (*left*), the peripheral palisading (*white arrow*) and patchy areas of keratinization (*black arrow*) are visible, whereas in the second (*right*), necrotic debris are seen in the center of masses of BCC. H&E ×100 o m

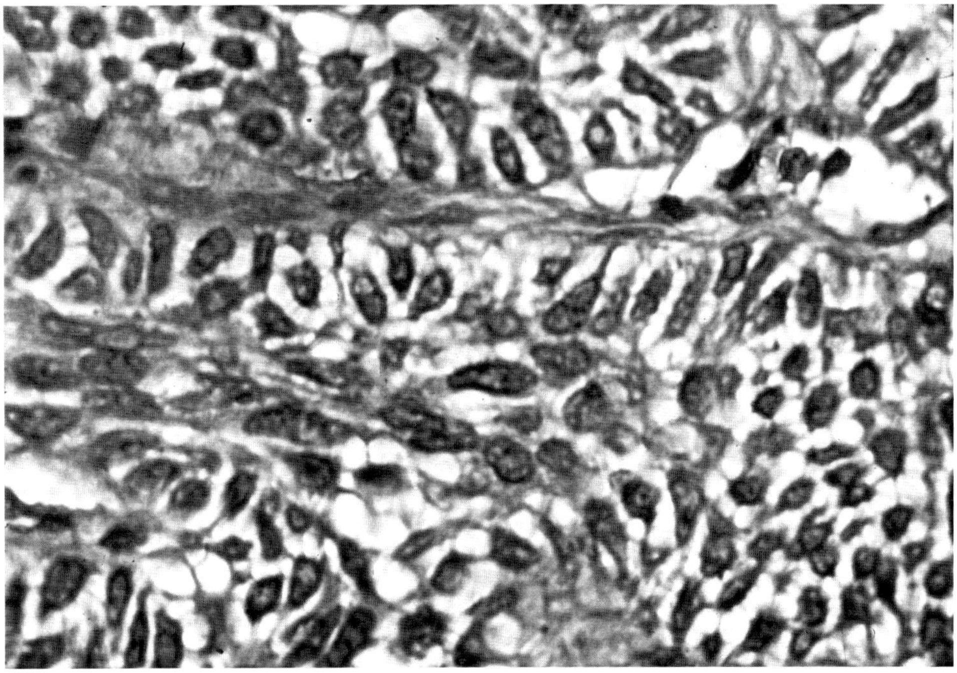

Fig. 6.56 Adamantinoid basal cell carcinoma. Note the angulated basaliomatous cells, clearly different from the current ones of BCC, surrounded by mucin. H&E ×400 o m

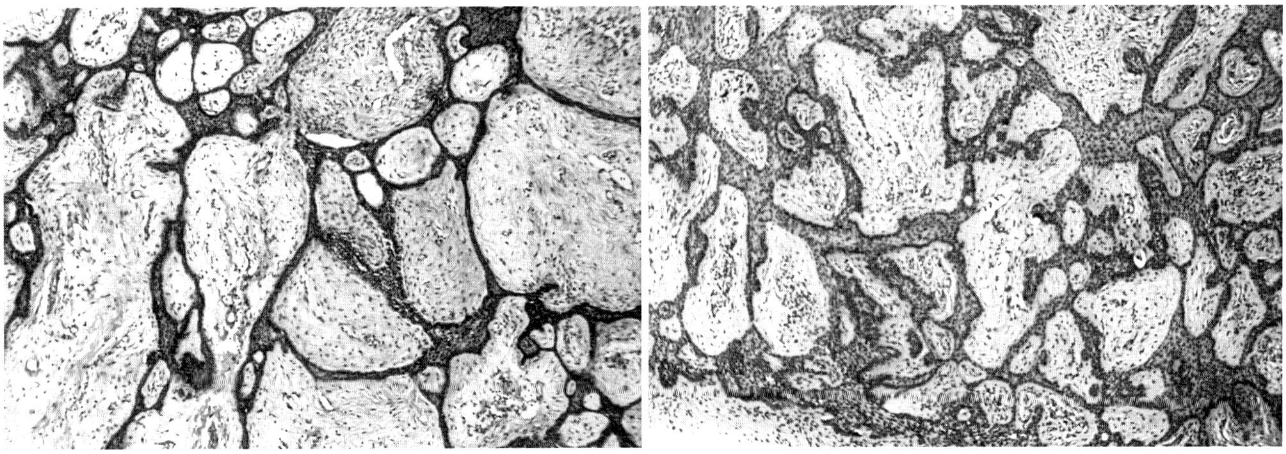

Fig. 6.57 Pinkus basal cell carcinoma. Note the cellular threads insinuating themselves among the thick fibrotic masses (*left*) and their expansion as neoplastic cords (*right*). H&E ×40; ×100 o m

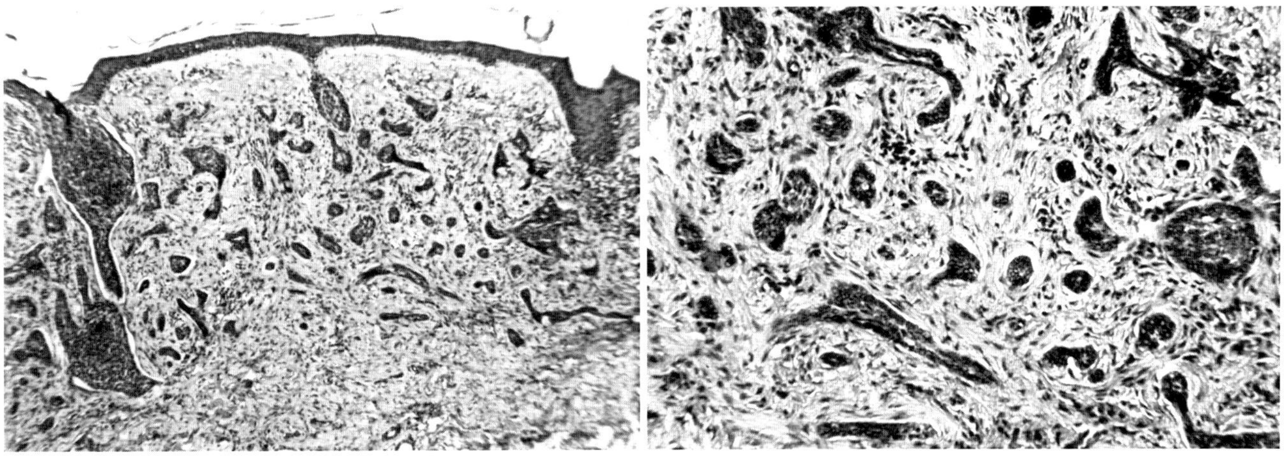

Fig. 6.58 Sclerosing basal cell carcinoma. (*Left*) Note the thread-like neoplastic cords with occasional palisading and peripheral cleft (*right*). These two features and the lack of cysts contribute to differentiate sclerosing BCC from desmoplastic trichoepithelioma. H&E ×40; ×100 o m

since trichoepithelioma is a benign malformative condition, whereas sclerosing BCC is a malignant proliferation with all the troubles these kind of lesions imply. In fact, the neoplastic cords of sclerosing BCC tends to infiltrate the surrounding tissues insidiously, in such a way that makes it difficult for the surgeon to delimit the lesion from the outside, preoperatively. This leads to incomplete resections and to a higher rate of postoperative recurrences, compared with other types of BCC. It is therefore a good practice to add in the report of a BCC, when the lesion warrants it, the qualificative "*sclerosing type*," in order to put the referring doctor on alert against unexpected reappearances of the excised lesion.

BCC associated with diverse hereditary or malformative conditions may present unusual details, not seen in the current forms of this lesion. For instance, in *Bazec* and *Gorlin syndromes* (p. 33), BCC appears at a much earlier age of the patient than usually does, and in the latter condition, BCC may appear on the palm of the hand, in association with keratotic pits. In other cases, the feature which distinguishes the lesion from a current BCC is its association with a determined entity, such as in *nevus sebaceous of Jadassohn*, of which BCC is a later component (Fig. 4.21).

At the beginning of the discussion of pilosebaceous neoplasias other than BCC, it should be remembered that from all the components of the pilosebaceous complex, the hair shaft is an inert structure devoid of vital activity; that the inner follicular sheath disappears early and spontaneously during the biological cycle of the hair; and that the glassy membrane of the outer follicular sheath is an acellular structure devoid of any proliferative potential. Therefore, the three elements of the pilar follicle from which neoplastic growths may be expected to arise are the lining epithelium of the follicular infundibulum, the trichilemma, and the hair matrix.

Dilated pore: This tumor, to which the name of its initial reporter L. Winer is frequently attached, is obviously derived from the follicular infundibulum, whose morphology it faithfully reproduces. The lesion appears V shaped, sending out toward the periphery epidermal projections of minimal invasive capacity (Fig. 6.59, left).

Follicular poroma or inverted follicular keratosis, a tumor not quite different from the above stated, is also supposedly originated in the follicular infundibulum. It shows a uniform thickening of the lining epithelium with a central keratinous structure resembling a miniature hair (Fig. 6.59, right).

Below dilated pore in Table 6.6, in an intermediate position between the follicular and the trichilemmal tumors, is trichoadenoma or Nikolowski's tumor. This appears as multiple tiny cavities which look like cross sections of follicular infundibuli. They are lined by a single row of clear cells yielding a strongly positive PAS reaction (Fig. 6.60).

Insofar as the adnexal tumors originated in the external sheath of the hair follicle or trichilemma are concerned, there is a series of these, ranging from benign to malignant in nature. The first in the series is "trichilemmoma." This is generally a solitary lesion located on the face and scalp, formed by a well-defined mass of large clear epithelial cells, delineated by a thin fibrous membrane. Trichilemmoma, as is the case of normal trichilemma, shows strong positivity to PAS, except in its central part which, after undergoing necrosis, is transformed into an amorphous mass (Fig. 6.61).

Keratinizing trichilemmoma is the next and also fully benign member of this series of tumors (Table 6.6). This lesion is, after BCC, the most frequent of the adnexal tumors. The high incidence of this lesion is masked, nevertheless, by the erroneous nomenclature used to designate it, which includes terms such as "pilar cyst" and "sebaceous cyst." Keratinizing trichilemmoma is *neither "a cyst*," since it is not a hollow, but a solid structure *nor contains sebum*, but keratin. The confusion about the nature of keratinizing trichilemmoma arises from considering it as a *retention cyst*, a lesion that occurs upon obstruction of the outlet of a hair follicle (p. 186).

Keratinizing trichilemmoma, known by the coloquial name of "wen," is not infrequently multiple, appearing on the scalp in the great majority of cases, although it may also be present in any area of the body where follicular infundibuli are present. Upon microscopic examination (Fig. 6.62), this lesion appears as a solid mass limited by a thin membrane lined by a mantle of large clear cells. These cells are similar to the ones of the common trichilemmoma, and in turn, to the ones of the trichilemma. The cells are projected to the center of the lesion, where they are abruptly transformed into hard keratin, *without the interposition of a granular layer*! In the center of the lesion, as frequently happens in tumors of pilar progeny, calcium deposit may be found (Fig. 6.62).

More aggressive members in the series of trichilemal tumors are the ones reported as "proliferating pilar cysts" [29], designated in this text as "proliferating trichilemmoma," and an overtly malignant member of the series is the "trichilemal malignant tumor."

Regarding the lowermost tumor in the column of the pilar tumors, (Table 6.6), that is, pilomatrixoma or "calcifying epithelioma of Malherbe" [30], the general consensus is that this lesion arises from the hair matrix. Its two characteristic microscopic elements are masses of anucleated cells, so-called shadow or ghost cells, and ribbons of small dark basophilic elements that outline these, redundantly called "basophilic cells" (Fig. 6.63).

Regarding the tumors of the sebaceous gland, there are a cystic and two solid varieties [31]. The first is steatocystoma, eventually originated on the excretory duct of that gland, at its merging point with the follicular infundibulum (see Fig. 6.52). The name "*steatocystoma*" is correct, since it adequately describes the *sebaceous* and *cystic* nature of the lesion (*steat* [G] fat+*cystoma* "cystic tumor"). It may be used specifically in connection with the multiple lesions in the hereditary steatocystoma multiplex syndrome. However, in order to point out to the analogy of the *solitary* steatocystoma with its similar lesion placed to its right in Table 6.6, in the column of the apocrine tumors, it is convenient to call both lesions "*cystomas*," the one on the left "*sebaceous*," and the one on the right "*apocrine*." As it was already explained, the excretory duct of the sebaceous gland ends, as the one of the apocrine duct does, in the follicular infundibulum (Fig. 6.52): this would explain the similar morphology of these two cystic lesions referred to here.

Sebaceous cystoma appears under the microscope as a simple cystic cavity with a peripheral membrane lined by squamous epithelium featuring intervening patches of sebaceous tissue (Fig. 6.64, left).

The two forms of solid sebaceous tumors are sebaceous adenoma and carcinoma. The incidence of the adenoma, which may be present in a solitary and a multiple form, as a component of the hereditary Muir-Torre syndrome, outnumbers sebaceous carcinoma.

Sebaceous adenoma: The sebaceous progeny of this lesion is already evident upon its low LM examination. Regarding sebaceous carcinoma, its microscopic diagnosis may offer considerable difficulties due to anaplastic changes which may deceive the observer about its true nature (Fig. 6.65).

Tubuloglandular Tumors

Tubuloglandular tumors occupy the right part of Table 6.6. The anatomic localization of these tumors may give a good hint to the microscopist regarding their apocrine or eccrine progeny: for instance, a tumor on the groin may most probably turn out to be of apocrine nature whereas a tumor on the plant of the foot is most probably eccrine.

Apocrine Tumors

The tumors in this column are headed by apocrine cystoma. This name replaces the confusing one, frequently given to this tumor, "apocrine hidrocystoma," a term which implies in its first part that the tumor is of *apocrine* nature, whereas in its second part suggests that it is of *eccrine* progeny (*hidros* [G] sweat). Apocrine cystoma was already comparatively mentioned in connection to its counterpart, *sebaceous* cystoma. Both are simple cystic structures, the one featuring patches of sebaceous tissue (Fig. 6.64, left) and the other areas of cylindric, apocrine epithelium (Fig. 6.64, center and right).

Below apocrine cystoma, there are several lesions, all of them characterized by the presence of rows of tall epidermal cells featuring the already mentioned "apocrine decapitation." As a prototypic one, tubular apocrine adenoma described by M. Landry and R. Winkelman [32] was selected. This is a cystic structure lined by a double-layered epithelium formed by a basal row of cuboidal cells overlaid by an upper one of cylindric elements displaying apocrine decapitation (Fig. 6.66).

The lesion may present a more proliferative tendency, throwing the epithelium into the central cavity and giving rise to an intracanalicular apocrine adenoma variety or spreading otherwise into the periphery, featuring the infiltrating apocrine adenoma.

The "nipple erosive adenomatosis" is a special form of tubular apocrine adenoma, known in breast pathology as "florid papillomatosis of the nipple" [33]. This lesion originates in the local apocrine glands of this organ and is covered by an eroded and crusted epidermis. The glands are lined by a double-layered epithelium with decapitation features, projecting folds toward the lumen of the tubule where they intercross, featuring "cart wheel" figures (Fig. 6.67).

Regarding Moll's gland cyst, this is a cystic adenoma of the modified apocrine glands of the eyelid, that is, Moll's glands.

Tubular adenocarcinoma is the malignant form of any of the mentioned apocrine glands, but the name also applies to malignant tumors of the eccrine glands (Table 6.6).

Eccrine Tumors

Upon glancing comparatively at Table 6.6, the absence of a cystoma as the uppermost lesion in the eccrine gland column will be noted. This one has been replaced by eccrine poroma, derived from the acrosyringum, that is, the structure through which the eccrine excretory duct opens onto the skin surface (see Fig. 6.52).

Eccrine poroma, described by H. Pinkus [34], is a lesion in direct continuation with the epidermis, formed by small monotonous round cells, spreading into the dermis and surrounding bulky masses of richly vascularized and edematous stroma very characteristic of this lesion (Fig. 6.68).

Intraepidermal poroma is a variety of eccrine poroma restricted to the epidermis (Fig. 6.69, left), whereas malignant eccrine poroma (Fig. 6.69, right) is the most aggressive variety of the lesion, with marked invasive potential.

In the line of the eccrine tumors exists a series of lesions supposedly derived from the excretory duct of the gland: these are the "syringomas" [35] (*syrinx* [G] a tube), all of them featuring a tubular character. The prototypic lesion here is the plain syringoma. This is predominantly localized on the face, showing under the microscope cross sections of excretory ducts of variable diameter, lined by single-cell layers of clear elements. The presence in the lumen of the tubules of droplets of inspissated secretion must be mentioned as a distinctive feature of the lesion (Fig. 6.70).

These cysts help to differentiate desmoplastic syringoma both from the sclerosing BCC which lacks these and from desmoplastic trichoepithelioma whose cysts contain laminated keratin.

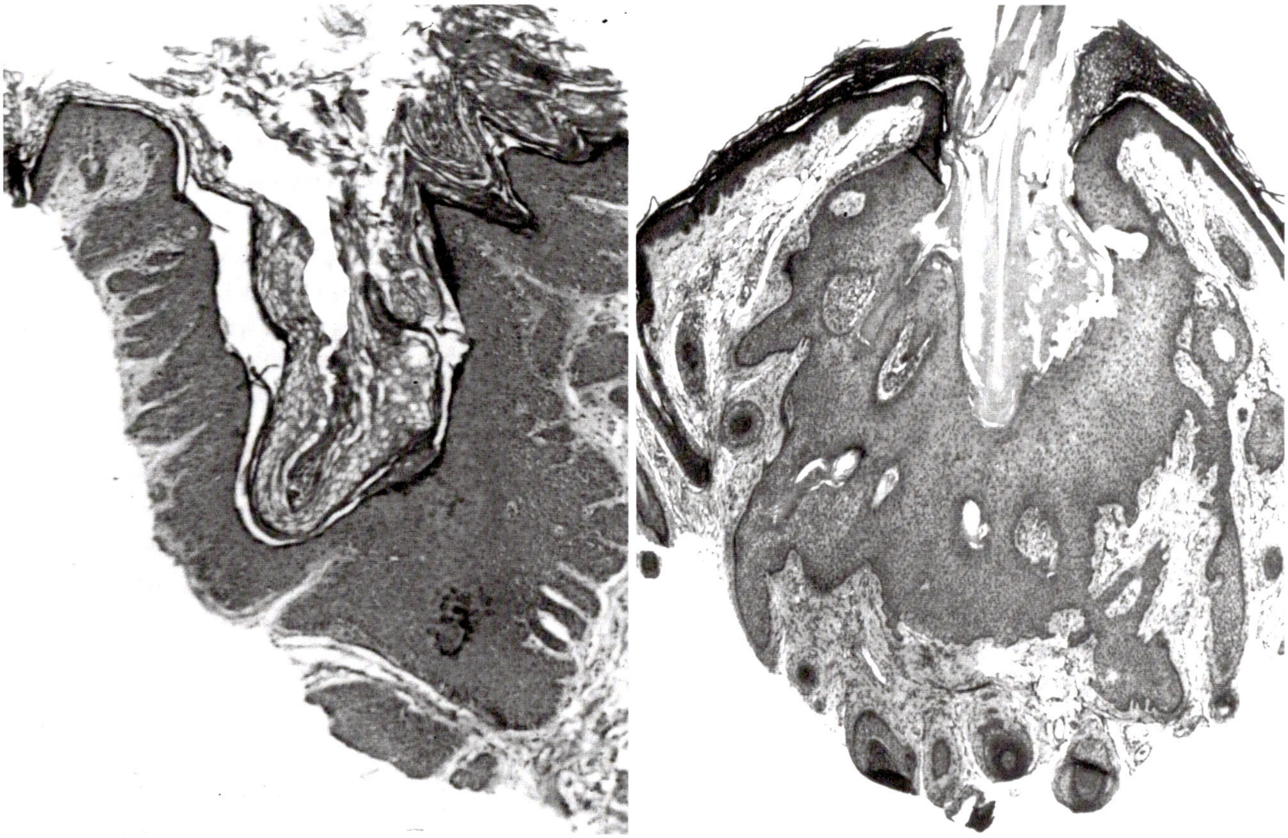

Fig. 6.59 Dilated pore and follicular poroma. Note in the first one (*left*) the thick epithelium which lines it and the digitations it projects toward the periphery. Observe in the second one (*right*) the uniform proliferation of the lining epithelium of the lesion and the presence in it of a rudimentary hair. H&E ×40 o m

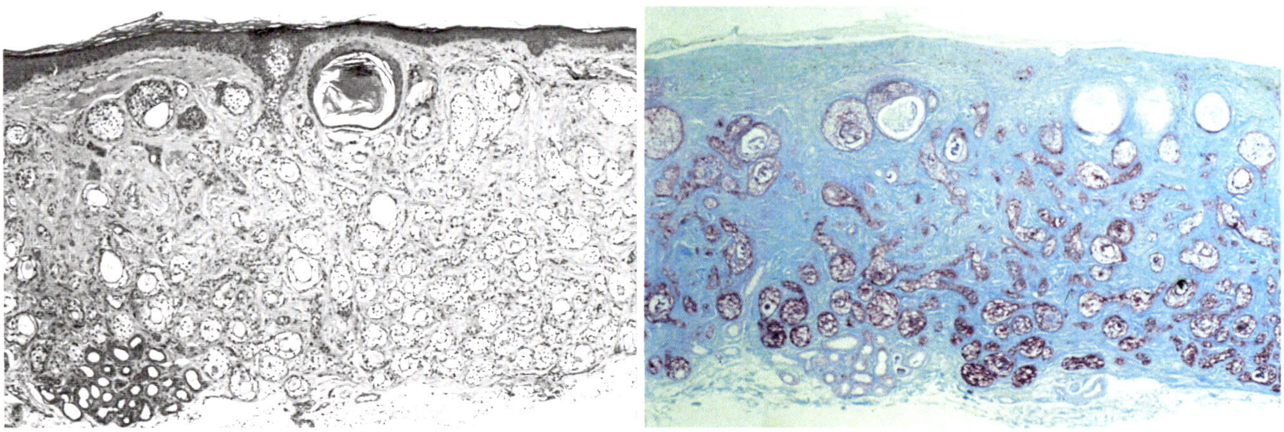

Fig. 6.60 Trichoadenoma. Note the numerous cavities lined by single rows of clear cells (*left*). These yield a strongly positive PAS reaction (*right*). H&E ×40; PAS ×40 o m

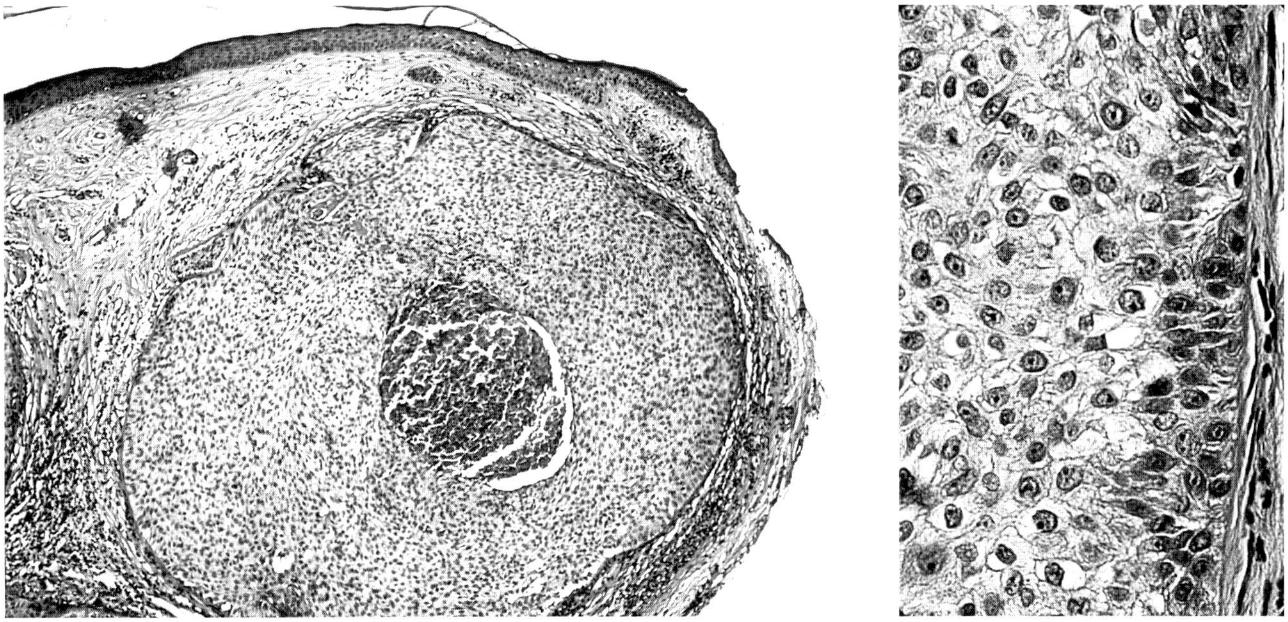

Fig. 6.61 Trichilemmoma. The tumor (*left*) has a uniform composition of large clear cells which yield a strongly positive PAS response. (*Right*) Observe the tumor wall at higher magnification. Note the large clear cells and the thin external membrane of the wall at the extreme right. H&E ×40; ×100 o m

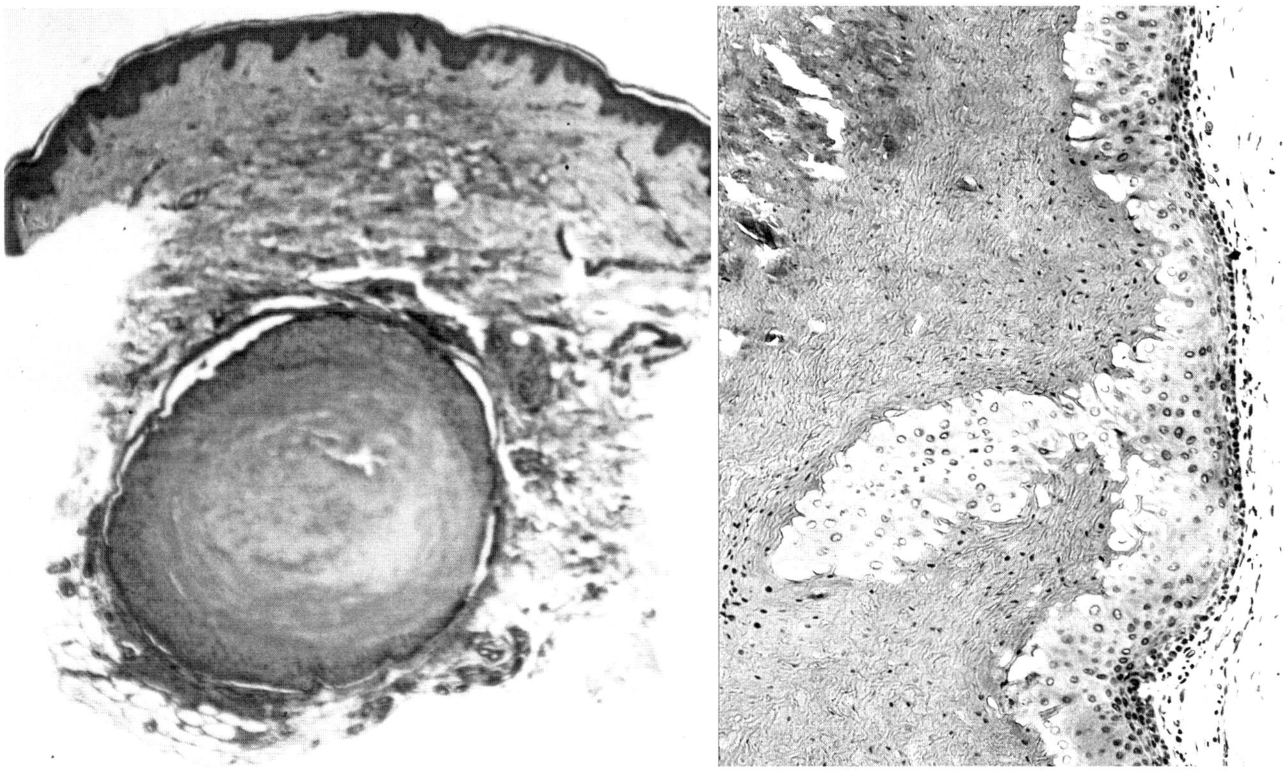

Fig. 6.62 Keratinizing trichilemmoma. At low magnification (*left*), the lesion, sharply delimited from the surrounding tissues, shows a solid aspect. At higher magnification (*right*), it appears lined by a mantle of large clear cells projected into its cavity, where they are transformed into solid keratin without interposition of a granular layer. Note the calcium deposits at the *left upper corner* of the figure. H&E ×40; ×400 o m

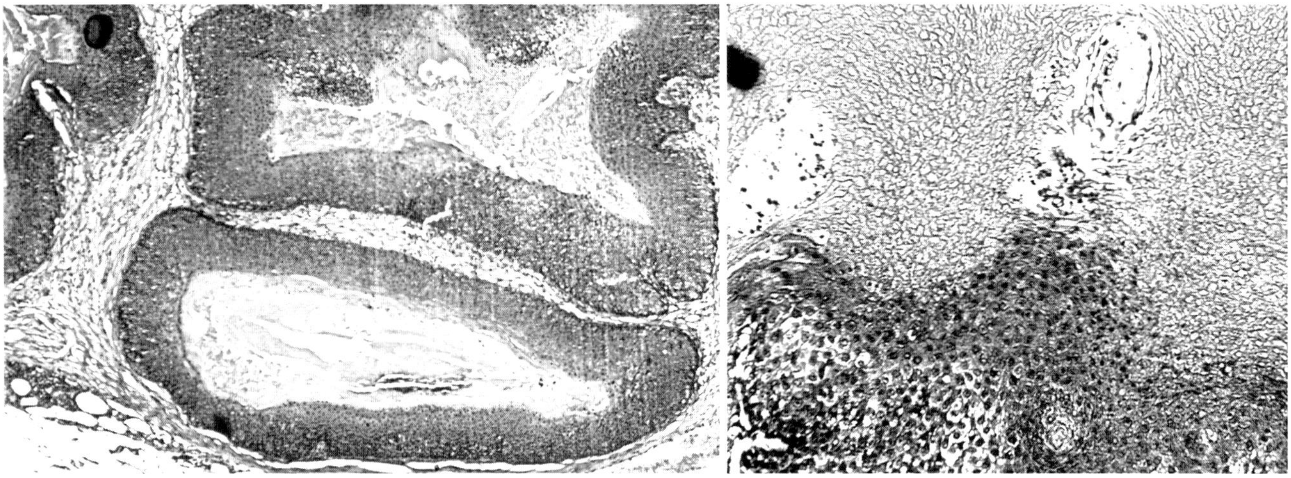

Fig. 6.63 Pilomatrixoma. (*Left*) The bands of "basophilic cells" are disposed around masses of anucleated "ghost cells." (*Right*) The picture illustrates the transition from the basophilic to the ghost cells of the lesion; note the lack of nuclei in the latter ones. H&E ×40; ×400 o m

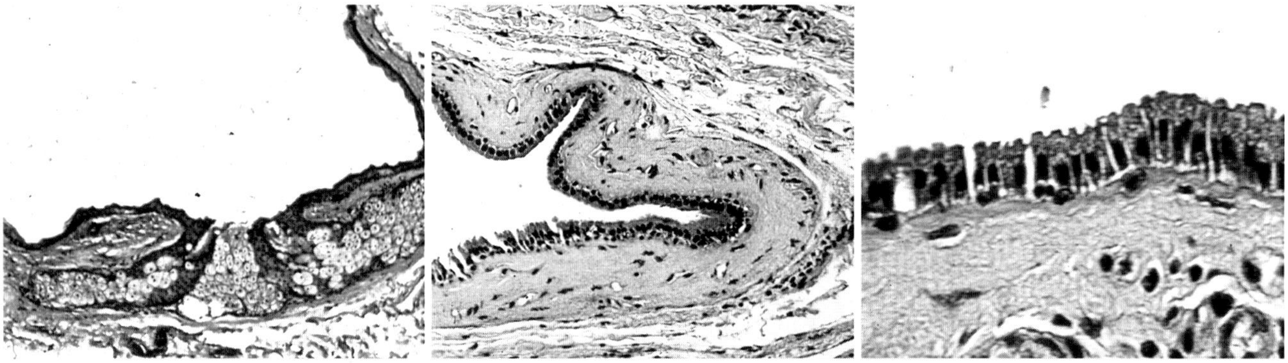

Fig. 6.64 Cystoma: sebaceous and apocrine. Note the simple cystic structure of both lesions (*left* and *center*). The one to the left features patches of sebaceous tissue on its wall, whereas the other (*center*) shows apocrine glands, presented at higher magnification to *the right*. H&E ×40; ×40; ×100 o m

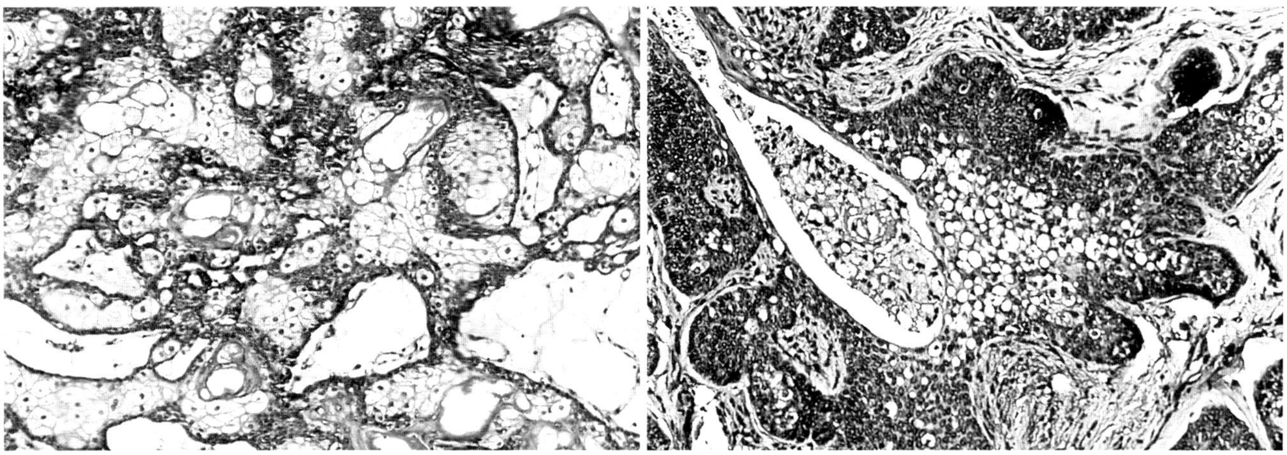

Fig. 6.65 Sebaceous adenoma and carcinoma. The progeny and diagnosis of the first (*left*) may be ascertained directly at low LM examination. In the case of the second one (*right*), the regressive changes in the lesion complicate its LM recognition, which may be observed in patchy areas with sebaceous differentiation. H&E ×40 o m

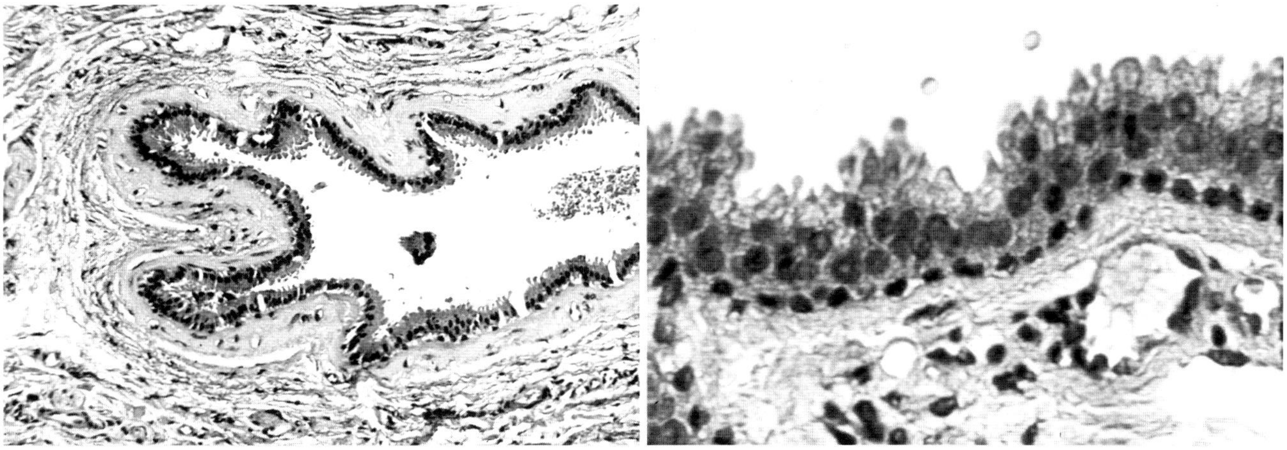

Fig. 6.66 Tubular apocrine adenoma. The lesion (*left*) presents a central cavity lined by a characteristic double-layered epithelium of cuboidal and cylindric cells. Note at higher magnification (*right*) the "decapitation features" on the free border of the epithelium. H&E ×40; ×400 o m

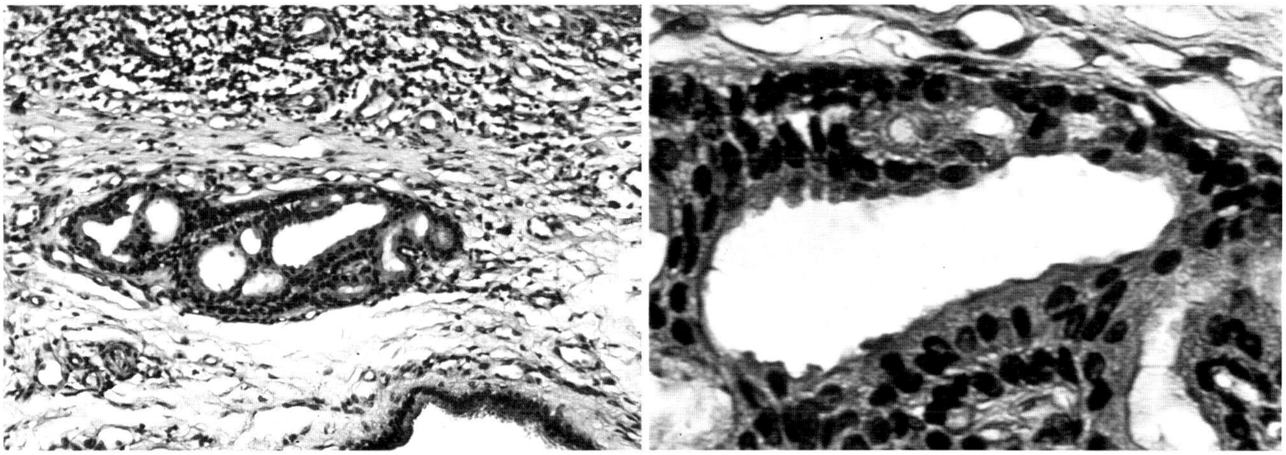

Fig. 6.67 Florid papillomatosis of the nipple. (*Left*) Observe the tubules lined by a double-layered epithelium thrown into the lumen and intercrossed with similar ones. Note at higher magnification (*right*) the secretory quality of the epithelium. H&E ×40, ×400 o m

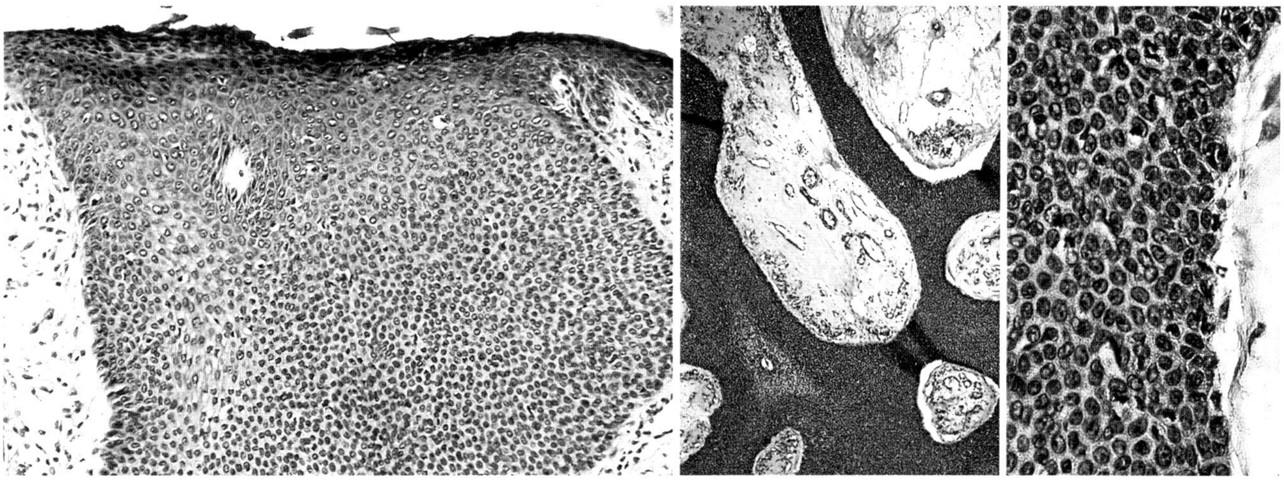

Fig. 6.68 Eccrine poroma. (*Left*) The lesion spreads out from the epidermis, with which it is in direct continuation. (*Center*) Upon its progression into the dermis the lesion surrounds bulky masses of edematous stroma. (*Right*) Note at higher magnification the monotonous character of the small, round cells of the tumor. H&E ×100; ×40; ×400 o m

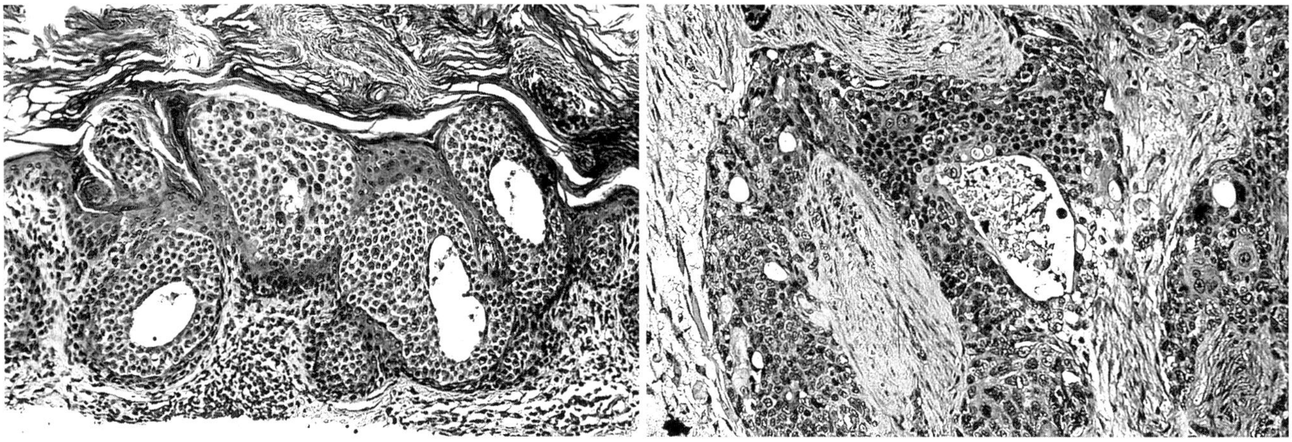

Fig. 6.69 Intraepidermal and malignant eccrine poroma. Note the intraepidermic position of the first one (*left*) formed by cystic cavities layered by mantles of small, uniform cells. Observe the dysplastic character of the second (*right*), which still maintains a cystic structure. H&E ×100 o m

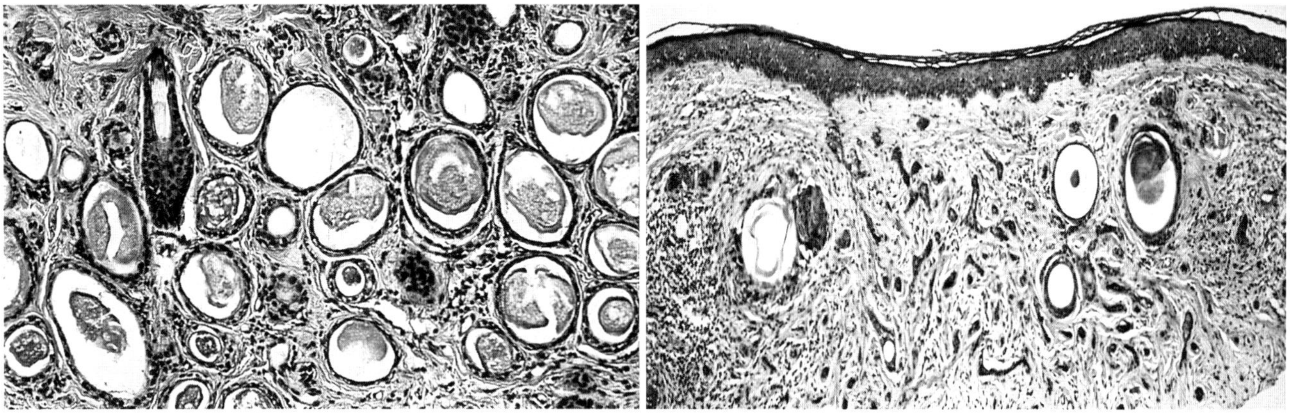

Fig. 6.70 Syringoma and desmoplastic syringoma. See in the first one (*left*) the large cystic cavities lined by a single layer of low clear cells and containing an homogeneous eosinophilic material, and in the second one (*right*) the tubules of the lesion compressed by the dense fibrous stroma into thread-like structures and occasionally expanded into cystic spaces containing the same material noted before. H&E ×100 o.m

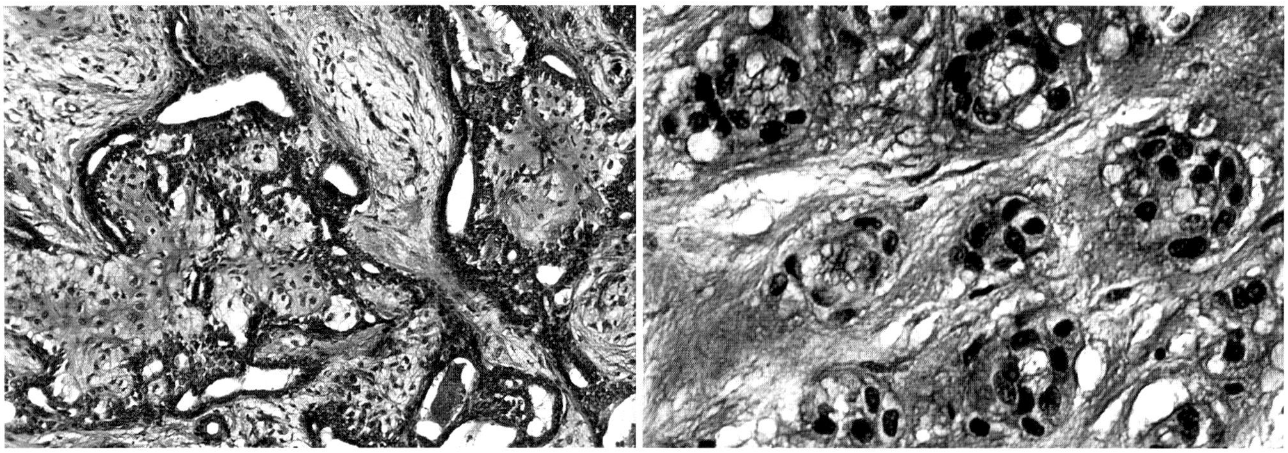

Fig. 6.71 Chondroid syringoma. (*Left*) Note the tubular elements of the lesion enmeshed in a cartilaginous matrix. (*Right*) Observe details of the lesion at higher magnification. PAS ×40; ×400 o m

The existence of a multiple, hereditary variety of syringoma must be mentioned, of microscopic features undistinguishable by LM from the plain syringoma discussed before.

Chondroid syringoma [36] shows a characteristic cartilaginous matrix (Fig. 6.71) which makes it closely similar under the microscope to mixed tumor of the salivary gland [37], a well-known tumor in general pathology.

Upon reviewing the pathology of syringomas, the existence of an aggressive variety of this lesion, "infiltrating syringoma," is worth mentioning. It is able to invade the surrounding tissues, as well as produce distant metastasis (Fig. 6.72).

Below the syringomas in Table 6.6 is the lesion described by E.D. Helwig as eccrine acrospiroma [38]. This name tends to be replaced by "clear cell hidroadenoma," which facilitates its comparison with its apocrine counterpart, *apocrine tubular adenoma*, positioned in the column at its left. The lesion appears formed by large clear cells with pyknotic, punctiform nuclei covering the wall of the secretory conducts as a single cellular layer (Fig. 6.73, left). Occasionally, these cells heap into papillary formations thrown into the cavity of the conducts (Fig. 6.73, right).

Tumors of the Secretory Coil

In this systematic review of the tubular adnexal tumors, the ones believed to be derived from the secretory coil of any of the two tubular glands should be discussed.

Cylindroma is the first of the duo. The origin of this tumor is controversial: whereas it is generally assumed to be of apocrine or eccrine nature, some opinions have been even exteriorized in favor of a pilar origin for it [39]. This lesion occurs most frequently on the scalp, in a solitary or a multiple, hereditary form. The last form, because of the hypertrophic deformation it produces on the patient's scalp, has been named "turban tumor." The microscopic picture of this lesion is striking, appearing as a solved jigsaw puzzle, with many interlocked, polygonal islets surrounded by a hyaline membrane. The islets are formed by small pyknotic elements located at the periphery and surrounding larger clear cells disposed in the center of the islets (Fig. 6.74).

Spiradenoma or eccrine spiradenoma [40] is the second member of this group, admittedly of eccrine origin. The circumstance that this lesion presents pain as a clinical symptom qualifies it as a member of the already mentioned group of painful tumors of the skin.

Under the microscope, spiradenoma is a densely cellular and sharply delimited lesion which not infrequently presents several smaller satellite lesions. The lesions are formed by tightly coiled cords with a dual cell population of dark and clear cells disposed around narrow and frequently branched ducts. These microscopic details are difficult to be discerned in the densely cellular central areas of the lesion but may be evident at the periphery, where the lesion shows a looser disposition (Fig. 6.75).

Neoplastic Mesenchymal Proliferations

The third Class of cutaneous neoplasias posted in Fig. 6.27 are the one of the mesenchymal or soft tissue tumors (Fig. 6.27). This Class contains five Subclasses which are the neoplasias of fibrohistiocytic, muscular, vascular, and adipose tissue, and the ones of peripheral nerves (Table 6.7). The Subclass of peripheral nerves is actually conventionally included in this Class since peripheral nerves cannot be considered as "soft tissue" [41].

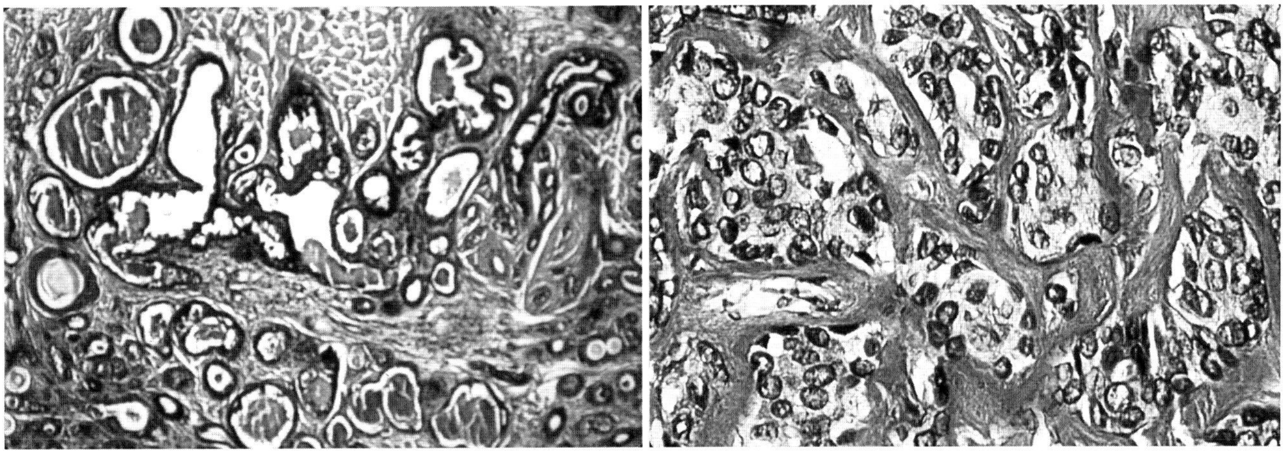

Fig. 6.72 Infiltrating syringoma. (*Left*) The lesion is in the process of actively invading the surrounding tissues. (*Right*) At higher magnification, the anaplastic character of the lesion is evident. H&E ×40; ×400 o m

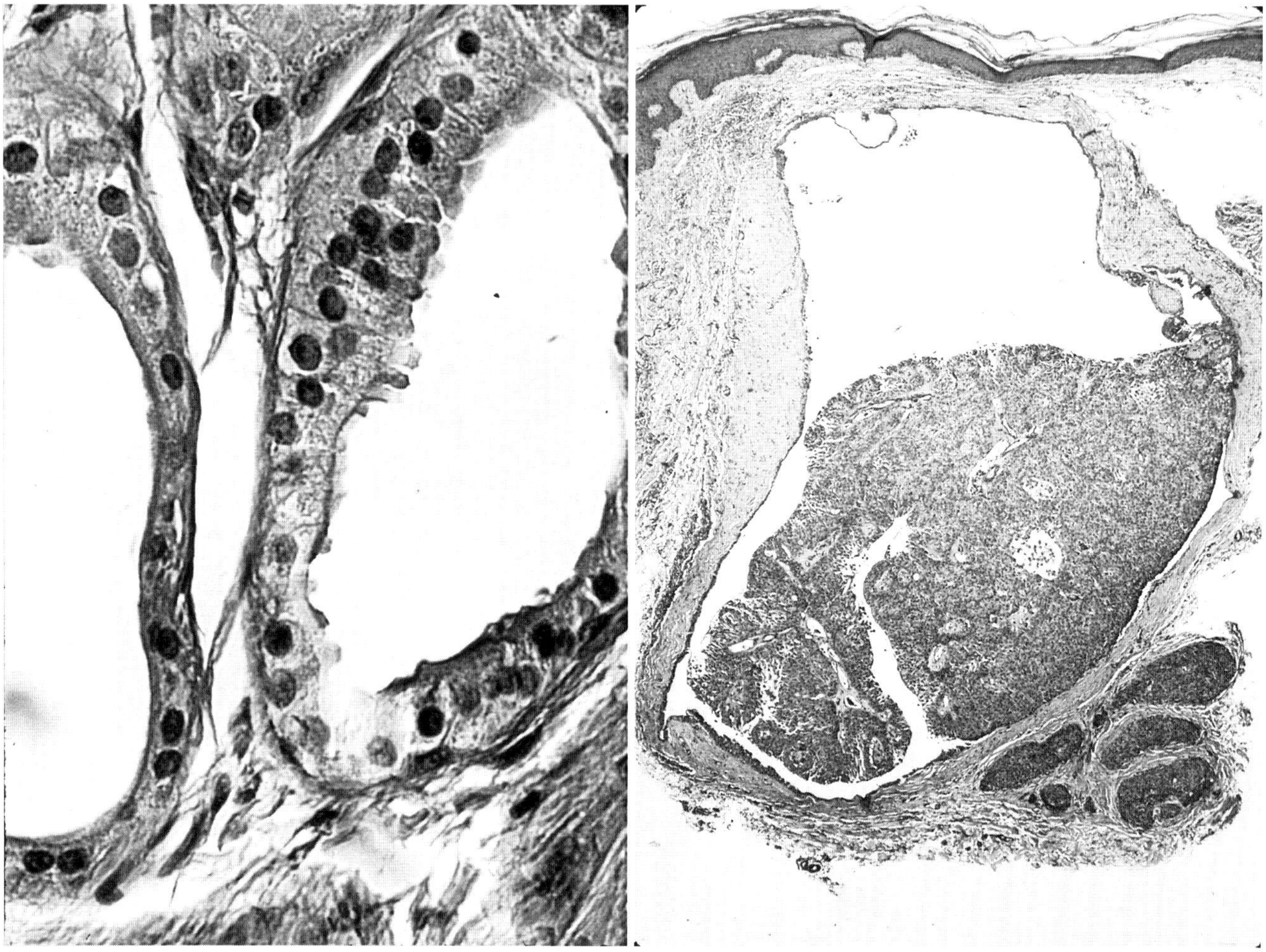

Fig. 6.73 Clear cell hidroadenoma. (*Left*) The clear cells lining the wall of the secretory duct are clearly discerned. (*Right*) The accumulation of the tumoral cells gives rise to an intracanalicular variety of this lesion. H&E ×400; ×40 o m

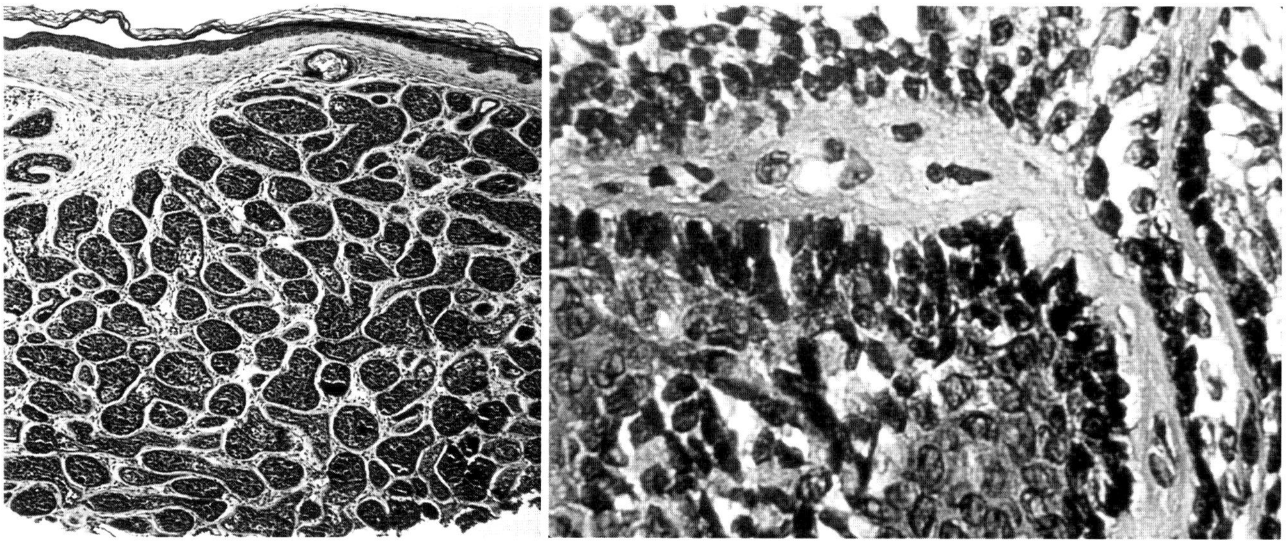

Fig. 6.74 Cylindroma. The striking microscopic picture of the lesion resembling a solved jigsaw puzzle is evident at low magnification (*left*). The composition of the tumoral islets formed by dark peripheral cells surrounding central masses of larger clear cells is visible at higher magnification (*right*). H&E ×40; ×400 o m

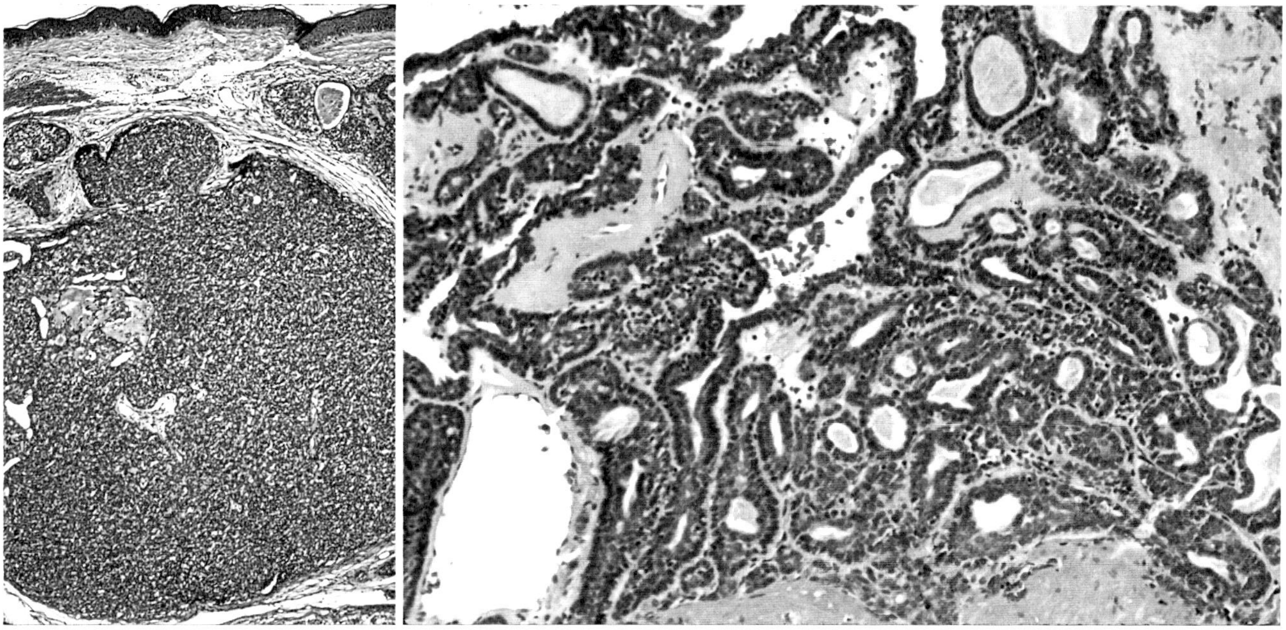

Fig. 6.75 Spiradenoma. Note the densely cellular and sharply delimited mass of the lesion and its satellites (*left*). At higher magnification, the dual cellular composition of the tubular structures of the lesion may be recognized (*right*). H&E ×40; ×400 o m

Fibrohistiocytic Neoplasias

The lesions subclassified as "fibrohistiocytic tumors" are formed by fibroblasts, fibrocytes, histiocytes, myofibroblasts, etc., as established by EM examination in combination with cell-marker studies and other techniques. Following their biological behavior, rather than their histologic composition, these tumors may be meaningfully separated into three Groups, which are those of benign tumors, tumors of intermediate malignancy, and malignant tumors. The ones of the first group are limited to local growth and do not recur after appropriate excision. The ones of the second Group display local infiltrating activity, and the ones of the third Group, that is, the *malignant* ones, have a potential for producing distant metastases. Table 6.8 presents pertinent examples of these three types of tumors.

Fibrohistiocytic Neoplasias: Benign

The prototypic and most common lesion in this Group is known as fibrohistiocytoma [42]. This lesion, which under early examination appeared as a fibrocytic proliferation, was initially reported as "fibroma simple" or dermatofibroma." Further studies revealed that it presented histiocytic features, evidenced by the presence of multinucleated foamy cells as well as by their phagocytic capacity. For this reason, its name was changed to "histiocytoma" or "fibrous histiocytoma." The latter designation was received with general approval, in spite of the fact that ultrastructural and other studies revealed in it a more variegated composition which included fibroblasts, myofibroblasts, fibrocytes, etc. (Fig. 6.76, center).

Table 6.7 Soft tissue tumors: Subclasses

Fibrohistiocytic
Muscular
Vascular
Adipose
Of peripheral nerves

Table 6.8 Fibrohistiocytic tumors: Groups and examples

Benign
Fibrohistiocytoma
Nevoxanthoendothelioma
Fibrous papule of the face
Nodular fasciitis
Of intermediate malignancy
Flat Dupuytren's disease
Nodular Dermatofibrosarcoma protuberans
Extra-abdominal desmoid tumor
Atypic fibroxanthoma
Malignant
Malignant fibrohistiocytoma

The names "sclerosing hemangioma" [43] and "nevoxanthoendothelioma" were alternatively proposed for fibrous histiocytomas with a strongly developed vascular framework or with a predominance of foamy cells, respectively. Prior to signing out a lesion as "nevoxanthoendothelioma," it is advisable for the pathologist to find out about the patient's blood lipoprotein values since neoplastic xanthomas cannot

Table 6.9 Summary of the differences between schwannoma and neurofibroma (see Fig. 6.95)

	Schwannoma	Neurofibroma
Appearance	Solitary dermal or subcutaneous nodule	Solitary or multiple, nodular or pendulous[a]
Predominant location	Head and limbs	Trunk and limbs
Age range	20–50 years	20–40 years; lower in NF1
Malignant transformation	Extremely rare in NF1	Possible in NF1
Gross detail	Nodular; with nerve fibers attached to its external surface	Spindle shaped
Microscopic detail	Encapsulated biphasic (Antoni A and B zones)	Nonencapsulated monophasic
Cellular composition	Formed by Schwann cells exclusively;	Formed by Schwann cells, mast cells, etc.
	Axons and mast cells absent	Axons present
	Verocay bodies present	Verocay bodies absent

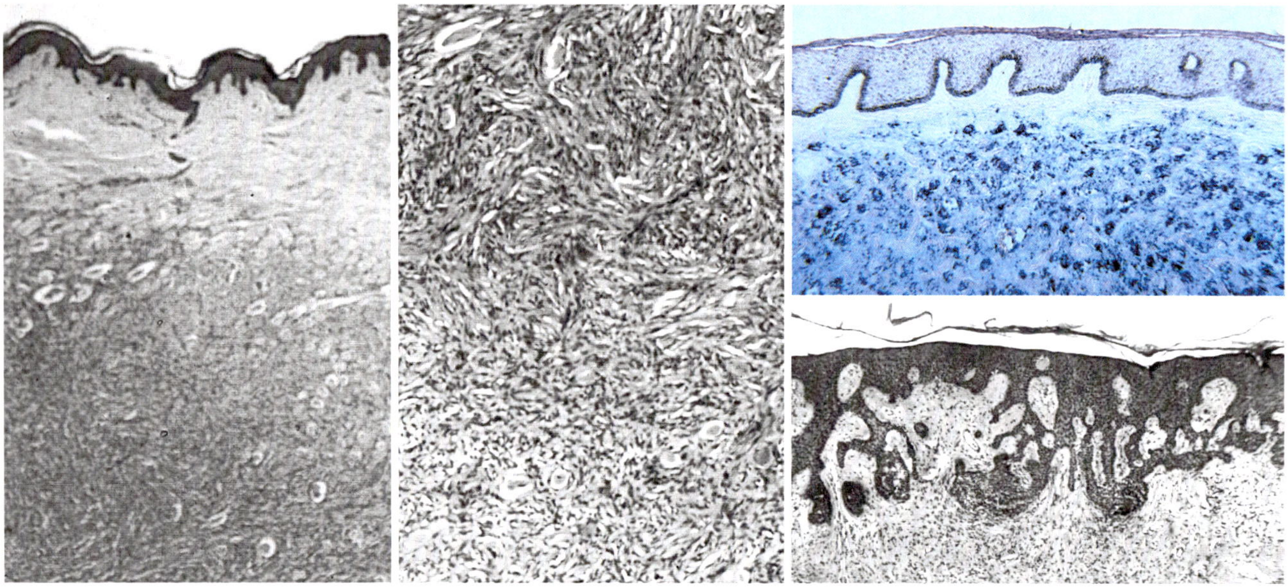

Fig. 6.76 Fibrous histiocytoma. (*Left*) Note the densely cellular texture of the lesion and its clear separation from the epidermis. The cellular composition of the lesion is shown at higher magnification (*center*). The combined application of Fontana-Masson and Perls stains (*upper right*) outlines the contour of the rete ridges in dark brown and simultaneously reveals the lesion's heavy load of hemosiderin (*upper right*). Deformed adnexae or, according to a different interpretation, BCC buds are found between the epidermis and the lesion (*lower right*). H&E ×40, H&E ×100; M/P ×40; H&E ×100 o m

be easily told apart under the microscope from the metabolic types associated to dyslipoproteinemias.

Fibrous histiocytomas appear most frequently as painless, solitary nodules or papules on the lower limbs (Fig. 6.76, left). Microscopic examination in early phases shows a predominant fibrohistiocytic population with accentuated pleomorphism and scattered multinucleated giant cells. In addition to these haphazardly disposed elements, a low amount of interstitial collagen can be found (Fig. 6.76, center). The lesion has unprecise limits and is generally located in the dermis, but it may also spread into the subcutaneous fat. The overlying epidermis appears distended and occasionally presents deformed adnexae. As already stated, this sometimes makes it impossible to tell these adnexal lesions apart from BCC buds (Fig. 6.76, right).

Fibrous histiocytomas involute through progressive collagen deposition as they are transformed into paucicellular, fibrotic nodules (Fig. 6.77, left).

Fibrous papule of the nose [44] is a lesion whose more accurate name should be "fibrous papule of the face" since it may also be found on other facial locations, for instance on the forehead (Fig. 6.77, left). Since this lesion shows a structure that closely resembles an involuted fibrous histiocytoma (Fig. 6.77, right), it is not unrealistic to consider it a small version of the latter. The same histopathologic disposition is found in acquired digital fibrokeratoma and even in epulis, although in this case the lesion, since sitting on the gingiva, is overlaid by a mucosal rather than a keratinizing epithelium. An increase in the vascular component transforms a fibrous papule of the face into an angiofibroma.

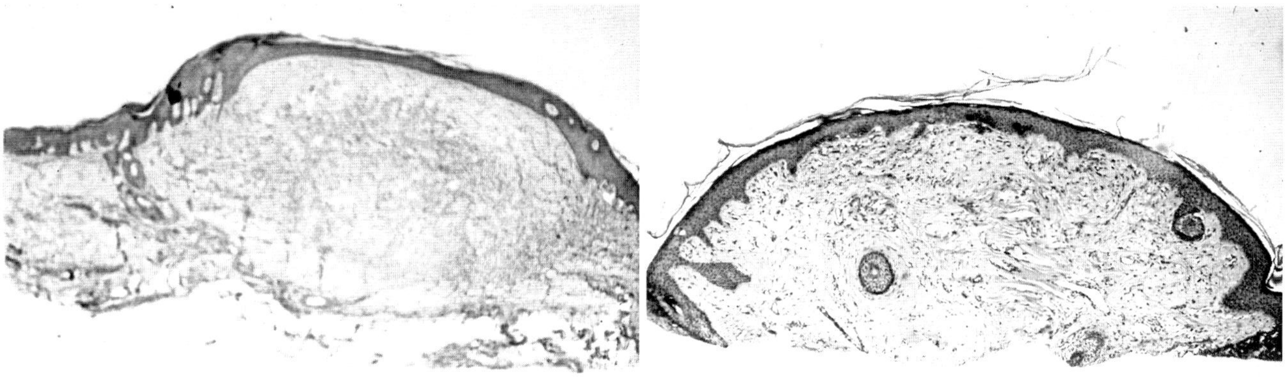

Fig. 6.77 Involuted fibrous histiocytoma and fibrous papule of the face. The microscopic picture of the first lesion (*left*) is similar to that of the second (*right*) insofar as both show a fibrotic core overlaid by a distended epidermis. H&E ×40 o m

Pigmented villonodular synovitis and giant cell tumor of tendon sheeth [45] are also examples of benign proliferative lesions developed in these cases from the fibrohistiocytic population in synovial cavities and around digital tendons. These two lesions are exteriorized as tiny, firm, and painless nodules in the interosseal spaces of hand and foot. These two lesions appear microscopically as ill-delimited masses of histiocytes with large numbers of multinucleated giant cells. These are loaded with hemosiderin granules, which impart to the lesion its typical brown discoloration (Fig. 6.78).

Nodular fasciitis [46] may also be mentioned in this context due to its fibrohistiocytic composition and its benign behavior. However, its deeper localization on the perimuscular fasciae and suspicion regarding its *reactive* rather than *neoplastic* pathogenesis tends to distance it taxonomically from this group of lesions.

Fibrohistiocytic Neoplasias of Intermediate Aggressivity

The fibrohistiocytic lesions of intermediate aggressivity may appear in a flat or a nodular manner.

Fibrohistiocytic Neoplasias of Intermediate Aggresivity: Flat

The flat forms of fibrohistiocytic neoplasias of intermediate agressivity are called – although improperly – "fasciitis." The three most important of them are palmar contracture or Dupuytren's diseases [47], plantar contracture or Ledderhose's disease, and the one described by F.d.l. Peyronie and currently known as Peyronie's disease, located, respectively, on the palm of the hand, the plant of the foot, and the intercavernous septum of the penis. Under the microscope, the three lesions are similar, appearing as bundles and sheaths of filiform elements with a low mitotic rate, although featuring atypias. These masses do not show clear limits but insinuate themselves in the surrounding fibrous stroma and fatty tissue (Fig. 6.79), making their surgical excision very problematic. These lesions are not supposed to produce distant metastasis, but due to their unremitting infiltration into the surrounding tissues, they are able to permanently incapacitate patients.

Fibrohistiocytic Neoplasias of Intermediate Aggresivity: Nodular Forms

Among the nodular varieties in the category of fibrohistiocytic proliferations of intermediate aggresivity, dermatofibrosarcoma protuberans [48] should be mentioned first. This lesion has a special significance for dermatologists since it was described by the head of the French school of dermatology, J. Darier, along with M. Ferrand. The peak incidence of this lesion occurs at middle age. It appears as a bulky mass of firm consistency, mainly on the trunk, neck, and proximal part of the extremities. Under the microscope, the lesion appears densely cellular, being formed by filiform elements in a whorly arrangement called "storiform" (Fig. 6.80). The term "storiform" derives from antiquity. A "*storia*" was a matt made of rope, sewn in a spiral shape and used in Roman household [49]. Storiform is an ill-chosen word, which could be replaced by "swirling," "whorled," or even comparatively, as proposed by some authors, by "nubecular," a term which in spite of its astronomic connotation is more down to earth than "storiform" as it does not require a Latin dictionary to decipher its meaning.

Bednar tumor [50], originally reported as a special form of neurofibroma, turned out to be a lesion of fibrohistiocytic nature close to a fibrous histiocytoma. It may be distinguished from the first at the grossing bench by dark brown bands visible on the cut surface of the specimen. Those bands are melanin deposits whose origin has still not been established (Fig. 6.81).

Extra-abdominal desmoid tumor [51]: This is another fibrohistiocytic tumor of moderate aggressivity. Although its primary localization is intra-abdominal, it may occasionally be found in an extra-abdominal position, bulging from underneath the skin of the abdominal wall of pregnant or puerperal women. The lesion is formed by intersecting bundles of thin spindle-shaped cell containing abundant interstitial collagen. It forms bulky masses that are hard to excise completely, which accounts for the high rate of postoperative recurrences.

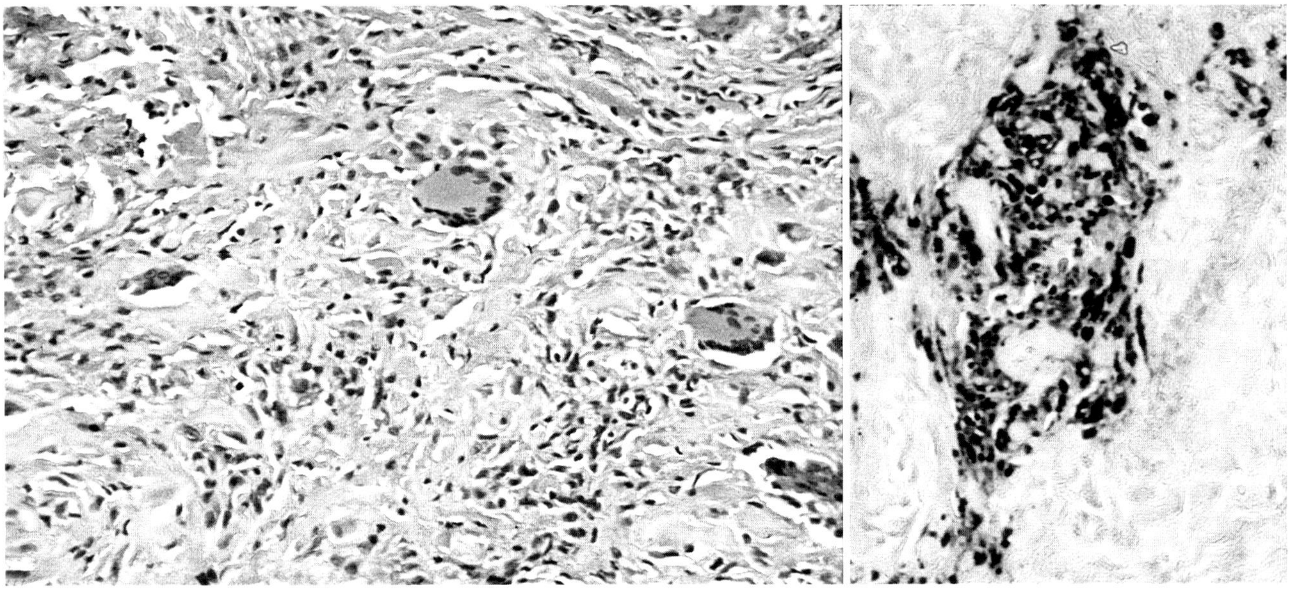

Fig. 6.78 Pigmented villonodular synovitis. Note the abundant giant cells over a background of epithelioid elements (*left*). The black granules correspond to hemosiderin (*right*). H&E ×100; M/P ×100 o m

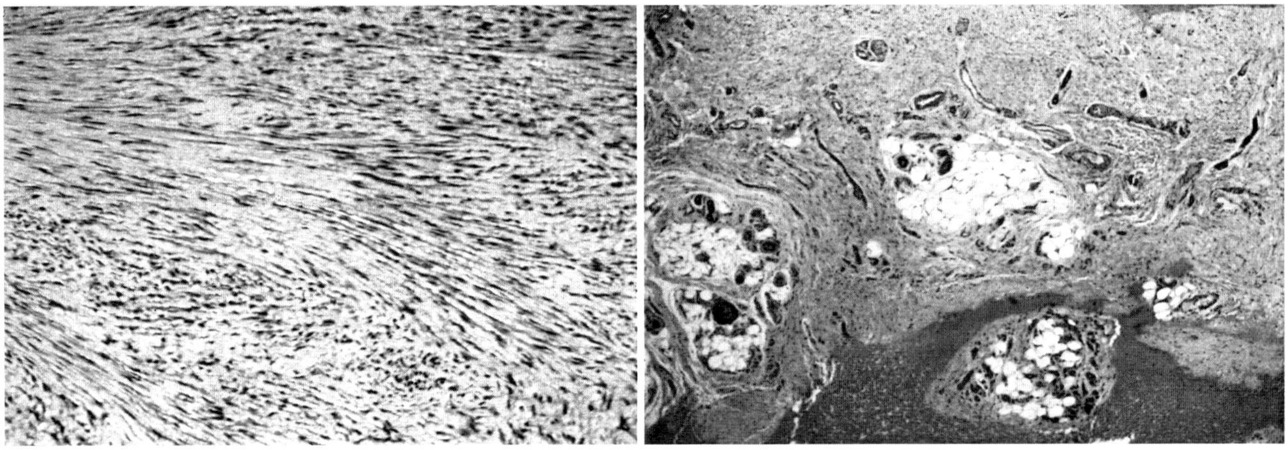

Fig. 6.79 Dupuytren's disease. The delicate filiform character of the lesion may be appreciated on the picture to the (*left*). The infiltrating character of the lesion toward the surrounding stroma and fatty tissue is demonstrated in the picture on the (*right*). H&E ×100 o m

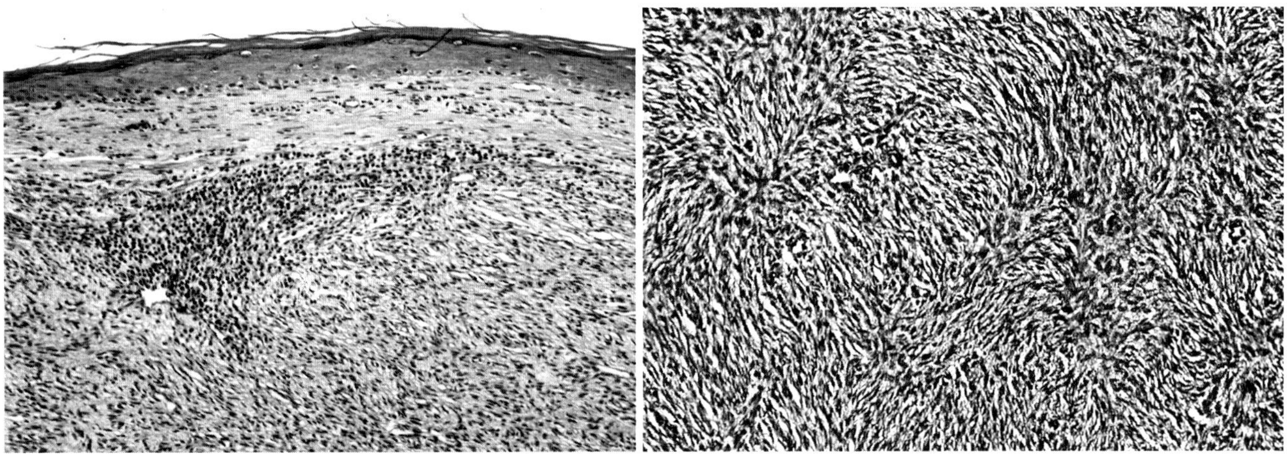

Fig. 6.80 Dermatofibrosarcoma protuberans. Note the high cellularity of the lesion, which at low magnification appears separated from the overlying epidermis (*left*). At higher magnification (*right*), the lesion appears formed by thin spindle-shaped elements arranged in a somewhat whorly pattern. H&E ×40; ×100 o m

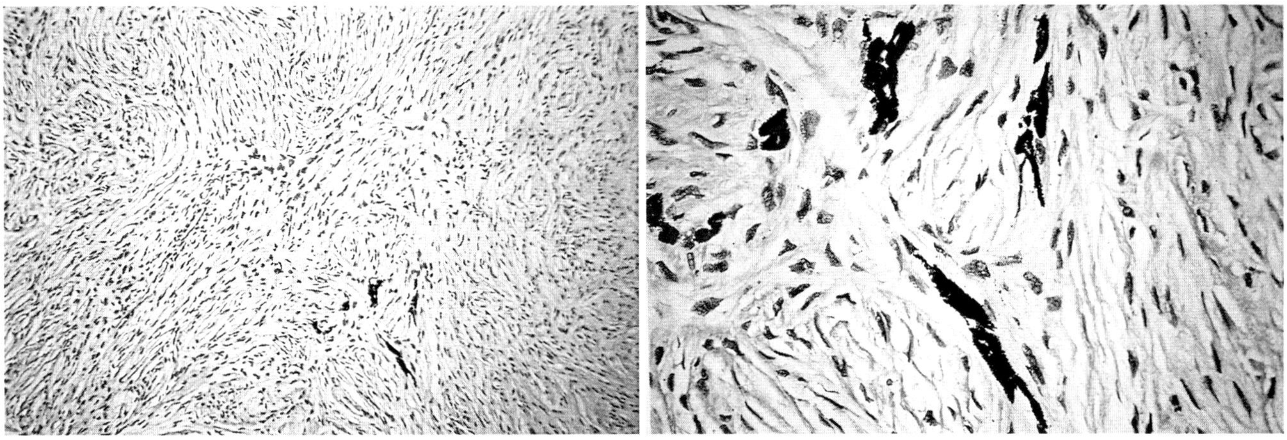

Fig. 6.81 Bednar tumor. (*Left*) Note the dense cellularity of the lesion, comparable to that of dermatofibrosarcoma protuberans, and also the melanin streaks. (*Right*) Higher magnification of the same lesion. H&E ×40; ×100 o m

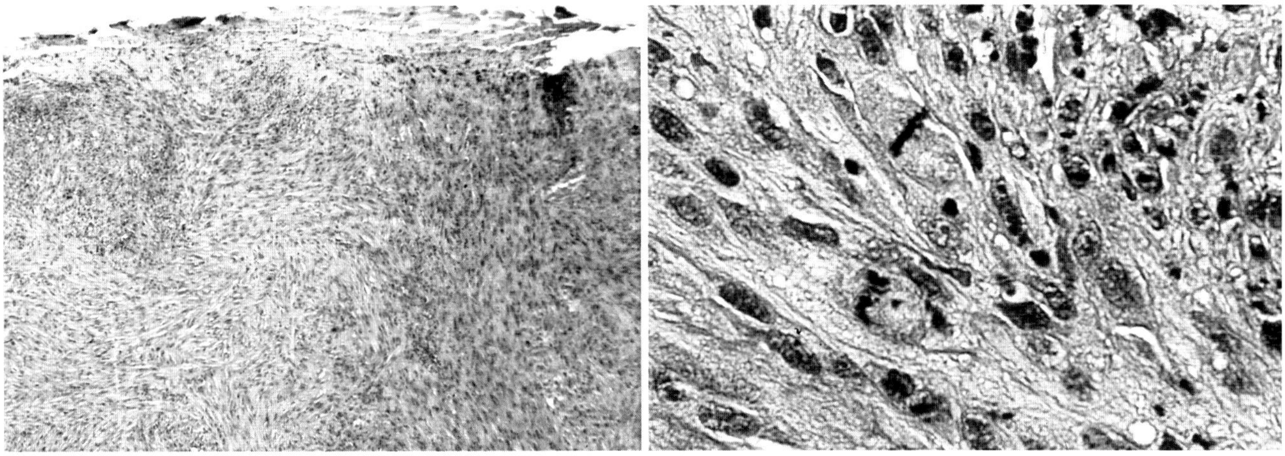

Fig. 6.82 Atypical fibroxanthoma. Note the high density of the lesion which in this case appears ulcerated (*left*). Observe the anaplastic character of the lesion and its high mitotic rate (*right*). H&E 40; ×400 o m

Atypical fibroxanthoma [52] is a lesion predominant in the aged population. It appears most frequently in areas exposed to actinic radiation, particularly the temporal region. Although from its microscopic aspect (Fig. 6.82), it may be considered a malignant fibrous histiocytoma, atypical fibroxanthoma proves to have a much more benign evolution than the former. This led to its classification into the group of lesions of moderate aggresivity.

Malignant Fibrohistiocytic Neoplasias

Malignant fibrous histiocytoma is the most frequent member of this group of lesions [53]. This assertion, however, is more pertinent to general pathology than to dermatopathology since primary malignant fibrous histiocytomas of the skin are of rare occurrence. This lesion appears most frequently on the inferior limbs of middle-aged persons, showing a clear male predominance. Although several histopathologic types occur, there is a constant pleomorphism in all varieties of this tumor, with anaplastic cellular elements and multinucleated giant cells often present in a whorled pattern (Fig. 6.83, left). Malignant fibrous histiocytoma is propagated by the blood to the lungs in the majority of cases but can also end up in liver and bones.

Fibrosarcoma [54] is the second member in the group of malignant fibrohistiocytic tumors. Following a long period of reevaluation, fibrosarcoma is today considered a lesion of much lower incidence than malignant fibrous histiocytoma. The most important clinical differences between these lesions are that the first one occurs in a younger population, and that it does not have the strong male predominance of the second. These clinical differences are also supported by microscopic distinctions. Fibrosarcoma shows a more organized structure than malignant fibrous histiocytoma: in contrast with the whorled structure of the latter, fibrosarcoma is formed by elongated cells organized as parallel bundles (Fig. 6.83, right), often perpendicular to a central one, forming characteristic "herring bone figures."

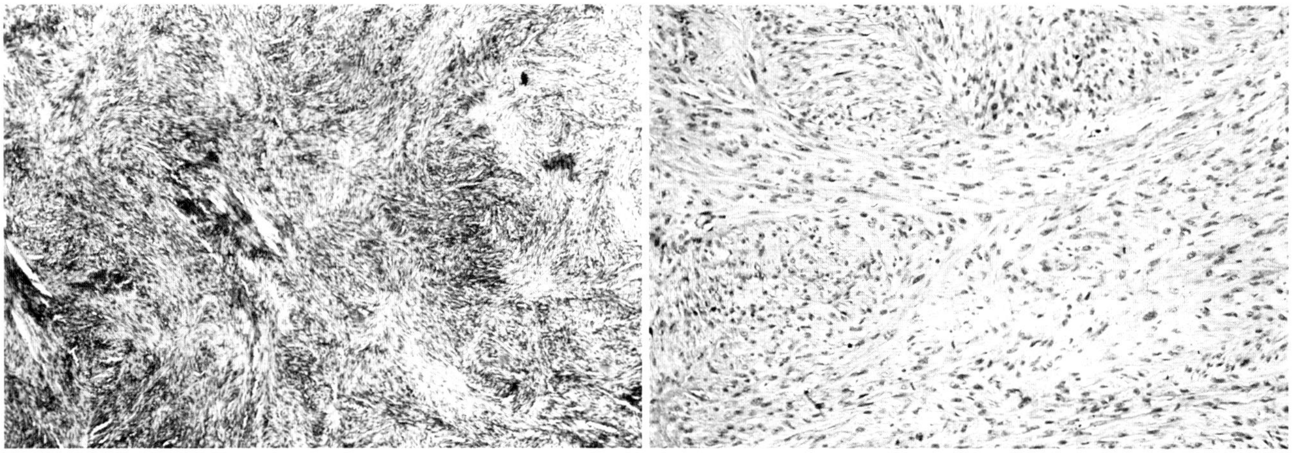

Fig. 6.83 Malignant fibrous histiocytoma and fibrosarcoma. The first lesion (*left*) presents a vague nodular structure being formed by bundles of spindle-shaped cells with pyknotic nuclei in a whorled disposition. The second lesion (*right*) features a more fascicular structure. H&E ×40; ×100, o m

Muscular Neoplasias

The most frequent and pertinent muscular tumors in dermatopathology derive from smooth muscle and are therefore called "leiomyomas" [55] (*leio* + myo [G] smooth + muscle). Tumors of striated muscle, "rhabdomyomas" (*rhabdo* + *myo* [G] striated + muscle), are of relative minor importance and shall be left aside in the coming discussion. The Subclass of the leiomyomas may be divided into two Groups, the *superficial* and the *deep*. Both Subclasses contain benign and malignant varieties [55].

A distinctive sign of some of the leiomyomas is *pain*, reason for which they integrate the already mentioned group of the painful tumors of the skin.

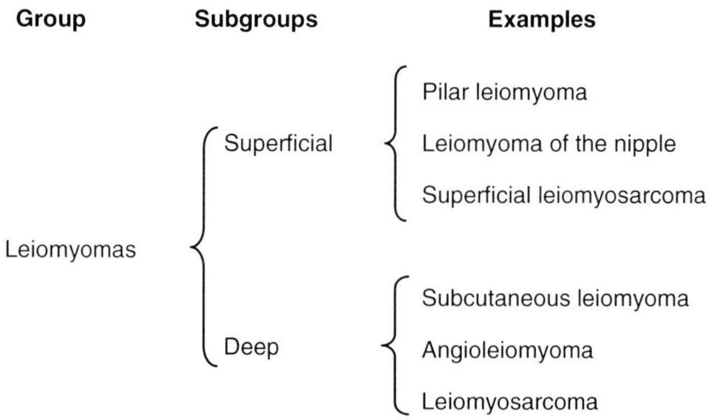

Fig. 6.84 Leiomyomas: subgroups and examples

Leiomyomas: Superficial

Superficial leiomyomas are derived from the arrector pilorum of pilosebaceous complexes, in which case they are called "pilar leiomyomas," or derived from the muscular fibers of the nipple or the dartos scrotum, being then known, collectively, as "genital leiomyomas" [56] (Fig. 6.84).

The superficial leiomyomas are formed by spindle-shaped cells with "cigar-shaped" nuclei featuring tiny perinuclear vacuoles. They form nodules sharply delimited from the surrounding stroma (Fig. 6.85, left). The absence of or very low level of mitotic activity of these lesions is the main feature that distinguishes them from superficial leiomyosarcoma, which is the malignant, albeit, very mild version of the lesions in this group.

Leiomyomas: Deep

Subcutaneous leiomyoma is a lesion of histologic composition similar to the superficial one, although often larger and featuring intervening fibrous septa. This lesion (Fig. 6.85, center and right) originates in the muscular wall of the blood vessels in the reticular dermis, and in spite of being well circumscribed, it may display some local infiltrating activity.

Deep leiomyosarcoma is a lesion which, in contrast to the superficial type, is of fully malignant character. Therefore, it deserves to be plainly called "leiomyosarcoma," without any reference to its level of occurrence in the skin. The microscopic image of this lesion may go from moderately differentiated to anaplastic, with large amounts of malignant cells (Fig. 6.86).

Vascular Tumors

Upon approaching the vascular tumors, it must be emphasized that the ones of lymphatic tissue are not considered to be *neoplasias* but rather *malformations* originated on lymphatic remnants [57]. For this reason, the neoplasias discussed in this subclass are all of blood vessels. These are grouped according to their origin as *endothelial* or *perivascular* [58] (Fig. 6.87).

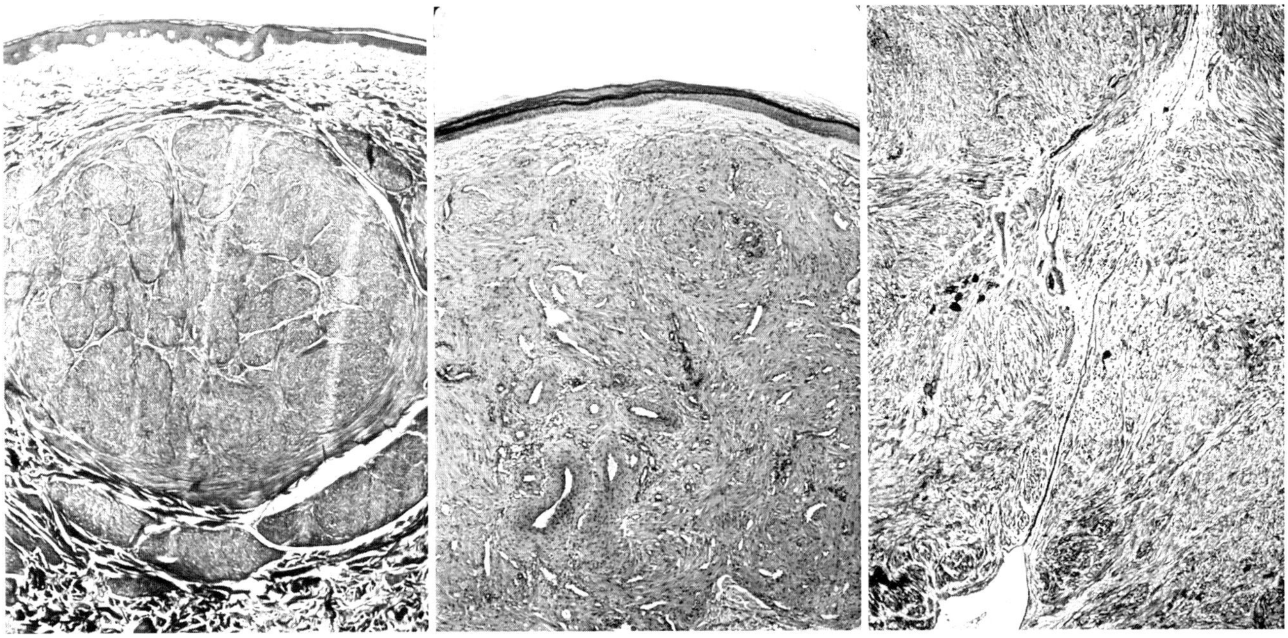

Fig. 6.85 Pilar leiomyoma, superficial angioleiomyoma, and subcutaneous leiomyoma. Pilar leiomyoma (*left*) is a solid lesion sharply separated from the surrounding stroma. Angioleiomyoma (*center*) appears as a solid lesion, formed in this case by sheaths of muscular cells disposed around the vessels of the reticular dermis. Subcutaneous leiomyoma (*right*) is arising from a midsized vessel. Tri ×40 o m

Fig. 6.86 Leiomyosarcoma. Note the anaplastic character of this lesion. H&E ×40; ×400 o m

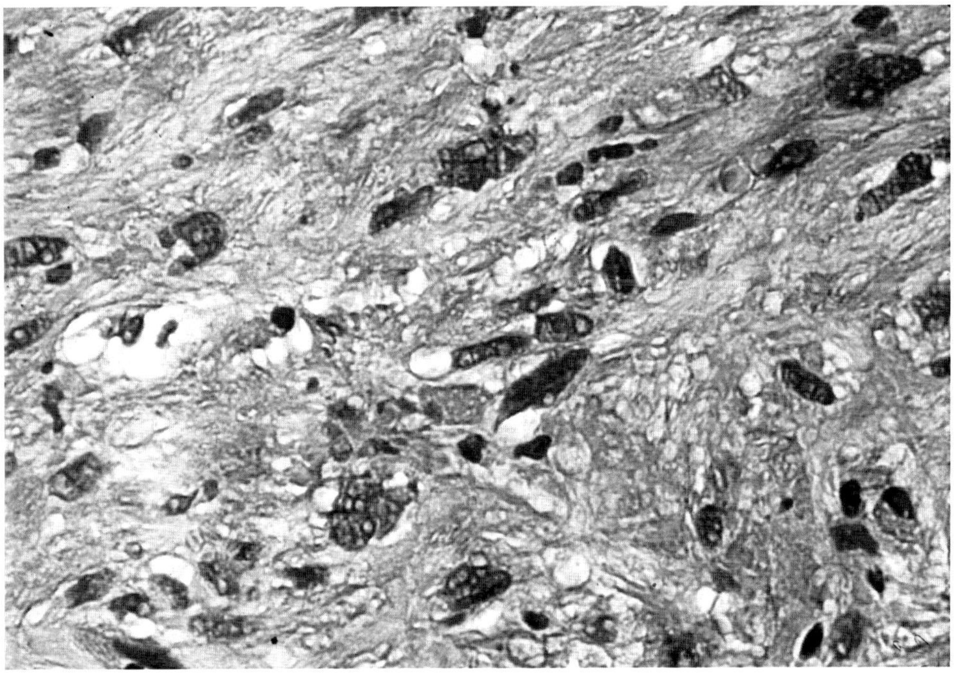

Vascular Tumors: Endothelial

Upon studying the group of endothelial tumors, their components may be separated into three Subgroups, that of benign, uncertain, or malignant behavior (Fig. 6.87).

Endothelial Tumors: Benign

The most frequent representative of the subgroup of endothelial neoplasias is pyogenic granuloma [59]. This lesion appears as an exophytic, painless, often ulcerated mass,

Group	Subgroups	Examples
Endothelial	Benign	Pyogenic granuloma
	Of uncertain behavior	Hemangioendothelioma (Dabska's tumor)
	Malignant	Angiosarcoma Kaposi sarcoma
Perivascular	Benign	Glomus tumor Hemangiopericytoma
	Malignant	Malignant Hemangiopericytoma

Fig. 6.87 Vascular tumors

most frequently located on fingers or toes. Microscopic examination reveals that pyogenic granuloma appears as a lobulated mass of endothelial cells found around dilated vascular channels, whose shape is often compared to deer staghorns (Fig. 6.88).

The epidermal ridges at the base of the lesion appear stretched, featuring "collarettes," not pathognomonic, but very characteristic of this lesion.

In spite of their clear differences, there is a tendency to incorrectly consider pyogenic granuloma equivalent to granulation tissue. The comparison of these lesions in Fig. 6.89 offers conclusive evidence of the differences between the former, a *vascular neoplasia*, and the latter, a *reactive vascular proliferation*, whose pathogenesis has already been discussed (p. 129).

The extirpation of a pyogenic granuloma is occasionally followed by the disturbing appearance of nodules around the area of surgery: these nodules, which may be regarded as metastatic growths, do not have any malignant implication and tend to disappear spontaneously [60].

Endothelial Tumors of Uncertain Behavior

There is a variety of endothelial growths which, due to their *potential* aggressivity, should be set aside from those of clearly benign character studied in the preceding section (Fig. 6.87). These lesions offer difficulties for their characterization due to the widely variable microscopic picture they present. They can be recognized, however, by their common tendency of growing within vascular spaces: they are called "hemangioendotheliomas" [61]. As an example, Dabska tumor should be mentioned. This lesion has a peak incidence in young individuals and an uncertain biological character, although it often proves to be of benign nature.

Endothelial Tumors: Malignant

As regards overtly malignant endothelial neoplasias, angiosarcoma should be the first to be mentioned [62] (Fig. 6.87). In spite of its low frequency, this tumor is of particular concern in dermatology because contrary to other sarcomas, it has a predominant incidence in the skin: its characteristic presentation is on the head of aged persons. Under LM, angiosarcoma features a widely variable picture, ranging from the most differentiated forms to the most anaplastic ones (Fig. 6.90).

Angiosarcoma is a lesion whose aggressivity is manifested locally, as well as by distant metastasis which predominantly affects the lymph nodes and the lungs.

Areas of the body affected by chronic lymphedema, such as the arms of patients following mastectomy with axillary dissection, may be the sites of apparition of malignant proliferations. Such lesions were reported as lymphangiosarcoma by F.W. Stewart and N. Treves in the syndrome which bears their names. However, today, lymphangiosarcoma is considered instead an *angiosarcoma* [63], similar in its characteristics to the above described.

Kaposi sarcoma is also included among the malignant endothelial proliferations (Fig. 6.91). Its classic form was described by M. Kaposi as a "*multiple malignant pigmented lesion*" in patients originated from the Mediterranean basin. An endemic lymphadenopathic form occurs in equatorial regions of Africa, whereas the form associated to immunodeficiency has spread worldwide as a result of the HIV/AIDS pandemic. In spite of the name's clear implication, today, there are doubts regarding the neoplastic character of Kaposi sarcoma [64].

The cutaneous lesions associated with the classic form of Kaposi sarcoma appear as macules, plaques, and nodules with a purple tinge. At the beginning of the AIDS pandemic, the microscopist had to learn to recognize the inconspicuous initial forms of the disease without the help of any ancillary technique. This condition is characterized by a mild proliferation of spindle-shaped elements with a sprinkle of mononuclear cells located around scant neoformed vessels (Fig. 6.91).

The fully developed lesion of Kaposi sarcoma (Fig. 6.92) features a clear nodular appearance and the presence of intersecting bundles of neoplastic spindle cells. The interstitial spaces in between them are filled with abundant red blood cells which impart a hemorrhagic character to the lesion. A characteristic detail of Kaposi sarcoma at this stage is the presence of eosinophilic globules, smaller in size than erythrocytes, and PAS positive [65].

Vascular Tumors: Perivascular

Perivascular or pericytic tumors may also be subgrouped as benign and malignant (Fig. 6.87).

Pericytic Tumors: Benign

The most common benign pericytic tumor is known as glomus tumor, more conveniently called "glomangioma" [66].

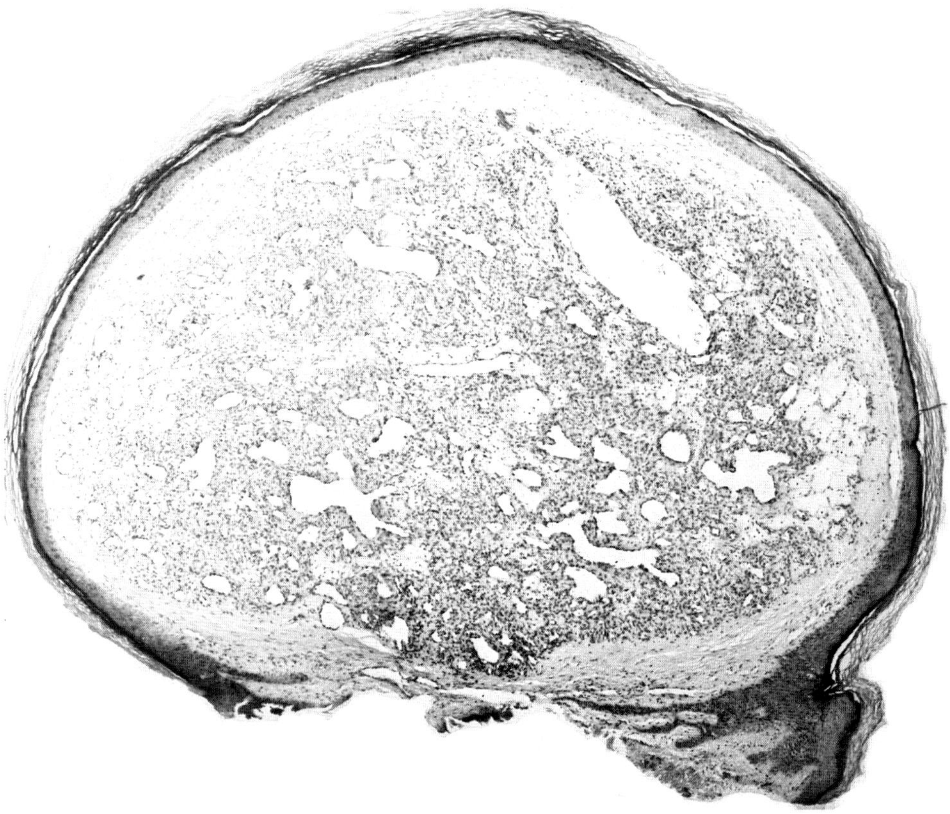

Fig. 6.88 Pyogenic granuloma. Note the exophytic character of the lesion along with its lobulated masses of cells disposed around irregularly dilated channels. H&E ×40 o m

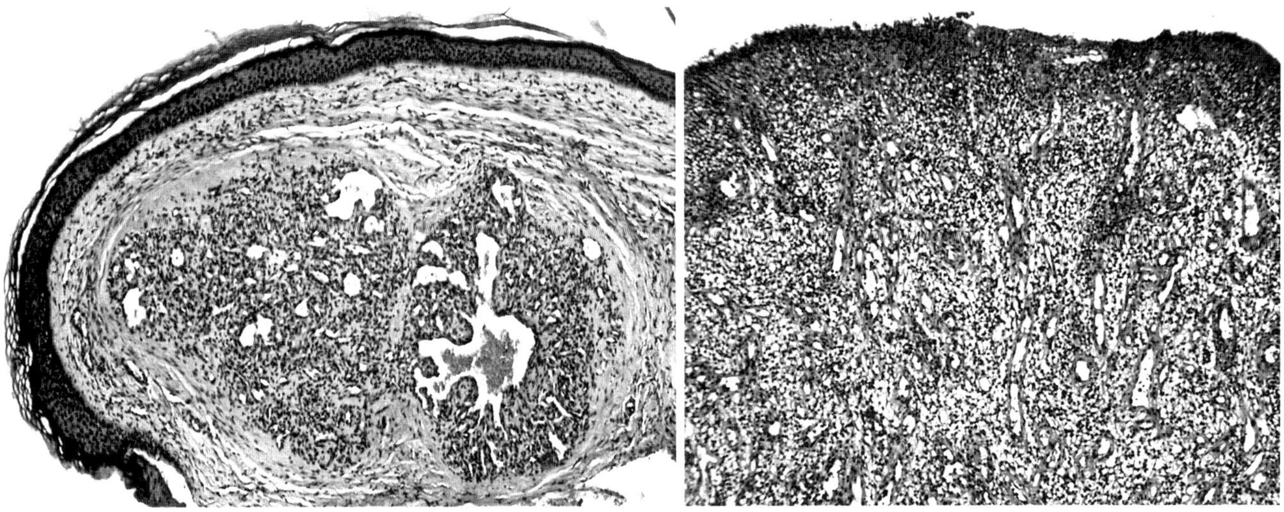

Fig. 6.89 Pyogenic granuloma and granulation tissue. Note the distended epidermis and the nodular structure with "staghorn" formations of pyogenic granuloma (*left*). In contrast, note the appearance on the neoformed vessels in the granulation tissue which ascend in parallel from the bottom toward the ulcerated external surface (*right*). H&E ×40 o m

According to P. Masson, who reported it in 1924, this lesion originates in the Sucquet-Hoyer thermoregulatory organs, mainly located in hands, fingers, peri- and subungual regions, etc. (p. 18).

Pericytes are essential components of these organs. These surround participating blood channels as subtle mantles, imparting to this lesion its characteristic organoid structure (Fig. 6.93). Glomus tumor sufferers may also experience attacks of lacinant pain, hence making this lesion another member of the group of painful tumors of the skin.

Vascular Neoplasias of Uncertain Biological Behavior

After glomus tumor, a second pericytic lesion was reported by P. Stout and M.R. Murray. They called it "hemangiopericytoma" [67]. These authors postulated a close relationship between glomus tumor (Fig. 6.94, left) and

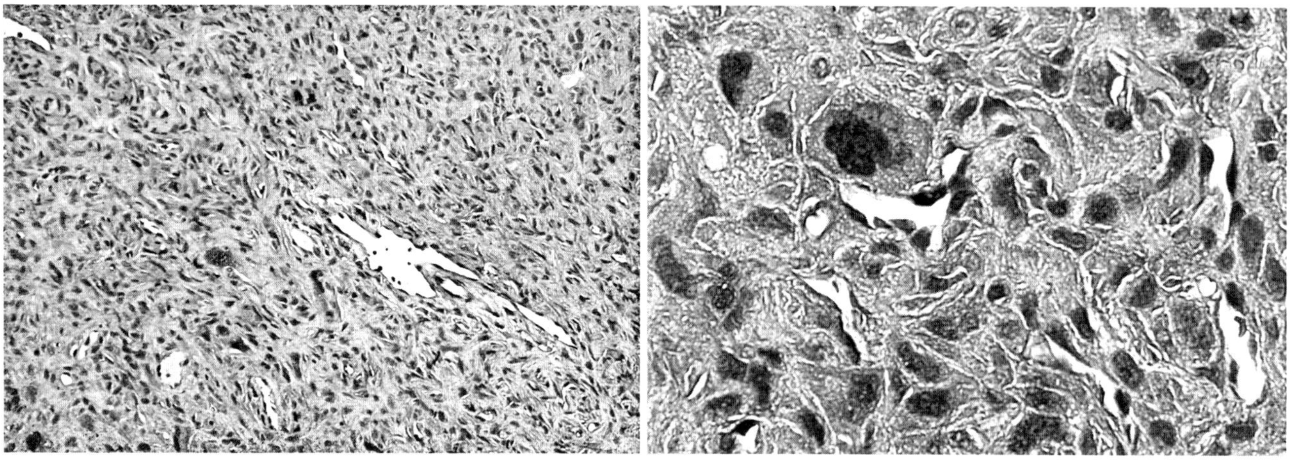

Fig. 6.90 Angiosarcoma: anaplastic. The lesion is composed of spindle-shaped cells, tightly surrounding irregular vascular spaces (*left*). At higher magnification, the syncytial and anaplastic character of the lesions are evident (*right*). Note the deeply stained and irregular nuclei as well as the interstitial clefts. H&E ×40; ×400 o m

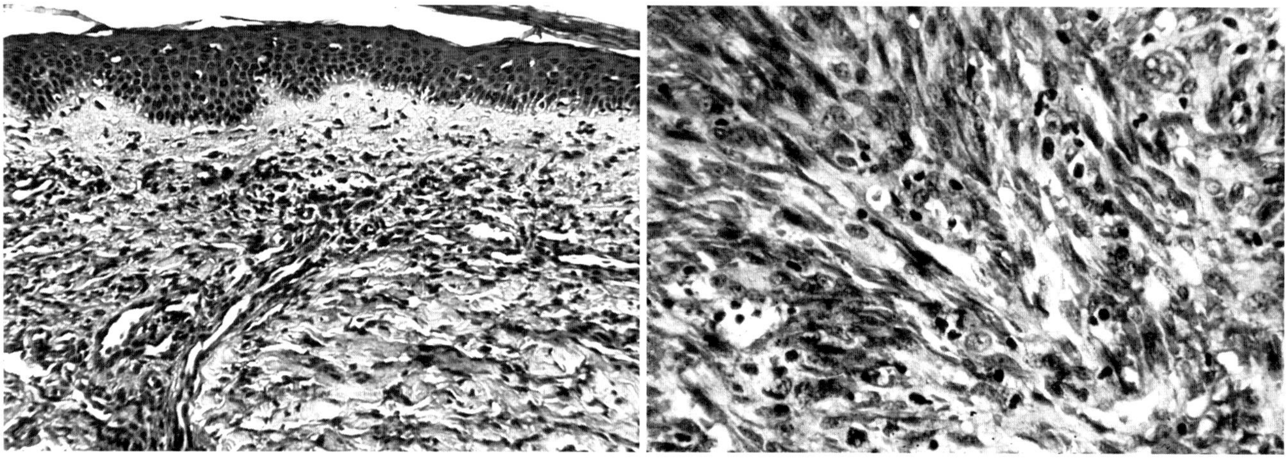

Fig. 6.91 Kaposi sarcoma: initial and moderately advanced lesion. The initial lesion (*left*) is formed by an inconspicuous proliferation of channels surrounded by spindle-shaped and mononuclear elements. A more advanced lesion (*right*) features a considerable proportion of atypical spindle-shaped elements with mononuclear cells disposed around dilated vessels. H&E ×40; ×100 o m

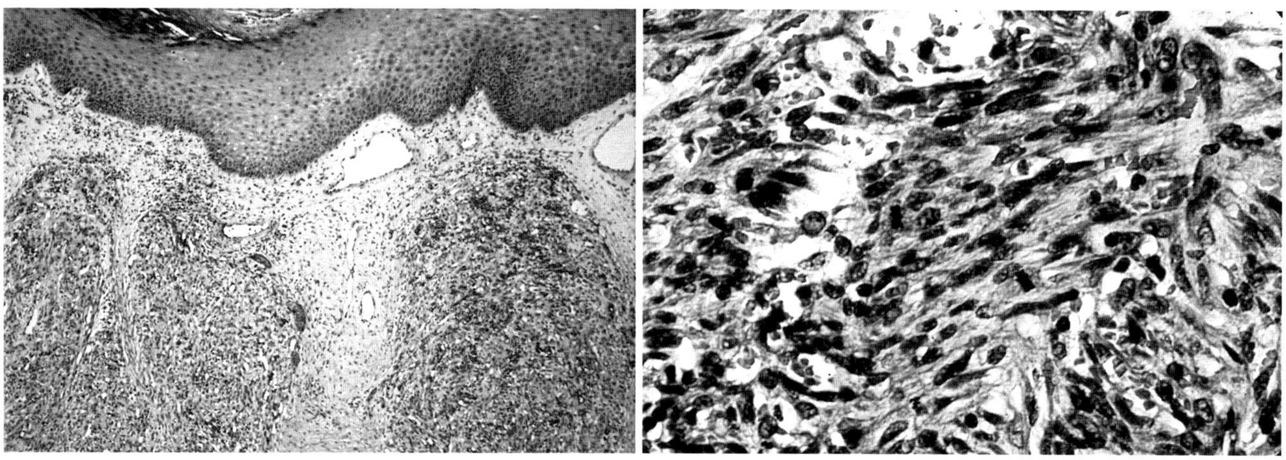

Fig. 6.92 Kaposi sarcoma: fully developed lesion. See details in the text. H&E ×40; ×100 o m

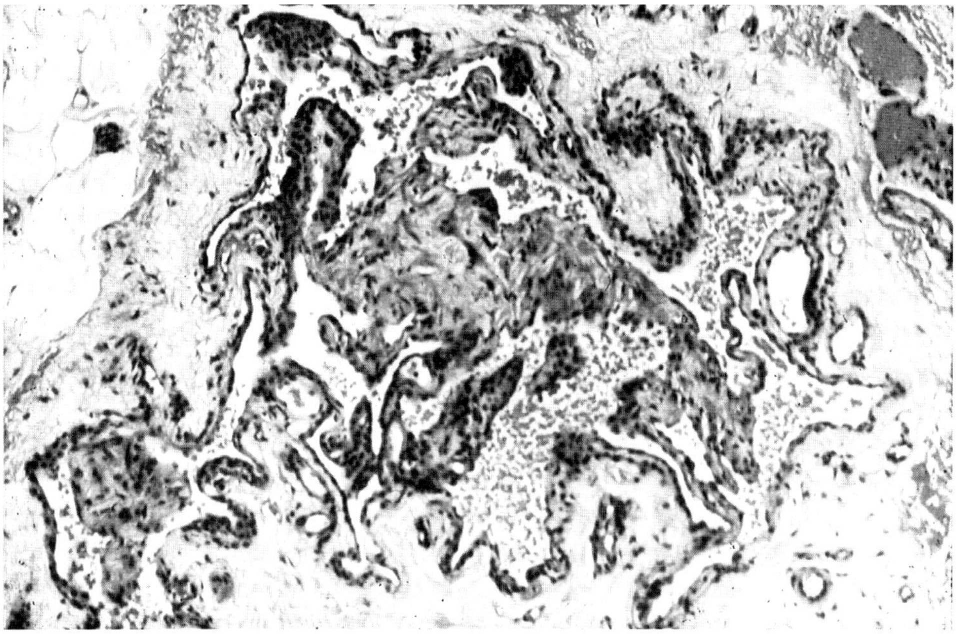

Fig. 6.93 Glomus tumor. See details in the text and on p. xxx. H&E ×40 o m

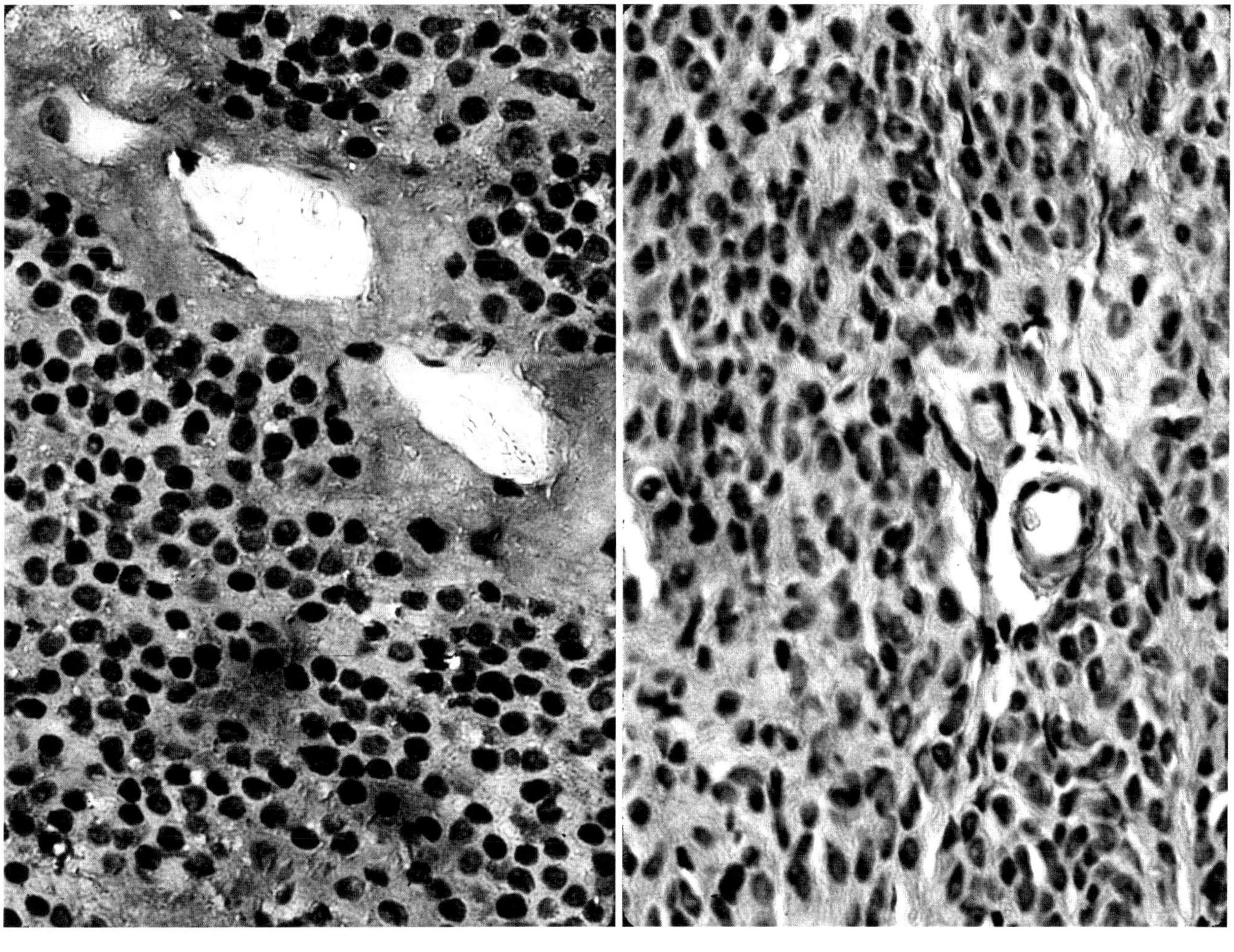

Fig 6.94 Glomus tumor and hemangiopericytoma. Compare the organized structure of the glomus tumor (*left*) with the disorganized one of the hemangiopericytoma whose cellular elements show an irregular and angulated contour (*right*). H&E ×100 o m

hemangiopericytoma (right), although considering the latter a more cellular lesion with a disorganized structure (Fig. 6.94).

The biological behavior of hemangiopericytoma cannot be predicted, and it must be accepted that there exist among them more and less aggressive forms.

Tumors of Adipose Tumors

Tumors of adipose tissue (Table 6.7) are scantly represented in textbooks of dermatology. This fact reflects the low interest that these lesions are given at the clinical level.

Lipomas may appear as solitary or multiple forms of benign or of variable aggresivity. A special mention is made of liposarcoma. It is an uncommon lesion in the field of dermatopathology, despite being one of the most frequent soft tissue tumors in general pathology. Its occasional presence in the skin is usually attributed to the tumor's propagation from deep-seated lesions.

The common lipoma, an encapsulated lesion formed by mature adipocytes, is currently considered of malformative nature. However, chromosomal anomalies in contrast suggest that they are true neoplasias [68].

Multiple lipomas may represent the cutaneous component of a hereditary multisystemic disorder. Multiple lipomas in a symmetric distribution give rise to the clinical picture of Madelung's disease.

Angiolipoma is a neoplasia of benign character formed by adipocytes combined with a variable proportion of blood vessels. This lesion has a predominant incidence in young individuals and is often painful, thus representing another member of the group of the painful tumors of the skin.

Tumors of Peripheral Nerves

Although peripheral nerve neoplasias are conventionally considered *soft tissue tumors*, important differences separate these from mesenchymal lesions. Three points should be emphasized in this regard. In the first place, neoplasias of peripheral nerves, contrary to soft tissue tumors, are frequently *heterogeneous* in their histologic composition. In the second place, they *tend to be associated with genetic disorders*. Third, these tumors present a peculiarity rarely observed in soft tissue tumors, as *they may progressively change their nature from benign into malignant forms* [69].

In this revision, the two most important of the peripheral nerve tumors, schwannoma and neurofibroma will be discussed. Three additional entities, neurothekeoma, acoustic neuroma, and granular cell tumor, shall be mentioned in the discussion. Although *amputation neuroma* and *Morton's neuroma* are frequently included with the peripheral nerve tumors, *they are really not tumors*, that is, neoplastic growths. Instead, they are cicatricial proliferations which enclose neural fibers. They have already been discussed elsewhere in this text along with other cicatricial lesions (Fig. 6.95).

Schwannoma [70]: This lesion is also called "neurinoma" and "neurilemmoma." This lesion is formed by the proliferation of Schwann cells in a nerve fascicle. The cellular proliferation may give rise to several forms of this tumor, from which only the conventional schwannoma should hereby be discussed. It summarizes all the microscopic details found in the other.

The microscopic examination of a schwannoma (Fig. 6.96) discloses an encapsulated mass with alternating areas of high and low cellular density, called "Antoni A" and "Antoni B zones," respectively. Antoni A zones show a fibrous background with scattered structures called "Verocay bodies," formed by clusters of staggered cells with dark nuclei appearing in parallel. Verocay bodies, along with the fibrous capsule and absence of mast cells, are the three most significative elements for the microscopic differentiation of schwannoma from neurofibroma. Antoni B zones have a myxoid appearance and show scant cellular elements; these zones supposedly represent areas of the tumor with necrotic degeneration.

Neurofibroma [71], either in its solitary or multiple form, grows diffusely, incorporating nervous fibers into its mass and giving the affected nerve a spindle-shaped contour (Fig. 6.95, bottom). Microscopic examination of the lesion (Fig. 6.97) reveals a structure formed by small, curled elements, wavy fibers, and scattered mast cells. The lesion appears clearly delimited from the surrounding stroma, although lacks a peripheral capsule.

Neurothekeoma [72]: This lesion appears as a lobulated mass containing abundant mucin and cellular elements which cannot be identified as Schwann cells or fibroblasts. Its name implies a neural origin, neuro + (thekeoma *theke* [G] a box or a sheath), and was assigned to it in order to emphasize its postulated perineural origin. *Neurothekeoma* has a special interest in dermatopathology insofar that it presents microscopic features that make it somehow similar if not identical to *Clark nevus*, which therefore, should be included in the list of differential diagnoses (p. 144).

Acoustic neuroma is a lesion essentially similar to a neurofibroma. It is hereby mentioned only because it constitutes an important element in the nosologic picture of NF2, in which it frequently appears bilaterally.

Granular cell tumor [73]: Based on its response to the trichrome staining procedure, this lesion was initially reported as a *muscular* tumor, reason for which it was called

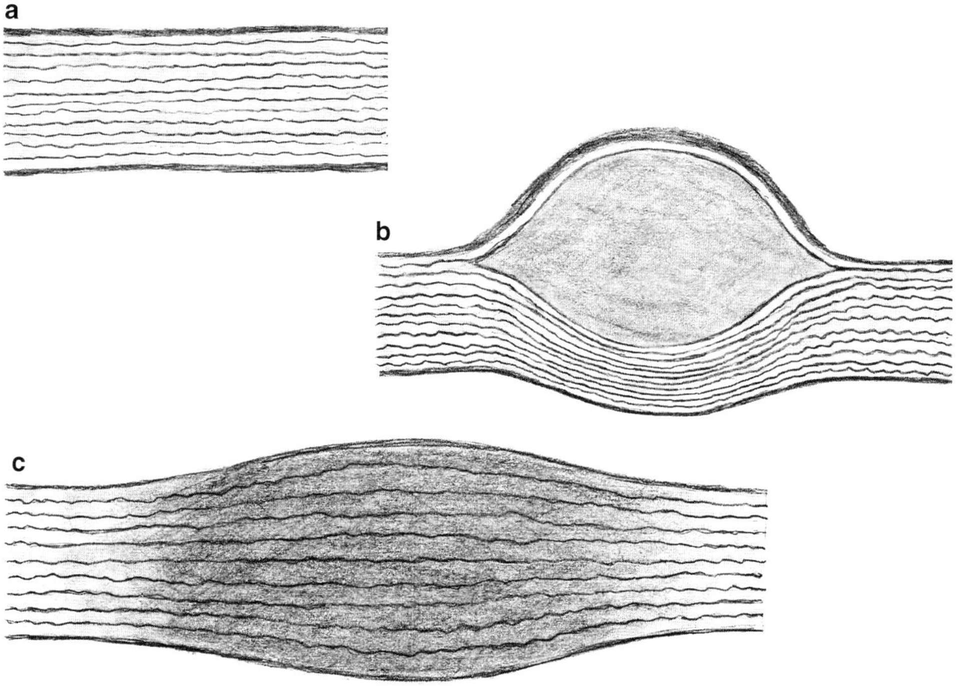

Fig. 6.95 Schematic representation of a nerve fascicle: a schwannoma and a neurofibroma. The nerve fascicle (**a**) is formed by a bundle of neural fibers (*light wavy lines*) surrounded by the perinerve (*heavier lines* at the periphery). Schwannoma (**b**) occurs as Schwann cells proliferate under the perinerve, pushing aside the nervous fibers, which appears compressed at the periphery overlaid by a fibrous capsule. The neurofibroma (**c**) results from a diffuse interstitial proliferation which incorporates all the present neural fibers in its body, giving rise to a spindle-shaped mass clearly different from the schwannoma, which is nodular (**b**, in the figure) and nonencapsulated

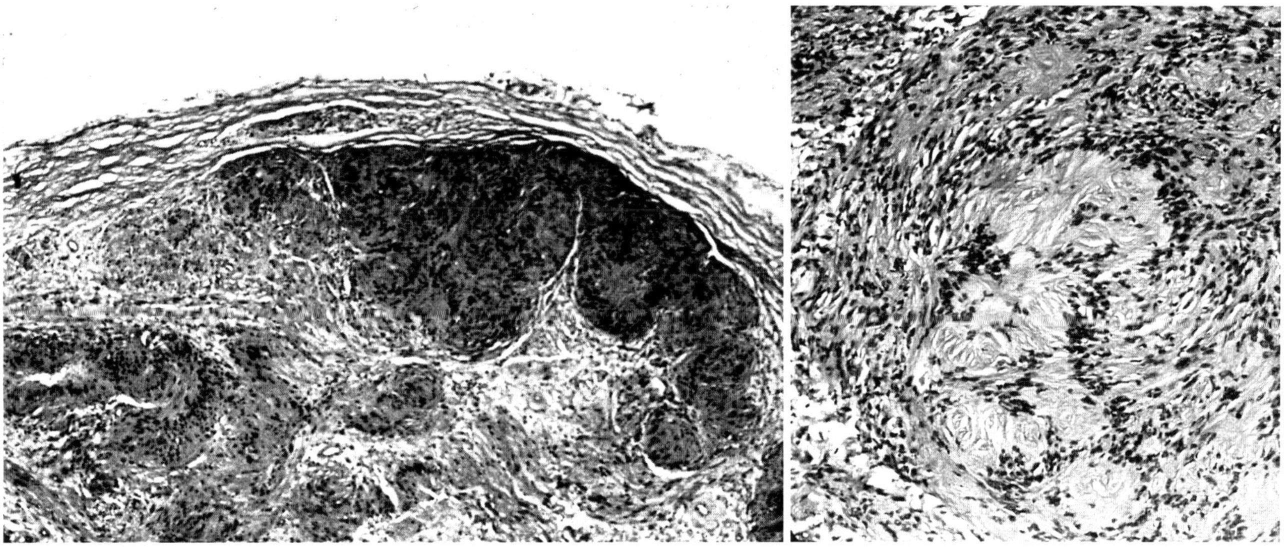

Fig. 6.96 Schwannoma. (*Left*) Note the fibrous capsule which surrounds the lesion. The deep stained Antoni A zones contrast with the myxoid, paucicellular, and faintly stained Antoni B zones. (*Right*) Verocay bodies shown at high magnification. H&E ×40; ×400 o m

"granular cell myoblastoma." After ultrastructural and other studies demonstrated the actual *nervous* nature of the lesion, its name was changed to the current one: "granular cell tumor." This name was based on the granular aspect of the cytoplasm in the tumoral cells, which, along with their characteristic punctiform nuclei, lend this lesion its characteristic appearance (Fig. 6.98).

Cutaneous Neoplasias of Extracutaneous Origin

The Class of the cutaneous neoplasias of extracutaneous origin (invasive tumors of the skin) (Fig. 6.27) may be separated into two Subclasses, according to the way their invasive tendency is manifested: in the first case, the epidermis is selectively invaded, and in the second, an indiscriminate

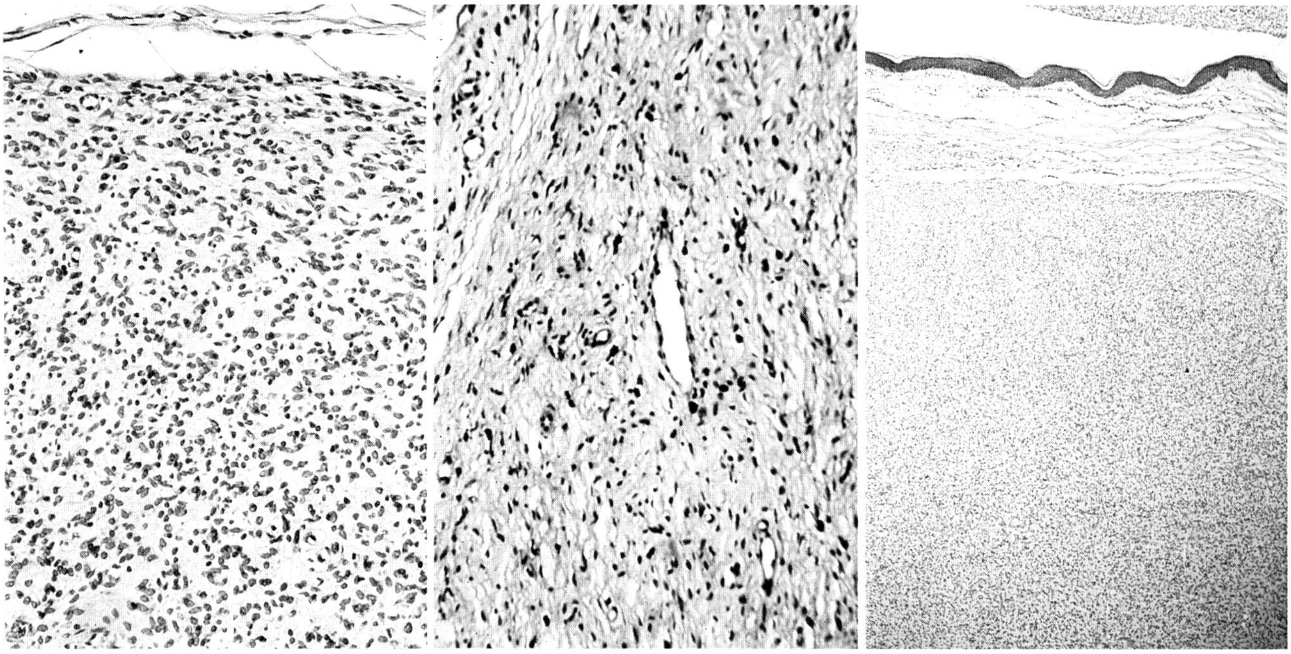

Fig. 6.97 Neurofibroma. (*Left*) Note the structure of the lesion formed by small, curled cells. (*Center*) The composition of the lesion may be observed at higher magnification. The use of toluidine blue as a staining reagent reveals purple metachromatic dots corresponding to numerous mast cells (*right*). The lesion is clearly separated from the surrounding stroma but devoid of a peripheral capsule. H&E ×40; ×100; ×100 o m

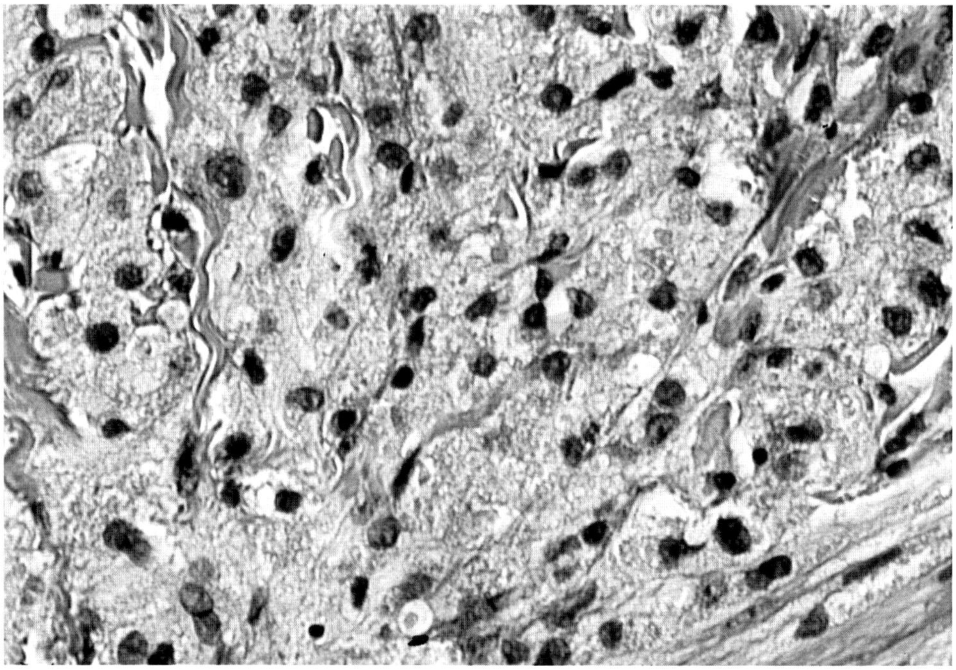

Fig. 6.98 Granular cell tumor. See text for details. Tri ×400 o m

invasion of the skin occur. In this latter case, four invasive patterns may be recognized, each listed as a Group: by contiguity, by infiltration of systemic processes, by metastasis, and by instrumental contamination (Fig. 6.99).

Epidermotrophic Neoplastic Invasions

Three conditions may be considered as examples in the first Subclass of selective epidermal invasion: intraepidermal carcinoma of Jadassohn, Paget's disease, and malignant

Subclass	Group	Example
Epidermotrophic		Jadassohn's intraepidermal carcinoma Paget's disease Superficially spreading malignant melanoma
Indiscriminate	By contiguity	Cancer "*en cuirasse*"
	By infiltration of systemic processes	Mycosis fungoides
	Metastatic invasions	Alopecia metastatica
	By instrumental contamination	Neoplastic implantation by needle biopsies

Fig. 6.99 Cutaneous neoplasias of extracutaneous origin

melanoma in the horizontal phase of *propagation* (Fig. 6.100).

Intraepidermal carcinoma of Jadassohn (Fig. 6.100, top): This condition is of historic importance because it first raised the possibility that a carcinoma could be propagated throughout the thickness of the epidermis [74]. The origin of the invasive cells in this lesion has not been determined, but the final result of the process is the infiltration of the epidermis by groups of anaplastic keratinocytes, clearly different from the normal ones, which form the background of the lesion.

Paget's disease [75] (Fig. 6.100, center): Contrary to the uncertainty about the origin of Jadassohn intraepidermal carcinoma, the origin of the invasive neoplasia in Paget's disease has been clarified and found to be an underlying carcinoma of the breast, which propagates along lactiferous ducts to the nipple, where it becomes apparent. Under the microscope, the neoplastic cells appear as clusters of large clear, mucin-containing elements with a high mitotic rate, clearly different from the surrounding keratinocytes. Subsequent to *Paget's disease*, extramammary Paget's disease [76] was also described. This condition, similar to the preceding one, appears in the skin on genital areas and supposedly originates in the duct of local apocrine glands.

Superficially spreading malignant melanoma (Fig. 6.100, bottom): This condition develops during the invasive process of malignant melanoma, offering a highly characteristic, previously described microscopic image.

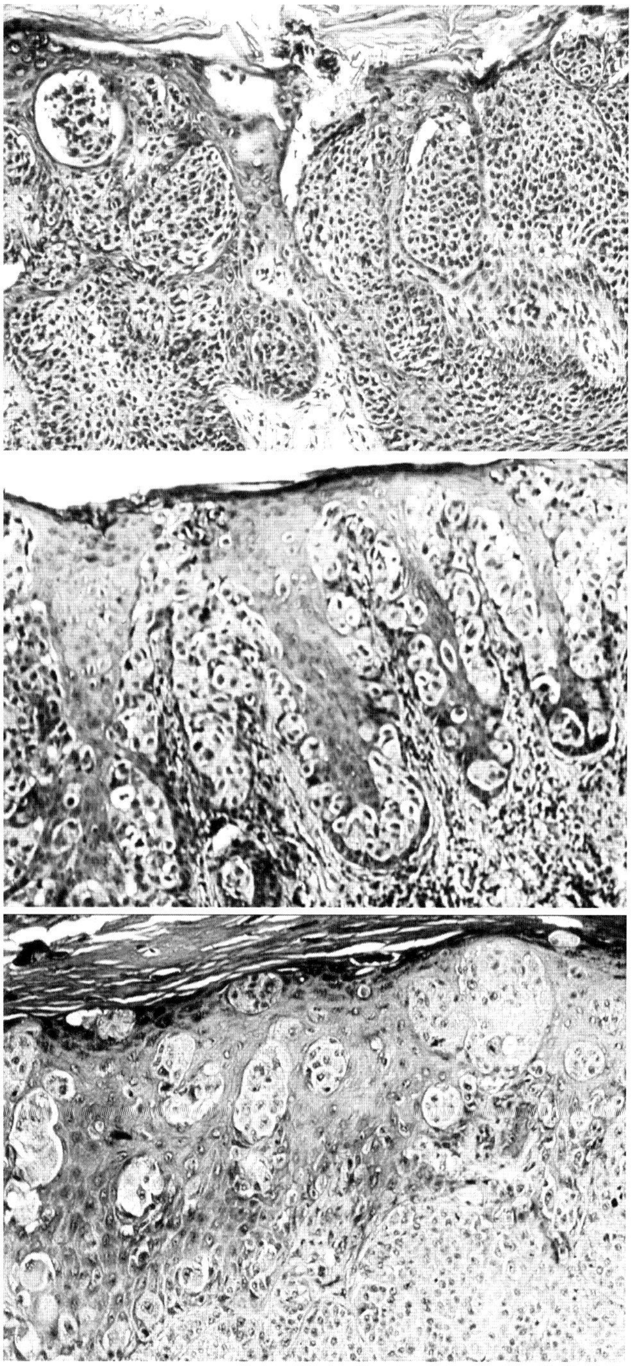

Fig. 6.100 Three instances of selective epidermal neoplastic invasion. From *top to bottom*, Jadassohn intraepidermal carcinoma; Paget's disease and malignant melanoma in the horizontal phase of propagation. See details in the text. H&E ×100; MC ×400; H&E ×100 o m

Indiscriminate Cutaneous Invasions

The skin is a frequent target of extracutaneous neoplastic proliferations, which may invade it; four pertinent instances of indiscriminated neoplastic invasion of the skin may be recognized (Fig. 6.99).

Neoplastic Invasions by Contiguity

A typical case in this group is that of skin invaded by contiguity by an underlying breast adenocarcinoma, propagated by lymphatic vessels and configurating the so-called cancer en cuirasse (Fig. 6.101).

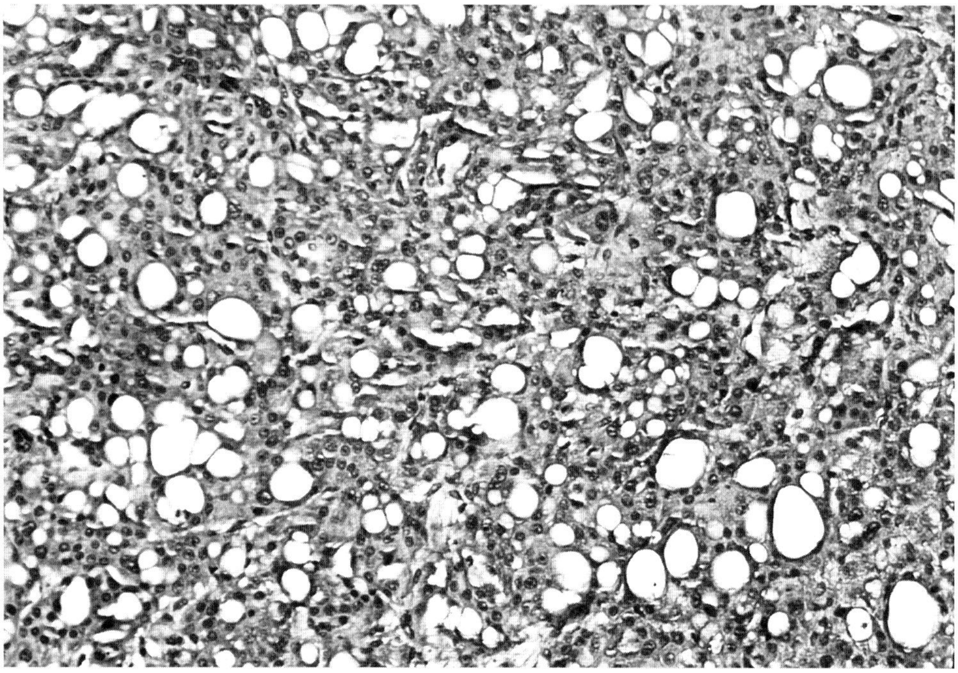

Fig. 6.101 Cancer en cuirasse. Note the diffuse infiltration of fatty tissue by the neoplastic process. H&E ×40 o m

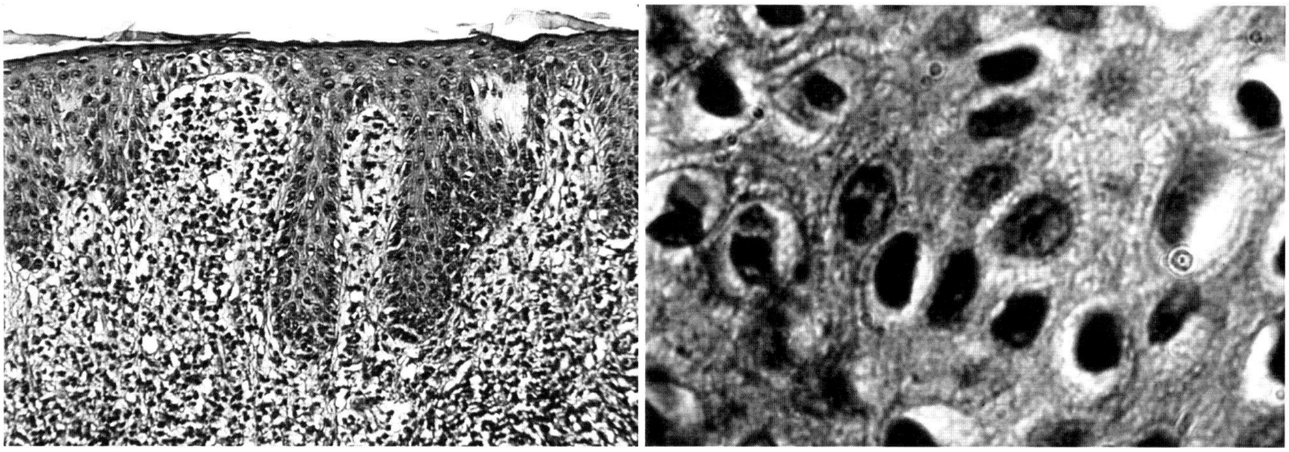

Fig. 6.102 Mycosis fungoides. Note to *the left* the dense character of the infiltrate located between the elongated ridges. Note also the lack of spongiosis in the epidermis. Observe to *the right* the atypical character of the lymphocytes, with hyperchromatic nuclei featuring prominent nucleoli. Contrast these with the keratinocytes in the same section surrounded by interstitial bridges. H&E ×100; ×1,000 o m

Cutaneous lesions of *Hodgkin's disease* in some rare cases may also be the result of direct propagation from subcutaneous foci. The possibility also exists that cutaneous propagation may be the result of a blockage of a lymphatic nodule with reflux of lymphatic circulation, which may carry back malignant cells into the skin.

Malignant Systemic Infiltration

The skin may suffer diffuse infiltrations by malignant lymphoproliferative processes. Of all of these, the most frequent and important is mycosis fungoides (MF) due to the malignant of T cells. While the initial forms of MF were already mentioned among the transitional inflammatory conditions, this section will touch upon the lesion's microscopic features as it advances from the most incipient form of the disease to the "patchy" or "plaque" form and, finally, to the "tumoral" form.

Microscopic examination reveals in all of these a dense cellular infiltrate in the dermis, which, however, displays the tendency to spread out into the epidermis (Fig. 6.102). This epidermotrophic tendency may cause the observer to underestimate that infiltrate and to consider it as a chronic dermatitis, instead. The *lack of spongiosis* is a diagnostic detail that weighs against an inflammatory exocytosis, pointing instead to MF.

The components of the MF infiltrate are irregular mononuclear and sometimes folded cells with hyperchromatic nuclei, featuring prominent nucleoli. The cells in which these details are most evident are called "Pautrier cells." Groups of these cells in the epidermis are the so-called Pautrier microabscesses (Fig. 6.103). These are primordial for the diagnosis of MF.

Sézary syndrome, which may be considered an advanced stage of MF, has the clinical appearance of a diffuse, intensely pruritic erythroderma with a moderate leukocytosis: its most important diagnostic feature are circulating Sézary cells, closely similar to the before-mentioned "mycosis cells."

In the case of the leukemias, the cutaneous manifestation generally follows the systemic ones. This facilitates the diagnosis of the infiltrates which eventually appear on the patient's skin. The microscopic examination of these infiltrates reveals atypical leukocytes similar to the circulating ones. A characteristic acute granulocytic leukemia is the "granulocytic sarcoma," formerly known under the name of "cloroma," in which the atypical elements of this condition are identified.

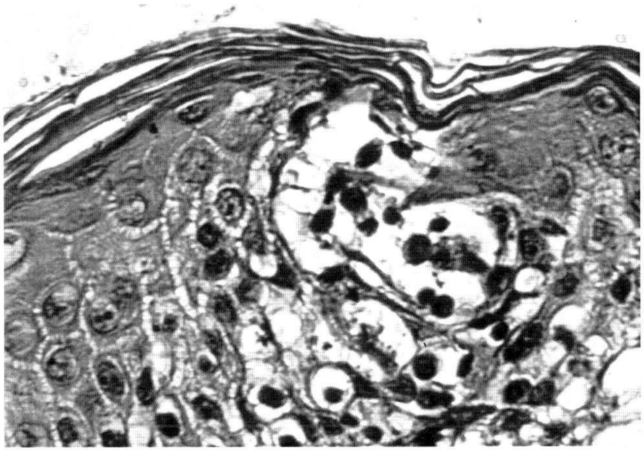

Fig. 6.103 Mycosis fungoides. Note the cluster of atypical lymphocytes within the epidermis, featuring a Pautrier microabscess. H&E ×400 o m

Metastasis

The appearance of a cutaneous metastasis is occasionally the first signal of the presence of a malignant neoplasia in a patient. Although this event may occur in every part of the body surface, the scalp is a frequent site for their localization. Microscopic examination frequently gives a fairly precise indication regarding the nature of the examined specimen. A particular example of a blood-borne metastasis is "alopecia metastatica." This lesion represents a metastasis from a distant adenocarcinoma, very often of the breast, which reaches the scalp. The lesion (Fig. 6.104) compresses the hairy skin above it causing a circumscribed loss of hair, which bears the above-mentioned name.

A metastasis which bears its own name is "Sister Mary Joseph nodule." This lesion corresponds to a blood-borne metastasis, generally from the pancreas or stomach. It is carried by the umbilical vessels and appears in the periumbilical region (Fig. 6.105, left). Contrasting that figure, Fig. 6.105, right, shows another adenocarcinoma metastatic to the scalp, this time from the kidney.

Instrumental Implantation

The performance of a surgical operation or even a restricted invasive procedure such as a needle biopsy may cause the implantation of tumoral cells, most frequently on the thoracic or abdominal wall as in the case featured in Fig. 6.106, of a pancreatic adenocarcinoma implanted in the abdominal wall.

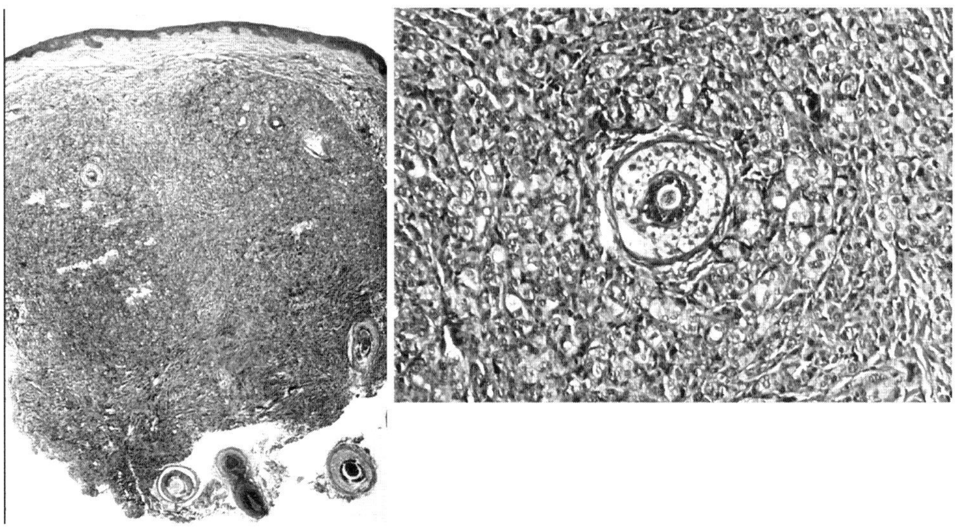

Fig. 6.104 Alopecia metastatica. (*Right*) Note the dense infiltrate in the scalp, as well as its lack of hair follicles. (*Left*) Observe the cross section of a hair follicle surrounded by neoplastic cells. H&E ×40; ×400 o m

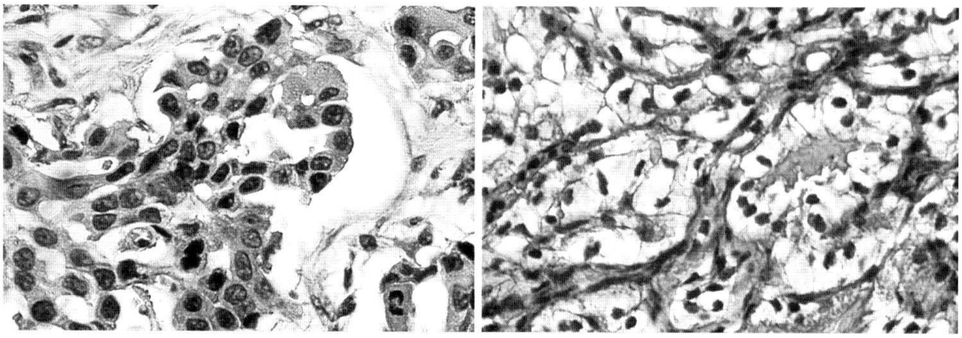

Fig. 6.105 Sister Mary Joseph nodule and metastatic kidney adenocarcinoma. The dermis of the first specimen (*left*) features a group of adenocarcinoma, mucus-containing cells appearing in a disorganized fashion. The lesion in the metastatic kidney adenocarcinoma (*right*) is formed by characteristic clear cells. H&E ×400 o m

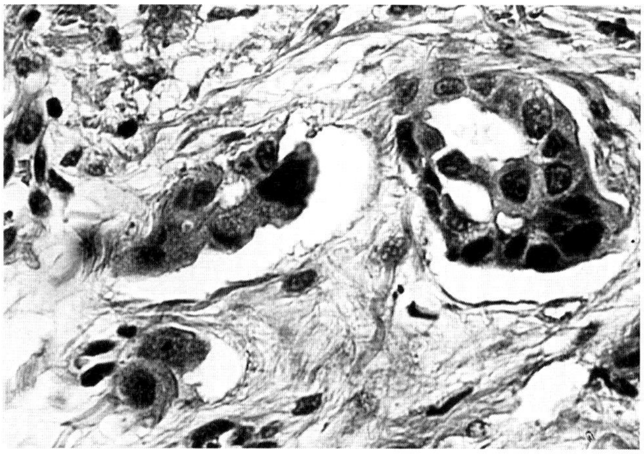

Fig. 6.106 Implant of a pancreatic adenocarcinoma on the abdominal wall after a needle biopsy. H&E ×400 o m

References

1. Pinkus H. In: Mehregan AH, Hashimoto K, editors. Pinkus' guide to dermatohistopathology, 5th ed. Norwalk: Appleton & Lange; 1991. p. 502–7.
2. Rosai J. Rosai and Ackerman surgical pathology. 9th ed. Edinburgh: Mosby; 2004. p. 1524–6.
3. Pinkus H. In: Mehregan AH, Hashimoto K, editors. Pinkus' guide to dermatohistopathology, 5th ed. Norwalk: Appleton & Lange; 1991. p. 424.
4. Lever WF, Schaumburg-Lever G. Histopathology of the skin. 7th ed. Philadelphia: J.B. Lipppincott Company; 1990. p. 411.
5. Braun-Falco O, Plewig G, Wolff HH, Burgdorf WHC. Dermatology. 2nd ed. Berlin: Springer; 2000. p. 54.
6. Lowy DR, Androphy EJ. In: Freedberg IM, et al., editors. Fitzpatrik dermatologia en medicina general, 5th ed. Buenos Aires: Editorial Medica Panamericana; 2001. p. 2632.
7. Kirnbauer R, Lenz P, Okun MM. In: Bologna JL, Jorizzo JL, Rapini RP, editors. Dermatology. Edinburgh: Mosby; 2003. p. 1222.
8. Lever WF, Schaumburg-Lever G. Histopathology of the skin. 7th ed. Philadelphia: J.B. Lipppincott Co.; 1990. p. 418.
9. Schwartz RA, Stoll HL. In: Freedberg IM, et al., editors. Fitzpatrik dermatologia en medicina general, 5th ed. Buenos Aires: Editorial Medica Panamericana; 2001. p. 873.
10. Braverman IM. Skin signs of systemic diseases. 3rd ed. Philadelphia: W.B. Saunders Co.; 1998. p. 53–5.
11. Ho VCY. In: Freedberg IM, et al., editors. Fitzpatrik dermatologia en medicina general, 5th ed. Buenos Aires: Editorial Medica Panamericana; 2001. p. 917.
12. Willis RA. Pathology of tumors. 2nd ed. London: Butterworth & Co Ltd; 1953. p. 1.
13. Lever WF, Schaumburg-Lever G. Histopathology of the skin. 7th ed. Philadelphia: J.B. Lipppincott Company; 1990. p. 553–4.
14. Pinkus H. In: Mehregan AH, Hashimoto K, editors. Pinkus' guide to dermatohistopathology, 5th ed. Norwalk: Appleton & Lange; 1991. p. 512.
15. Lever WF, Schaumburg-Lever G. Histopathology of the skin. 7th ed. Philadelphia: J.B. Lipppincott Company; 1990. p. 556–7.
16. Braun-Falco O, Plewig G, Wolff HH, Burgdorf WHC. Dermatology. 2nd ed. Berlin: Springer; 2000. p. 1465.
17. James WD, Berger TG, Elston DM, editors. Andrews' diseases of the skin. 10th ed. Pennsylvania: W.B. Saunders; 2006. p. 687.
18. Nestle FO, Kerl H. In: Bologna JL, Jorizzo JL, Rapini RP, et al., editors. Dermatology. Edinburgh: Mosby; 2003. p. 1805.
19. Lever WF, Schaumburg-Lever G. Histopathology of the skin. 7th ed. Philadelphia: J.B. Lipppincott Company; 1990. p. 791–2.
20. Rosai J. Rosai and Ackerman surgical pathology. 9th ed. Edinburgh: Mosby; 2004. p. 174–5.
21. Nestle FO, Karl H. In: Bologna JL, Jorizzo JL. Rapini RP, et al., editors. Dermatology. Edinburgh: Mosby; 2003. p. 1795.
22. Mooi WJ, Krausz T. Biopsy pathology of melanocytic disorders. London: Chapman & Hall Medical; 1992. p. 186–210.
23. Mooi WJ, Krausz T. Biopsy pathology of melanocytic disorders. London: Chapman & Hall Medical; 1992. p. 178–83.
24. Rosai J. Rosai and Ackerman surgical pathology. 9th ed. Edinburgh: Mosby; 2004. p. 177–9.
25. Hashimoto K, Lever WF. Appendage tumors of the skin. Springfield: Charles C Thomas; 1968. p. 1.
26. Pinkus H. In: Mehregan AH, Hashimoto K, editors. Pinkus' guide to dermatohistopathology, 5th ed. Norwalk: Appleton & Lange; 1991. p. 583.
27. Pinkus H. In: Mehregan AH, Hashimoto K, editors. Pinkus' guide to dermatohistopathology, 5th ed. Norwalk: Appleton & Lange; 1991. p. 589.
28. Lever WF, Schaumburg-Lever G. Histopathology of the skin. 7th ed. Philadelphia: J.B. Lipppincott Company; 1990. p. 628.
29. Lever WF, Schaumburg-Lever G. Histopathology of the skin. 7th ed. Philadelphia: J.B. Lipppincott Company; 1990. p. 589.
30. Lever WF, Schaumburg-Lever G. Histopathology of the skin. 7th ed. Philadelphia: J.B. Lipppincott Company; 1990. p. 587–9.
31. Lever WF, Schaumburg-Lever G. Histopathology of the skin. 7th ed. Philadelphia: J.B. Lipppincott Company; 1990. p. 538.
32. Lever WF, Schaumburg-Lever G. Histopathology of the skin. 7th ed. Philadelphia: J.B. Lipppincott Company; 1990. p. 604–5.
33. Rosen PP, Oberman HA. In: Rosai J, editor. Atlas of tumor pathology, 3rd series, Fascicle 7. Washington, D.C.: Armed Forces Institute of Pathology; 1993. p. 78–86.
34. Pinkus H. In: Mehregan AH, Hashimoto K, editors. Pinkus' guide to dermatohistopathology, 5th ed. Norwalk: Appleton & Lange; 1991. p. 569.

35. Lever WF, Schaumburg-Lever G. Histopathology of the skin. 7th ed. Philadelphia: J.B. Lipppincott Company; 1990. p. 609–11.
36. Kersting W. In: Graham JH, Johnson WC, Helwig EB, editors. Dermal pathology. Hagerstown: Harper & Row; 1972. p. 526–7.
37. Ellis GL. Auclair PL. In: Rosai J, editor. Atlas of tumor pathology, 3rd series, fascicle 17. Washington, D.C.: Armed Forces Institute of Pathology; 1996. p. 39–57.
38. Lever WF, Schaumburg-Lever G. Histopathology of the skin. 7th ed. Philadelphia: J.B. Lipppincott Company; 1990. p. 616–7.
39. Rosai J. Rosai and Ackerman surgical pathology. 9th ed. Edinburgh: Mosby; 2004. p. 142.
40. Kersting W. In: Graham JH, Johnson WE, Helwig EB, editors. Dermal pathology. Hagerstown: Harper & Row; 1972. p. 511–3.
41. Enzinger FM, Weiss SW. Soft tissue tumors. 3rd ed. St. Louis: Mosby; 1995. p. 1.
42. Enzinger FM, Weiss SW. Soft tissue tumors. 3rd ed. St. Louis: Mosby; 1995. p. 293.
43. Pinkus H. In: Mehregan AH, Hashimoto K, editors. Pinkus' guide to dermatohistopathology, 5th ed. Norwalk: Appleton & Lange; 1991. p. 333.
44. Lever WF, Schaumburg-Lever G. Histopathology of the skin. 7th ed. Philadelphia: J.B. Lipppincott Company; 1990. p. 666.
45. Rosai J. Rosai and Ackerman surgical pathology. 9th ed. Edinburgh: Mosby; 2004. p. 2205–7.
46. Enzinger FM, Weiss SW. Soft tissue tumors. 3rd ed. St. Louis: Mosby; 1995. p. 167–73.
47. James WD, Berger TG, Elston DM, editors. Andrews' diseases of the skin. 10th ed. Pennsylvania: W.B. Saunders; 2006. p. 604–5.
48. Braun-Falco O, Plewig G, Wolff HH, Burgdorf WHC. Dermatology. 2nd ed. Berlin: Springer; 2000. p. 1563.
49. Hajdu SI. Pathology of soft tissue tumors. Philadelphia: Lea & Febiger; 1979. p. 83.
50. Rosai J. Rosai and Ackerman surgical pathology. 9th ed. Edinburgh: Mosby; 2004. p. 184.
51. Enzinger FM, Weiss SW. Soft tissue tumors. 3rd ed. St. Louis: Mosby; 1995. p. 211–20.
52. Enzinger FM, Weiss SW. Soft tissue tumors. 3rd ed. St.Louis: Mosby; 1995. p. 352–5.
53. Enzinger FM, Weiss SW. Soft tissue tumors. 3rd ed. St.Louis: Mosby; 1995. p. 355–77.
54. Enzinger FM, Weiss SW. Soft tissue tumors. 3rd ed. St.Louis: Mosby; 1995. p. 269–80.
55. Lazar AJF, Murphy GF, In: Kumar V, Abbas AK, Fausto N, Aster JC, editors. Robbins and Cotran pathologic basis of disease, 8th ed. Philadelphia: Saunders Elsevier; 2010. p. 1254.
56. Lever WF, Schaumburg-Lever G. Histopathology of the skin. 7th ed. Philadelphia: J.B. Lipppincott Company; 1990. p. 728.
57. Enzinger FM, Weiss SW. Soft tissue tumors. 3rd ed. St.Louis: Mosby; 1995. p. 679.
58. Enzinger FM, Weiss SW. Soft tissue tumors. 3rd ed. St.Louis: Mosby; 1995. p. 701.
59. Rosai J. Rosai and Ackerman surgical pathology. 9th ed. Edinburgh: Mosby; 2004. p. 190–1.
60. Lever WF, Schaumburg-Lever G. Histopathology of the skin. 7th ed. Philadelphia: J.B. Lipppincott Company; 1990. p. 695.
61. Enzinger FM, Weiss SW. Soft tissue tumors. 3rd ed. St.Louis: Mosby; 1995. p. 627–40.
62. Lever WF, Schaumburg-Lever G. Histopathology of the skin. 7th ed. Philadelphia: J.B. Lipppincott Company; 1990. p. 708–10.
63. Rosen PP, Oberman HA. In: Rosai J, editors. Atlas of tumor pathology, 3rd series, fascicle 7. Washington, D.C.: Armed Forces Institute of Pathology; 1993. p. 328.
64. Lever WF, Schaumburg-Lever G. Histopathology of the skin. 7th ed. Philadelphia: J.B. Lipppincott Company; 1990. p. 707.
65. Rosai J. Rosai and Ackerman surgical pathology. 9th ed. Edinburgh: Mosby; 2004. p. 193.
66. Enzinger FM, Weiss SW. Soft tissue tumors. 3rd ed. St.Louis: Mosby; 1995. p. 702–13.
67. Braun-Falco O, Plewig G, Wolff HH, Burgdorf WHC. Dermatology. 2nd ed. Berlin: Springer; 2000. p. 1581.
68. Klempson RL, Fletcher CDM, Evans HL, Hendrikson ML, Sibley RK, In: Rosai J (Ed). Atlas of tumor pathology, 3rd series, fascicle 30. Washington, D.C.: Armed Forces Institute of Pathology; 1993. p. 189–94.
69. Scheithauer BW, Woodruff JM, Erlandson RA. In: Rosai J, editor. Atlas of tumor pathology, 3rd series, fascicle 24. Washington, D.C.: Armed Forces Institute of Pathology; 1997. p. 1.
70. Scheithauer BW, Woodruff JM, Erlandson RA. In: Rosai J, editor. Atlas of tumor pathology, 3rd series, fascicle 24. Washington, D.C.: Armed Forces Institute of Pathology; 1997. p. 105–70.
71. Scheithauer BW, Woodruff JM, Erlandson RA. In: Rosai J, editor. Atlas of tumor pathology, 3rd series, fascicle 24. Washington, D.C.: Armed Forces Institute of Pathology; 1999. p. 177–216.
72. Scheithauer BW, Woodruff JM, Erlandson RA. In: Rosai J, editor. Atlas of tumor pathology, 3rd series, fascicle 24. Washington, D.C.: Armed Forces Institute of Pathology; 1999. p. 236–48.
73. Rosai J. Rosai and Ackerman surgical pathology. 9th ed. Edinburgh: Mosby; 2004. p. 2317–20.
74. Pinkus H. In: Mehregan AH, Hashimoto K, editors. Pinkus' guide to dermatohistopathology, 5th ed. Norwalk: Appleton & Lange; 1991. p. 596.
75. Pinkus H. In: Mehregan AH, Hashimoto K, editors. Pinkus' guide to dermatohistopathology, 5th ed. Norwalk: Appleton & Lange; 1991. p. 597.
76. Rosai J. Rosai and Ackerman surgical pathology. 9th ed. Edinburgh: Mosby; 2004. p. 145–7.

7 Miscellaneous Cutaneous Lesions

A number of cutaneous lesions exist which do not quite fit into any of the four previously postulated divisions of this classification. Whereas in some cases, these lesions correspond to mild or sporadic conditions which do not significantly impact on the patient's life, in other cases, they are manifestations of altered biological cycles or other situations that may have more serious consequences.

The great etiopathogenic disparity of these lesions prevents them from being worked out in a progressive and orderly fashion and from being logically distributed into the already available niches of the devised taxonomic system, as has been done in the previous four divisions. Instead, following a rather practical approach, these lesions are accommodated into a simplified seventh Division with five Classes and several Groups of miscellaneous lesions as shown in Fig. 7.1. This provides a well-rounded closure to the hereby proposed classification system.

Lesions Caused by Dysregulated Fibroblastic Activity

This Class includes three Groups of lesions, each resulting from the faulty production of a substance normally synthesized by fibroblasts: collagen, mucin, and elastin (Fig. 7.1).

Lesions Caused by Faulty Collagen Production

Among the lesions in this Group, there are some which occur *selectively* in the skin and others which are manifested in a *systemic* fashion, affecting the skin as well as other internal organs. Keloid formation should be mentioned first.

Keloid (*kelis* + *oid*) [G] (claw + similar) is due to uncontrolled, focal fibroblastic activity, often triggered by a wound or by the presence of a foreign body, which leads to the production of large amounts of collagen (Fig. 7.2). Contrary to the already discussed *hypertrophic scar* in which excessive production of collagen stops spontaneously at a certain point, in the case of keloid, collagen production continues uninterruptedly, leading to the formation of bulky masses of fibrotic material. The predominance of keloid among dark-skinned people hints toward the existence of genetic factors in the production of this lesion.

The exaggerated production of collagen may lead to more diffuse forms of cutaneous sclerosis: this process basically occurs in two conditions, morphea and scleroderma [1].

Morphea (*morphe* [G] form of figure) is a process of cutaneous localization, whereas scleroderma or systemic sclerosis involves the cutaneous as other systems, including the digestive, the respiratory, and the urinary. The histologic pictures of morphea and scleroderma are closely similar, to the point that they cannot be told apart under the

Classes	Groups
Caused by dysregulated fibroblastic activity	With faulty production of collagen With faulty production of mucin With faulty production of elastic fibers
Cutaneous deposits	Of endogenous material Of exogenous material
Metaplasias Degradative processes	Involutions Degenerations Atrophies
Cysts	Retention cysts Implantation cysts

Fig. 7.1 Miscellaneous lesions: Classes and Groups

E. Zappi, E.A. Zappi, *Dermatopathology*,
DOI 10.1007/978-1-4471-2894-6_7, © Springer-Verlag London 2013

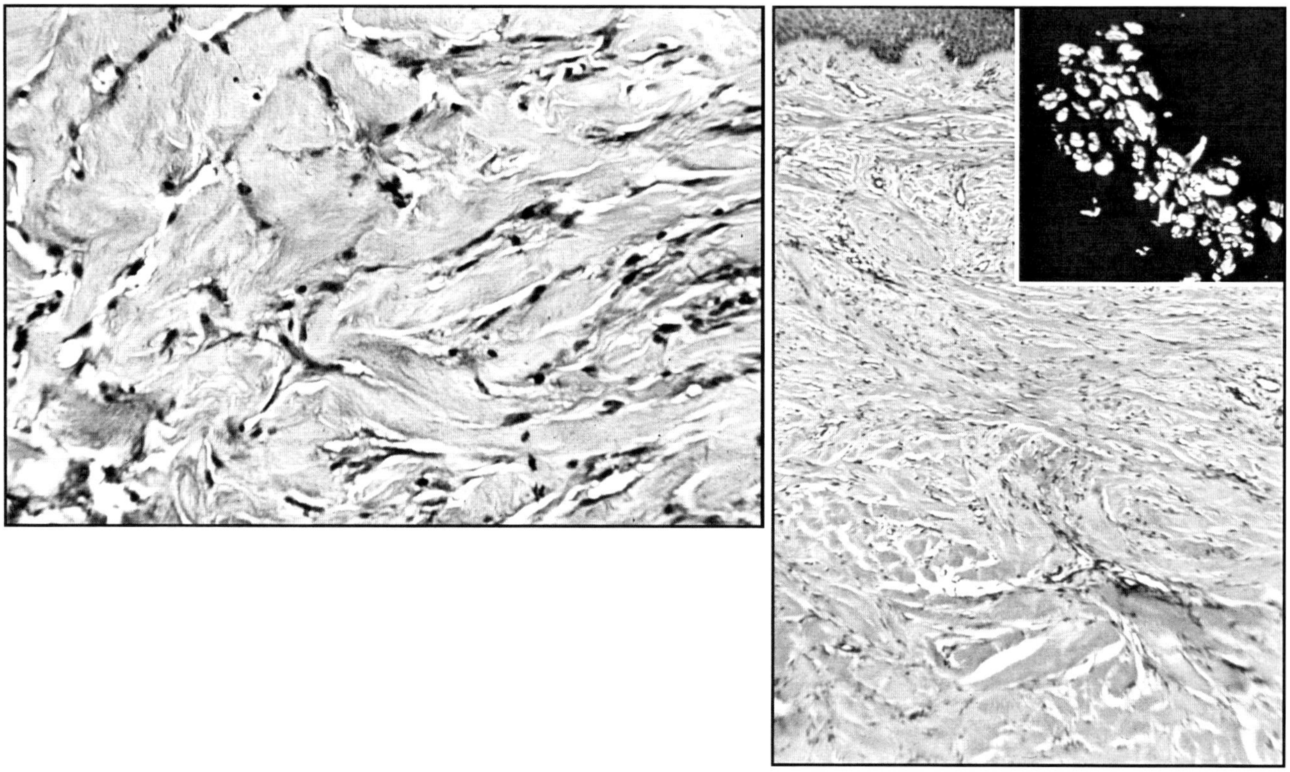

Fig. 7.2 Keloid. (*Left*) Note the absence of the longitudinal striations of normal collagen fibers. This, as well as their characteristic, "glassy straps" are indications of the abnormal quality of the collagen generated in this condition. (*Right*) Keloid formed around a cluster of foreign body. The latter are better visualized under polarized light. (*inset*) H&E ×100; ×40; ×1,000 polarized light o m

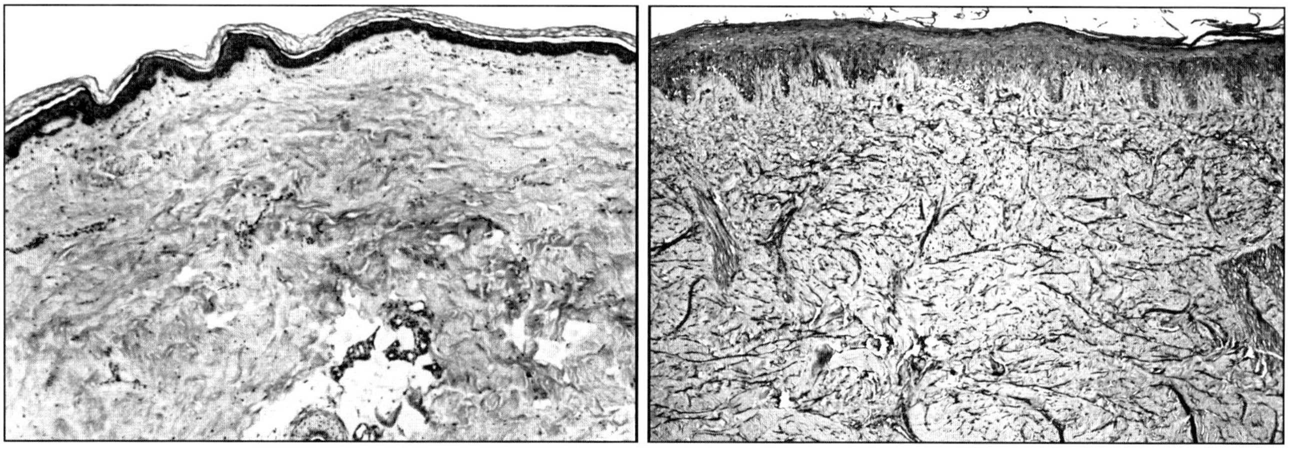

Fig. 7.3 Morphea. (*Left*) Note the homogenization of the dermis, in which structural distinctions between the papillary and the reticular layer are obliterated. In the same fashion, the spreading of the collagen into the fatty tissue erases differences between the dermis and the subcutaneous panniculus. Besides, the increase of collagen causes a relative diminution of the reticulin network, as can be observed upon examination of tissue sections stained by an appropriate technique (*right*). H&E; ETG ×100 o m

microscope (Fig. 7.2). Both lesions are characterized by the presence of a faintly eosinophylic and homogeneous abnormal collagen, which spreads downward into the dermis surrounding sweat gland coils and fat lobules and erasing the boundaries between the various levels of the skin. "Morphea *en coup de sabre*" is a particular type of this condition exteriorized as a deep groove running from the scalp to the face, as if produced by a blow with a saber. In spite of its peculiar form of presentation, its microscopic picture does not differ from that of the common form of morphea (see below), except for an irreversible alopecia in the area of the scalp affected (Fig. 7.3).

Scleredema: This disorder is of unknown origin. It causes a diffuse thickening of the skin due to the combined increase

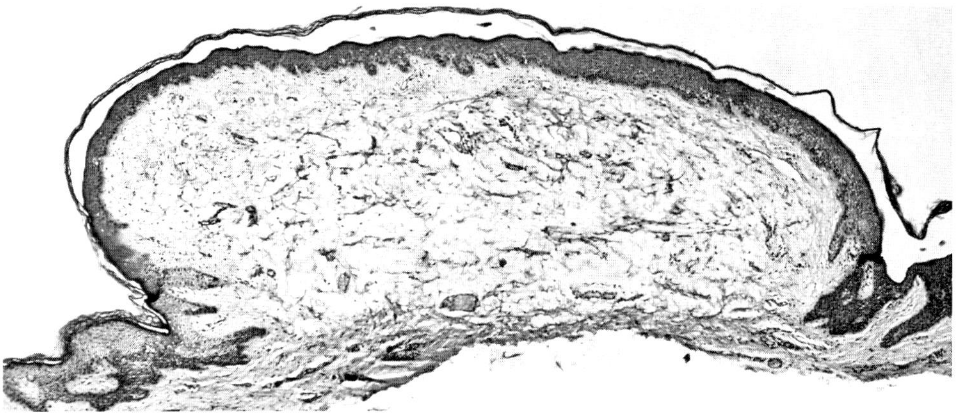

Fig. 7.4 Myxoid papule of the skin. The lesion consists of a mass of mucin with scant star-shaped cells and fibrillar elements, overlaid by a distended epidermis. TB ×100 o m

of collagen with mucin and associated substances [2]. From this point of view, it may be considered a condition intermediate between the ones in the above Class and others in the Class that follows.

Lesions Caused by Faulty Mucin Production

As in the case of collagen, deposits of mucin may occur in localized or generalized fashion, thus respectively called localized or systemic mucinosis. Hypothyroidism may be manifested in one form or the other, that is, as a systemic mucinosis, "generalized myxedema" or as a localized mucin deposition, as in pretibial myxedema [3].

Myxoid papule of the skin is a minimal form of mucinosis, devoid of any significant pathology. It is a frequent incidental finding in the dermatopathology laboratory (Fig. 7.4). Upon staining with toluidine blue, the material inside the lesion yields a metachromatic reaction (p. 194) appearing as a purple discoloration.

Lesions Caused by Faulty Elastin Production

Elastofibroma dorsi (assuming that this is an uncontrolled local proliferation of elastic fibers, and not a malformative lesion, as it may be alternatively argued) is a lesion of a characteristic localization on the tip of the scapula. It is usually seen in aged patients. Microscopic examination of the lesion reveals a highly disorganized structure, caused by the presence of clumps of elastic fibers, intermingled with the normal components of the dermis. In an advanced stage, the elastic fibers undergo fractionation and agglomeration, being transformed into amorphous masses of elastic tissue (Fig. 7.5).

Elastotic degeneration, a condition somehow pertinent to this Subgroup of lesions is more conveniently discussed below, along with *degenerative* processes.

Cutaneous Deposits

The lesions considered in this Group are deposits in the skin of *endogenous* or *exogenous* material. Unlike in the lesions already discussed in Chap. 5, these deposits do not elicit any *foreign body reaction.*

Cutaneous Deposits, Endogenous

Calcifications: Calcium, normally present in an ionized, soluble form in the blood, may be deposited in tissues under three circumstances: (a) alterations of tissues which favor its deposition in these, (b) electrolytic imbalances and hypercalcemia, or (c) unknown circumstances. These three forms of calcification are respectively called *dystrophic*, *metastasic*, and *idiopathic* (Table 7.1).

Whereas the last two forms of calcification exposed in Table 7.1 have only a marginal interest in this discussion, the first, that is, the *dystrophic* calcifications are worth a short discussion, since they are associated to several conditions pertaining to the realm of dermatopathology.

Dystrophic calcifications are associated with alteration of the tissues which occur in scleroderma and, in particular, in acrosclerosis. In this condition, *calcifications* combined with other symptoms give rise to the entity known as "CREST" [4], an acrostic formed as shown below:

Calcinosis cutis
Raynaud phenomenon
Esophageal dysphagia
Sclerodactyly periungual
Teleangiectasis

Microscopic examination of a dystrophic calcification presents calcium as subtle granules in the dermis, along with diffuse deposits of this material in the subcutaneous tissue. The calcium deposits, characteristic of the adnexal tumors of pilar progeny, and even of the calcific nodules of the scrotum – ultimately associated to steatocystoma

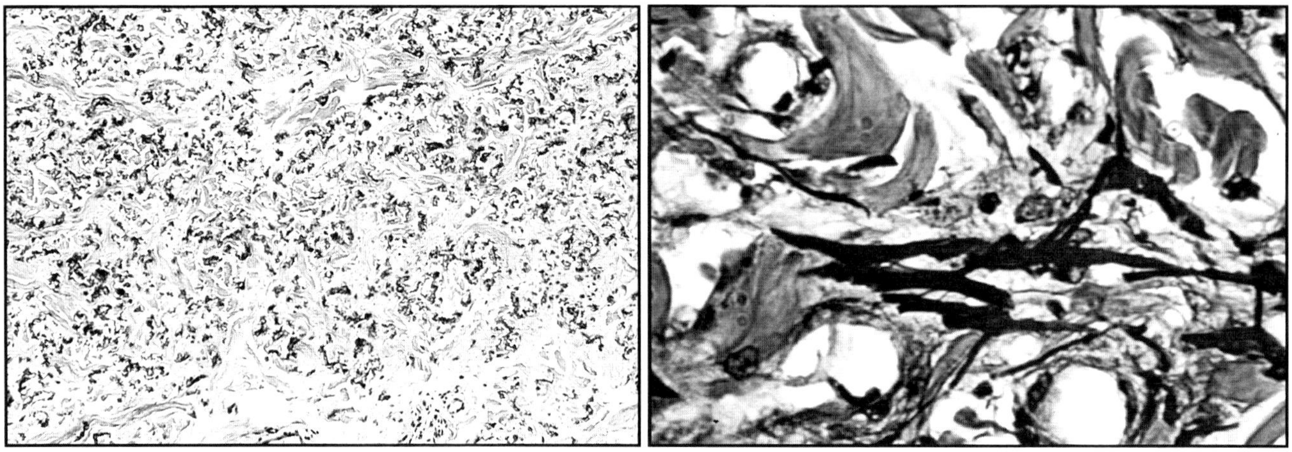

Fig. 7.5 Elastofibroma dorsi. (*Left*) Note the profound disruption of the area due to the presence of clumps of irregular elastic fibers. (*Right*) H&E ×40; ETG ×400 o m

Table 7.1 Calcification, forms, and examples

Dystrophic
In scleroderma
In CREST syndrome
In scars
Metastasic
In primary hyperparathyroidism
In chronic renal insufficiency
In cases of bone destruction
Idiopathic

Table 7.2 Amyloidosis: general classification

Primary
Systemic
Amyloidosis systemic
Amyloidosis systemic, myeloma-associated
Cutaneous
Lichen amyloidosus
Amyloidosis, nodular
Secondary

multiplex – could eventually be regarded as examples of *dystrophic calcifications* in abnormal or devitalized tissues, instead of considering them simply as idiopathic calcifications.

Amyloidosis generally refers to disorders in the course of which amyloid deposits occur in the tissues. The term "amyloid" was introduced by R. Virchow, who recognized its presence by the violet discoloration developed – as in the case of starch – (*amyl + oid* [G] starch-like) when a weak acid solution is applied onto a tissue previously treated with Lugol tincture.

Two main types of amyloidosis may be recognized: primary and secondary. Secondary amyloidosis, the so called wear and tear amyloidosis [5], is associated to chronic inflammatory processes which lead to the deposition of a proteinaceous material identified as an acute-phase protein, in several organs such as the spleen, kidney, and liver, *but not on the skin*. Because of its extracutaneous character, secondary amyloidosis does not need to be included in this discussion (Table 7.2).

Primary amyloidosis may be separated, for the purpose of its study, into systemic and cutaneous forms.

Systemic amyloidosis (SA): This condition involves mesenchymatous structures such as the myocardium and vessel walls, the tongue, and the dermis. SA is actually a plasma cell dyscrasia with a very unfavorable prognosis. It is so closely associated to multiple myeloma, that it is customary to separate it in the clinic as being, *associated* or *not*, with multiple myeloma. The amyloid deposits are formed by IgG light chains, or fragments of these, admixed with a "P non-fibrillar component." Amyloid appears under LM as amorphous and fissured, faintly eosinophilic masses distributed in the dermis and subcutaneous tissue. This material is also selectively deposited on the vessel wall, disrupting their structure and allowing the outward passage of red blood cells, which are found in the extravascular space. This explains the presence on the skin of SA patients of tiny petechiae the so called pinch purpura, a characteristic manifestation of this condition. Bence-Jones protein formed by IgG light chain fragments is found regularly in the urine of patients with multiple myeloma (Fig. 7.6).

Cutaneous amyloidosis: The two main forms of cutaneous amyloidosis are lichen amyloidosus and nodular amyloidosis. The fibrillar material deposited in these two particular conditions seems to be mainly derived from the keratinocytes overlying the lesion [6].

Lichen amyloidosus is a condition which presents particular interest in dermatology, since it is the only form of amyloidosis of exclusive cutaneous distribution. It presents a microscopic picture characterized by discrete deposits of this material occupying the dermal papillae, in an interstitial and perivascular disposition (Fig. 7.6).

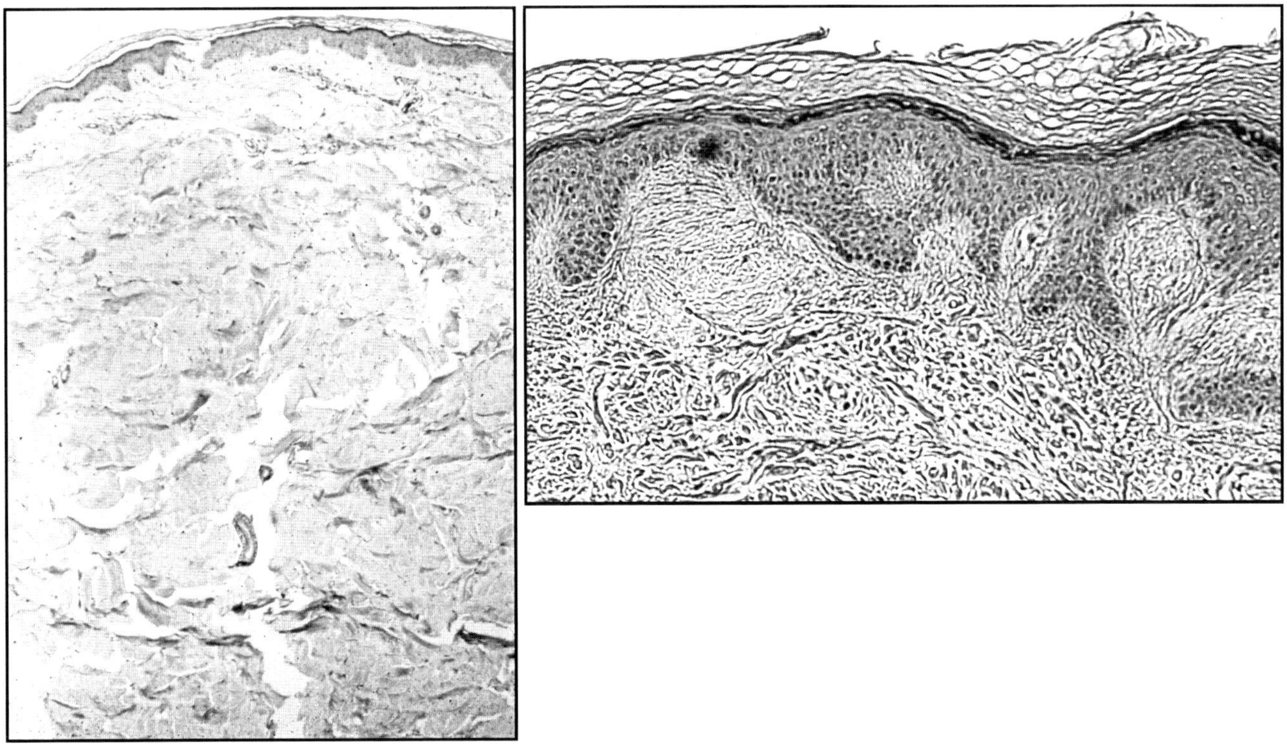

Fig. 7.6 Systemic amyloidosis and lichen amyloidosus. (*Left*) Note the homogeneous and fissurated masses of amyloid in the dermis and subcutaneous tissue in systemic amyloidosis. (*Right*) In lichen amyloidosus discrete masses of this material are seen, occupying dermal papillae. H&E ×40; ×100 o m

Table 7.3 Conditions associated to the presence of exogenous material

Ochronosis, exogenous
Argiria
Silicone deposits
Tattoos

Localized nodular amyloidosis is the least frequent of the primary amyloidosis. This is a condition which, in spite of its predominantly cutaneous distribution, presents a microscopic picture more consistent with that of the systemic form of amyloidosis.

Cutaneous Deposits, Exogenous

The lesions caused by the deposit of exogenous material form a list of entities which includes among others, the ones mentioned in Table 7.3.

Ochronosis, exogenous: Contrary to the previously mentioned *endogenous ochronosis*, which is associated to a MDwCR (p. 35), exogenous ochronosis is due to the local application of products based on hydroquinone, which lead to the accumulation of homogentisic acid. As in the case of endogenous ochronosis, this material is well tolerated by the patients, on which it does not cause major harm than an external brown pigmentation.

Argiria, caused by the prolonged ingestion of silver salts, leads also to a generalized bluish discoloration in the patient.

Silicone: Silicone oil is currently administrated as a "filler" with corrective purposes in the case of depressed scars and other conditions. Due to the inertness of this material, same is tolerated indefinitely without eliciting a foreign body reaction from the host (Fig. 7.7). The very popular practice of tattooing is responsible for the introduction of a series of pigments into the body. These are generally well tolerated, although occasionally may give rise to foreign body – or immune reactions.

Metaplasias

Metaplasia ([G] = *transformation*) is the transformation of a differentiated tissue into another under the persistent influence of an irritative stimulus. A very illustrative example of this phenomenon is the change of the cylindrical pseudostratified bronchial epithelium into a squamous stratified form.

Whereas in that case, the irritative agent responsible for the metaplasia can be easily determined; in other cases, it is hard to be ascertained. This is the case of the changes undergone by the nonspecific stroma surrounding a syringoma which turns it into a cartilaginous tissue, giving rise to the

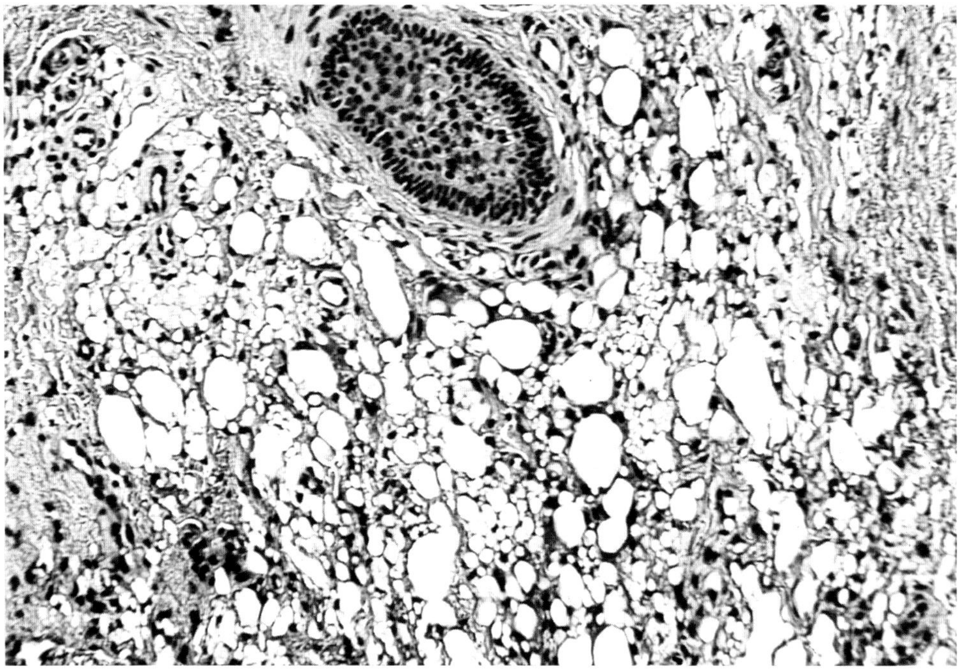

Fig 7.7 Silicone oil 5 years after its injection in the skin. Note the silicone oil droplets in the tissue without eliciting any inflammatory or foreign body reaction. H&E ×l00 o m

"chondroid syringoma" (p. 157). Another valid example of metaplasia is the transformation into bone of a calcific deposit in another adnexal tumor, that is, a pilomatrixoma (p. 150). In this regard, it must be remembered, though, that bone formation can only be considered to occur upon the development of bone marrow in the affected tissue.

Degredative Process

In this class, three types of lesions may be recognized. These are involutions, degenerations, and atrophies.

Involutions

The characteristic of involutions or involutive processes is that, after an initial phase, the affected organ may be able to regain its original condition and function. This cycle is particularly evident in some cases of hair loss or alopecia (p. 111).

Alopecia, nonscarring: Faced with a specimen to which the tentative clinical impression "*alopecia*" has been attached, the microscopist must first verify if that specimen actually pertains to a hairy region of the body. If this is so, the next step of the work-up, usually accomplished with ease, is to determine if the alopecia is of the *scarring type* – as the one discussed previously, or of the *nonscarring type.* In the latter case several diagnostic possibilities are opened.

Alopecia areata (*area* [L] a court, a limited space) is a not infrequent condition of undetermined cause [7], characterized by a solitary or multiple, well-delimited patch of hair loss, mainly on the face. Spread out cases of alopecia areata may involve the entire head (alopecia totalis) or even the entire body (alopecia universalis). Microscopic examination reveals in the lesion the generalized presence of hair follicles in telogen, with a mild round-cell infiltrate surrounding the individual hair follicles, which may lack the sebaceous component.

In regard to "alopecia areata," the term "*pseudopelade*" should be clarified. *Alopecia areata* – the classic type of nonscarring alopecia – has always been known as "pelade" by the French school of dermatology. At one point, however, it was thought that a type of *pelade* existed, which, contrary to the classic one, had scarring features, reason for which the entity was called "pseudopelade." The assumption did not materialize and the idea was dropped, but the term "pseudopelade" persisted and had been used by people who are fond of complicating matters, in place of the straightforward term "*scarring alopecia*" which perfectly describes that type of lesion.

Male type of alopecia, seen in female patients, is ultimately associated to hormonal imbalance. It carries this name because the pattern of hair loss is that usually seen in alopecia in male patients. Its microscopic examination shows the combination of telogen hair follicles surrounded by hypertrophic sebaceous glands.

Undue traction on hair shafts leads to traction alopecia of several types.

Telogen effluvium is another type of nonscarring alopecia which occurs suddenly and massively. It is often associated with infectious processes, but other times occurs after mentally stressful situations [8], following mysterious psychosomatic mechanisms.

Generally, some mentioned cases of nonscarring alopecias, particularly telogen effluvium, may regress. This is in contrast to the cases of scarring alopecias which, once settled, are of a definitive character.

Degenerations

Along sustained unfavorable conditions such as anoxia or steady solar radiation, cutaneous tissues may lose their original structure and properties, although without being transformed into another type of tissue, but rather into informal masses of material.

The most frequent and important of the degenerative processes is actinic degeneration or "elastosis," so called because of the changes elastic fibers undergo under steady solar radiation. In that case, these fibers change their shape and are transformed into thickened and irregular threads disposed as clumps or as masses of a lead-blue discoloration (Fig. 7.8).

Elastosis is not a lesion in itself but a component of many lesions, in some of which, as that in Favre-Racouchot syndrome, it is an outstanding feature.

Lichen sclerosus et atrophicus (LSEA) is a condition whose etiology has still not been settled. Since its lesions have been recognized by EM to be due to the degeneration of collagen [9], LSEA may be incorporated to the group of cutaneous degeneration. This disorder appears on the trunk and perineum, predominantly of female patients. The lesions appear as flattened areas of a whitish discoloration with punctiform depressions corresponding to atrophic hair follicles. These lesions may be intensely pruritic or otherwise cause no major trouble to the patient: at any rate, and to the contrary of erythroplasia Queyrat which arises in comparable anatomic regions, no propensity to malignant degeneration is recognized in LSEA.

After an initial inflammatory phase of heavy round infiltration of the deep dermis, the whole dermis in LSEA is transformed into a broad band of homogeneous, faintly eosinophilic and acellular material. The lesion presents extreme atrophy of the epidermis, which is reduced to a few keratin scales separated from the dermis, without interposition of the germinal layer, by an empty space: atrophic hair follicles are regularly noted in the lesion (Fig. 7.9).

The variations of LSEA, kraurosis vulvae (*krau* + *osis* [G] dry + condition) and balanitis xerotica obliterans, a degenerative condition starting as a dry (xeros [G] dry) and obliterant (*obliterans* [L]) process found on the prepuce and glans penis of male patients, feature the same histologic picture as LSEA.

Atrophies

The final phase of all inflammatory cutaneous processes which do not lead to scarring, as well as the senile cutaneous

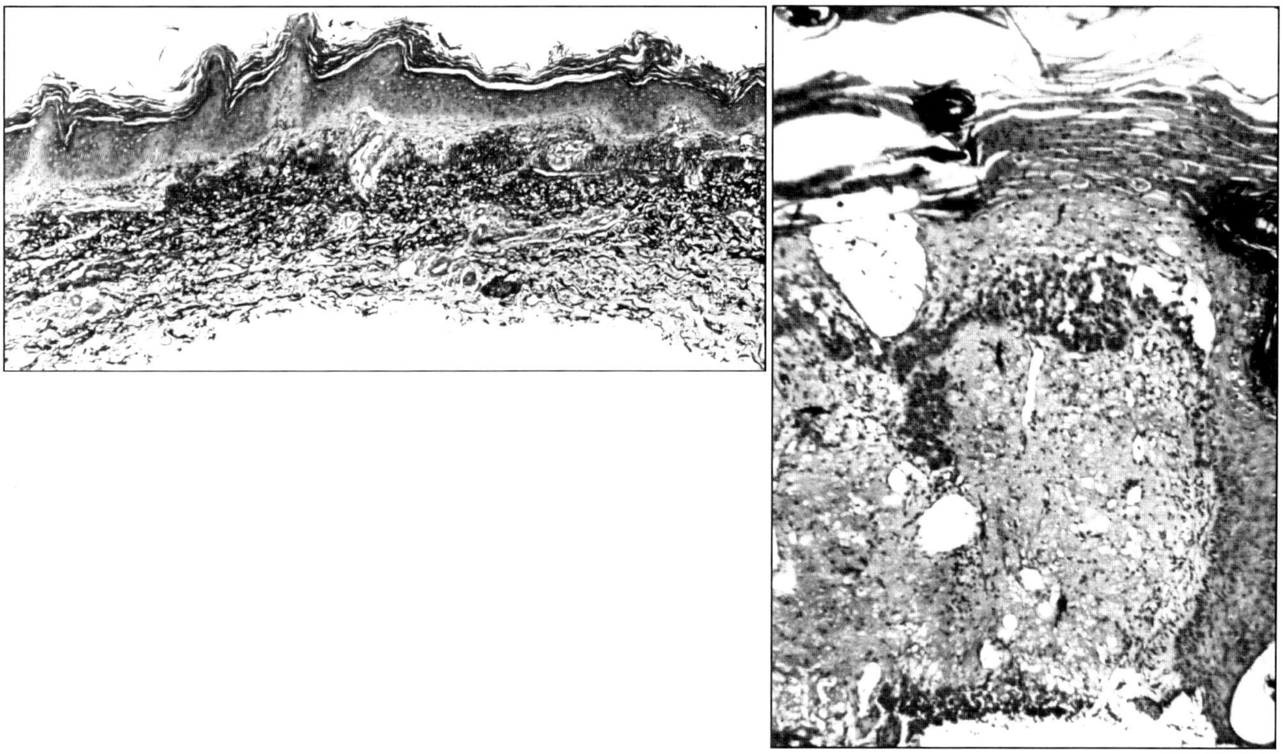

Fig. 7.8 Skin with elastotic degeneration. (*Left*) Note the altered network of elastic tissue in the superficial dermis and (*right*) its transformation into a solid mass. EvG ×40; ×100 o m

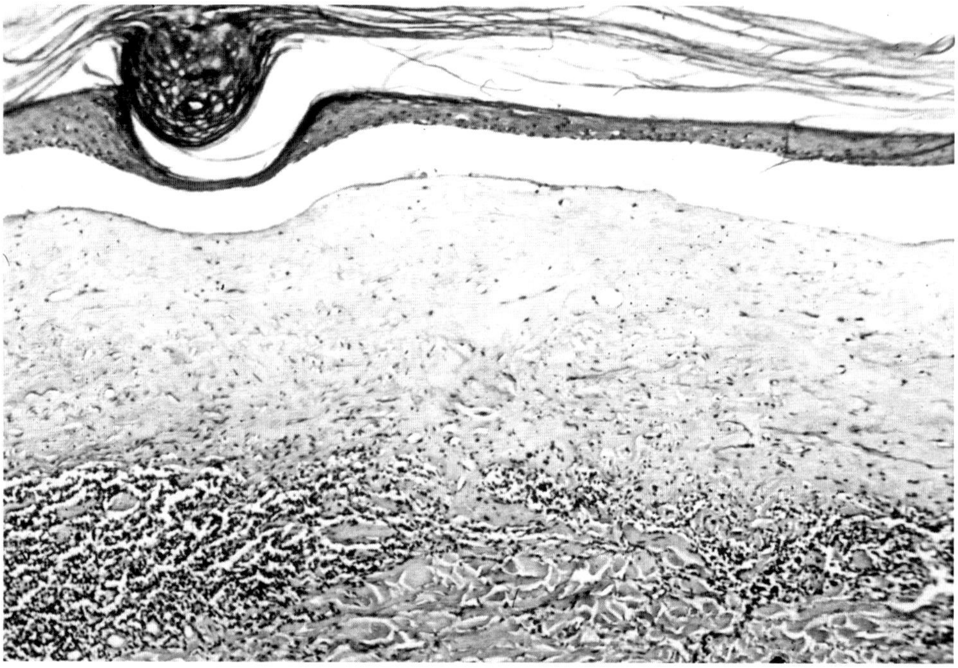

Fig. 7.9 Lichen sclerosus et atrophicus. See details in the text. H&E ×100 o m

transformation of the skin, may be considered expressions of irreversible atrophy.

Acquired Cysts

According to the definition of a "cyst" as an empty space surrounded by its own capsule (p. 40), two types of cysts are recognized in this text: the congenital and the acquired. The congenital or embryonic cysts are of malformative nature and have been discussed along with other malformative lesions in Chap. 4; the retention cysts shall be examined in this coming section.

Retention Cysts

Acquired cysts occur during postuterine life and are – with the exception of the "implantation cyst" – of a retentive quality. They occur following the occlusion of the outlet of cutaneous recesses, mainly follicular infundibuli. After this, the space behind undergo dilatation due to the accumulation of shed keratin scales and fluid secretion, frequently reaching sizable volumes (Fig. 7.10).

Figure 7.11 helps to understand the differences between a retention cyst and a *trichilemmoma* or "a wen," with which it is frequently mistaken.

A "comedo" (*comedo* [L] a glutton) is an infected retention cyst, and a "mucocele"is a cystic dilatation of a minor salivary gland located beneath the mucosa of the oral cavity.

Implantation Cyst

Contrary to the retention cysts, implantation cysts originate from tiny fragments of viable epidermis imported during surgical or traumatic events into the dermis, where they grow in a cystic fashion. They are easily distinguished from retention cysts by the thick layer of normal epidermis lining their wall, instead of the distended one of the former, and by the fact that they are found deep in the dermis (Fig. 7.12).

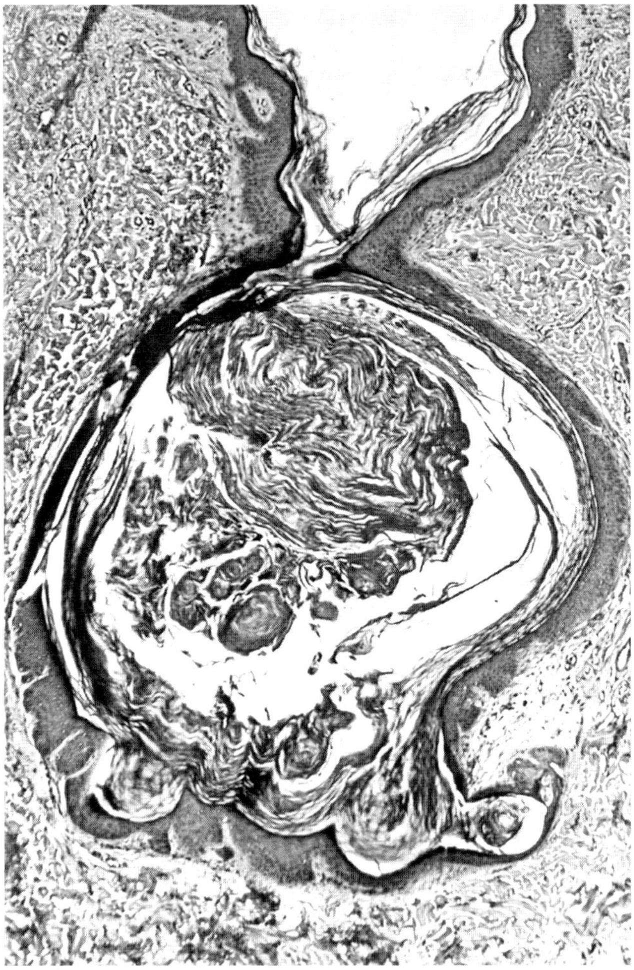

Fig. 7.10 Retention cysts. A retention cyst is shown formed after occlusion of a follicular infundibulum, enclosing keratin scales. H&E ×40 o m. See for comparison a retention cyst formed upon occlusion of a sudoriparous gland in Fig. 5.85

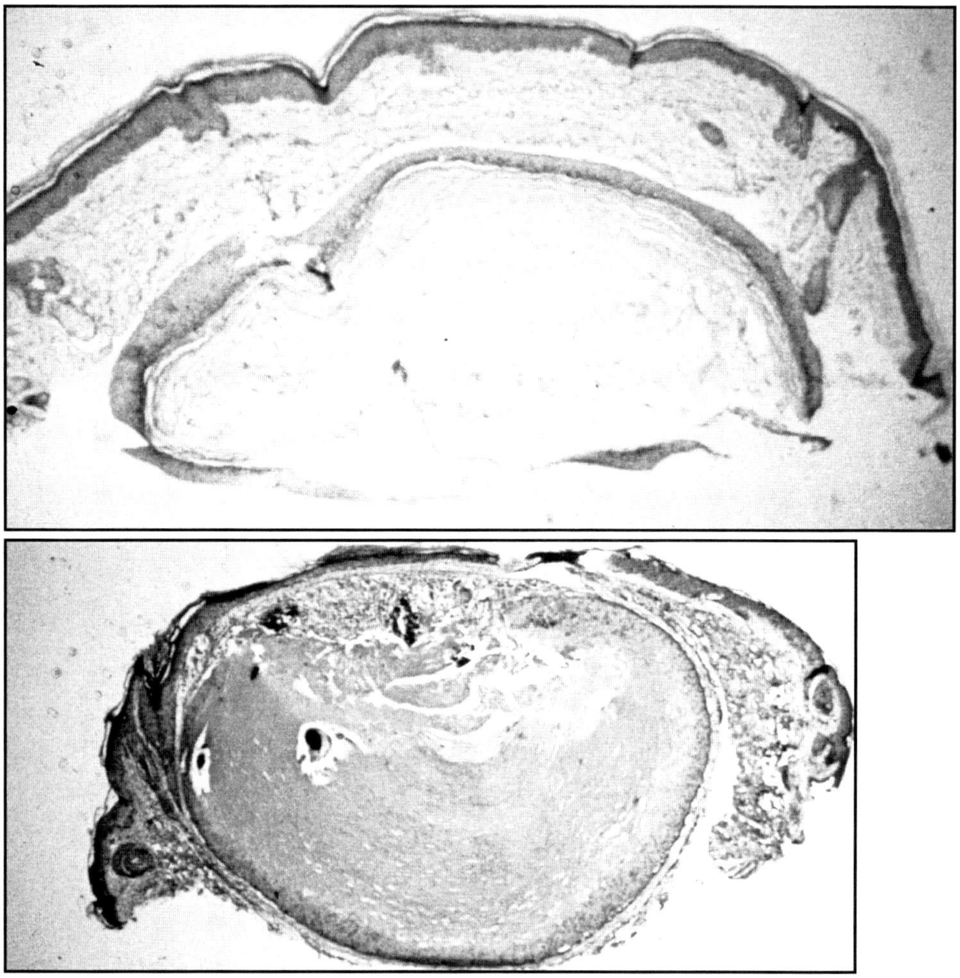

Fig. 7.11 Comparative picture of a retention cyst and a trichilemmoma. The retention cyst (*above*) is in this particular case an empty cavity, which may be secondarily filled with keratin scales, whereas the trichilemmoma (*below*) is an adnexal tumor. This one arises from the trichilemma, generating an exaggerated amount of keratin. Note the solid quality of the trichilemmoma compared with the empty one of the retention cyst. H&E ×40 o m

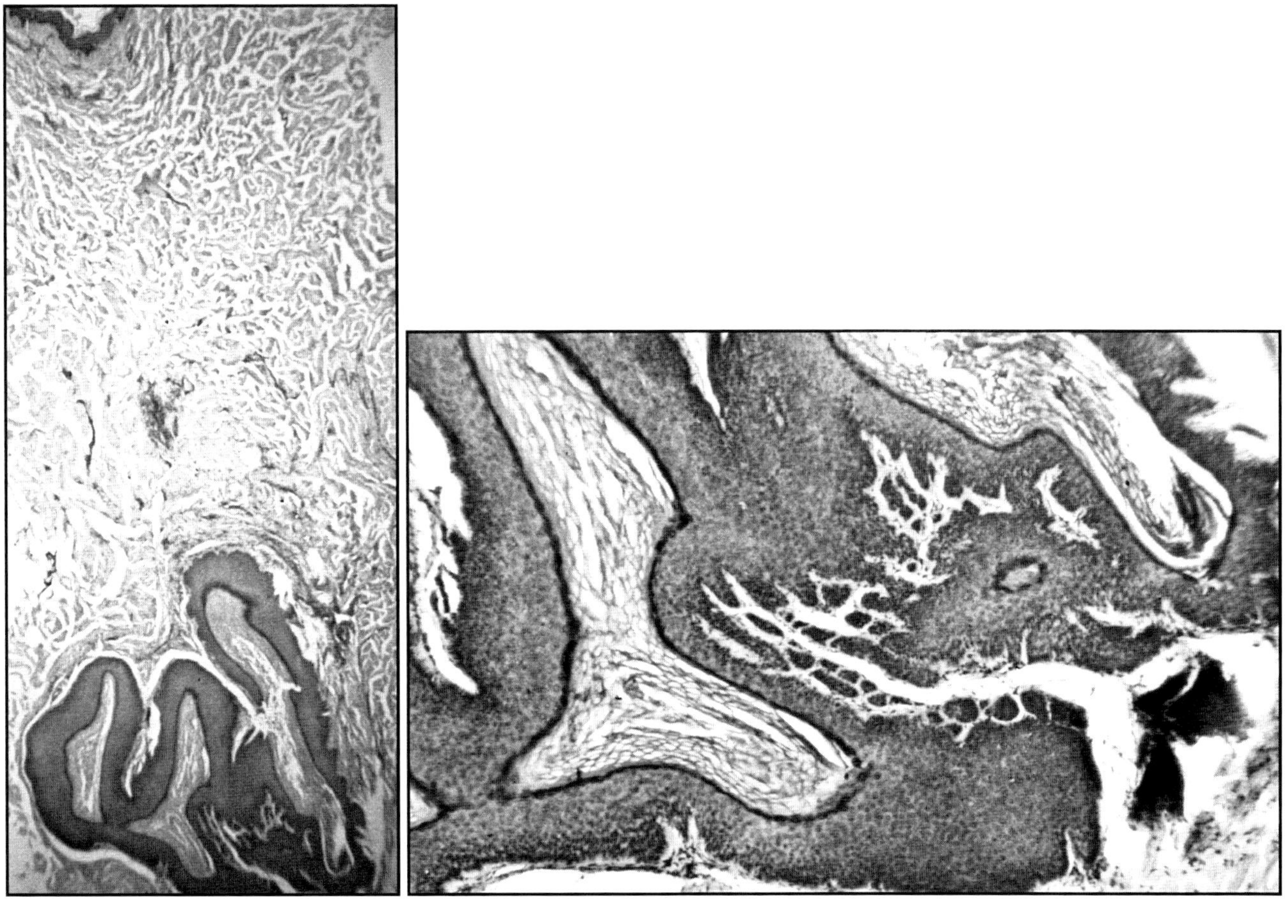

Fig. 7.12 Implantation cyst. (*Left*) Note the thick epidermis lining the cavity of the three cysts in the figure, and their deep location within the dermis, which appears scarred. (*Right*) Higher magnification of the cysts to show details of their wall. H&E ×40; ×100 o m

References

1. Lever WF, Schaumburg-Lever G. Histopathology of the skin. 7th ed. Philadelphia: Lippincott; 1990. p. 514.
2. Lever WF, Schaumburg-Lever G. Histopathology of the skin. 7th ed. Philadelphia: Lippincott; 1990. p. 475.
3. Braun-Falco O, Plewig G, Wolff HH, Burgdorf WHC. Dermatology. 2nd ed. Berlin: Springer; 2000. p. 1290.
4. James WD, Berger TG, Elston MD, editors. Andrews' diseases of the skin, 10th ed. Pennsylvania: W.B. Saunders; 2006. p. 172.
5. Braun-Falco O, Plewig G, Wolff HH, Burgdorf WHC. Dermatology. 2nd ed. Berlin: Springer; 2000. p. 1285.
6. Breathnach SM. In: Freedberg IM, et al., editors. Fitzpatrik dermatologia en medicina general, 5th ed. Buenos Aires: Editorial Medica Panamericana; 2001. p. 1855.
7. Rook A, Dauber R. Diseases of the hair and scalp. Oxford: Blackwell Scientific Publications; 1982. p. 272–3.
8. Mehregan AH, Hashimoto K, editors. Pinkus' guide to dermatohistopathology, 5th ed. Norwalk: Appleton-Lange; 1991. p. 715.
9. Lever WF, Schaumburg-Lever G. Histopathology of the skin. 7th ed. Philadelphia: Lippincott; 1990. p. 308.

Abbreviations

Ab	Antibody
Ag	Antigen
AIDS	Acquired immunodeficiency syndrome
AMH	Atypical melanocytic hyperplasia
APC	Antibody presenting cell
aut dom	Autosomal dominant
aut irreg dom	Autosomal irregular dominant
aut rec	Autosomal recessive
BCC	Basal cell carcinoma
BCIE	Bullous congenital ichthyosiform erythroderma
BM	Basement membrane
BMZ	Basement membrane zone
BPAg 1	Bullous pemphigoid Ag 1
BPAg 2	Bullous pemphigoid Ag 2
BW	Bowen disease
C	Complement
CBDCh	Chronic bullous disease of childhood
D	Dalton
DH	Dermatitis herpetiformis
DLE	Discoid lupus erythematosus
DOPA	Dioxyphenylalanina
EB	Epidermolysis bullosa
EBA	Epidermolysis bullosa acquisita
EED	Erythema elevatum diutinum
EM	Electron microscopy
EMu	Erythema multiforme
FB	Foreign body
FS chain	Secretory chain
G	Greek
GAG	Glycosaminoglycan
GF	Granuloma faciale
GI	Gastrointestinal
GP	Glycoprotein
GMS	Grocott methenamine silver stain
H&E	Hematoxylin/eosin
HLA	Human leukocyte antigen
HDCwCR	Hereditary disorder of control with cutaneous repercussion
HDCwCR	Hereditary disorders of control with cutaneous repercussion
HMEwCR	Hereditary metabolic errors with cutaneous repercussion
HPDwCP	Hereditary polysystemic disorder with cutaneous participation
HSV	Herpes simplex virus
HPV	Human papilloma virus
HT	Hereditary transmission
IC	Immunocomplex
IDN	Nevocytic nevus
IF	Immunofluorescence
IFM	Immunofluorescent mapping
IgA	Immunoglobulin A
IgD	Immunoglobulin D
IgE	Immunoglobulin E
IgG	Immunoglobulin G
IgM	Immunoglobulin M
ILVEN	Inflammatory linear verrucous epidermal nevus
IM	Immunocomplex
KD	Kilo Dalton
L	Latin
LD	Lamina densa
LIgAD	Linear IgA dermatosis
LAMB	
LC	Langerhans cell
LD	Lamina densa
LE	Lupus erythematosus
LEOPARD	
LL	Lamina lucida
LM	Light microscopy
LMa	Lentigo maligna
LMM	Lentigo maligna melanoma
LP	Lichen planus
LS	Lentigo simplex
LSC	Lichen simplex chronicus
MC	Mucicarmine
MF	Mycosis fungoides

E. Zappi, E.A. Zappi, *Dermatopathology*,
DOI 10.1007/978-1-4471-2894-6, © Springer-Verlag London 2013

M/P	Melanin/Perls stain
MW	Molecular weight
NBCIE	Non bullous congenital ichthyosiform erythroderma
NF	Neurofibromatosis
nm	Nanometer
NMM	Nevocytic malignant melanoma
NND	Nevocytic nevus dysplastic
PAS	Periodic acid/Schiff reagent
PF	Pemphigus foliaceous
PG	Proteoglycans
PLC	Pityriasis lichenoides chronica
PLEVA	Pityriasis lichenoides et varioliformis acuta
PM	Plasma membrane
PV	Pemphigus vulgaris
RDEP	Reactive dermoepidermal proliferation
RES	Reticuloendothelial system
SB	Subepidermal bulla
SES	Subepidermal space
SJS	Steven Johnson syndrome
SLDS	Sublamina densa space
SLE	Systemic lupus erythematosus
SQC	Squamous cell carcinoma
SSS	Scalded skin syndrome
SSSS	Staphylococcal scalded skin syndrome
TAD	Transient acantholytic dermatosis
tb	Tuberculosis
T_C cell	T cytotoxic cell
T_H cell	T helper cell
TRI	Masson trichromic stain
UV	Ultraviolet
VV	Verruca vulgaris
VZV	Varicella zoster virus
WS	Warthin-Starry stain
x-ld	X-linked dominant
Ø	Macrophage

Glossary

Accessory proteins (AP) Proteoglycan molecules which help in many biological processes. Some, as the filaggrins, are strictly intracellular; others, as the cadherins are transmembranous, whereas a third type as laminin or fibronectin are extracellular.

Adherent glycoproteins Filamentous elements of the BM frequently associated to type IV collagen.

Anaphylotoxina Low MW peptides with a strong inflammatory action generated by the splitting of C3 and CS.

Antibodies Family of proteins found in the fraction gamma of the electrophoretic spectrum of serum. Since these are originated along immunologic processes, the members of this family are defined as "immunoglobulins." Igs combine specifically with their corresponding Ag and are adaptors of primordial importance in the acquired immunoresponse. The specific function of Abs is to eliminate structures "foreign" to the organism: viruses, microbes, cells, etc. Abs get attached to them by their specific receptors, and bind them to C and macrophages, in order to destroy them. The chemical structure of Ab is discussed under "immunoglobulins."

Antigens Ag are (1.) substances able to elicit the production of Abs and (2.) to combine specifically with them.

Apoptosis or cellular death Operative process in embryonic development and remodeling, as well as in extrauterine life. It is involved in eliminating worn out, superfluous, or risky elements. Apoptosis is based on the activation of the caspases system, which leads to cellular death through DNA fragmentation and elimination of its residues without eliciting any inflammatory reaction.

Argentaffinity Is the property displayed by certain argyrophilic cells (see below) after being impregnated with silver salts, of reducing silver to its metallic form, without the help of external agent.

Argirophylia Is the property displayed by certain cells of allowing the passage through their external membranes of silver salt solution which impregnate them. The silver in these salts may then be reduced to its metallic form by external agents.

Cadherins Accessory proteins able to go through the cellular membrane. The name of these substances implies their Ca^{++} dependency in order to fulfill their functions.

Complement system One of the sequentially activated systems in the blood. C consists of about 20 factors, most of which are proteolytic enzymes, designated by C followed by a digit which indicates the precise identity of the factor. The activation of the C system occurs following the classic or the alternative pathway, in the first case by contact of ICs with C1, and in the second, by microbial or other foreign particles in contact with other elements of the system. The main purpose in both cases is to stimulate C3, the key element of the system. After this, the sequential triggering of the rest of the system follows, with liberation of active agents which help the C system fulfill its main functions of cytolysis, cellular activation, and opsonization.

Cytokines Small-sized, very active proteins involved as intercellular messengers in immune and nonimmune processes.

Cytoskeleton Eukaryotic cells possess a fibrous scaffold formed by three types of fibers, microtubules, actin fibers, and intermediary fibers.

C1-activated inhibitor Element normally present in the organism, which inhibits the effects of activated C1, thus preventing the extemporary or excessive activity of the whole C system.

Desmoplasia Changes in tissues that, because of the increase of their fibroblastic components and collagen deposition, become similar in aspect and composition to tendons and ligaments.

Dystrophic A structure which as a consequence of previous alterations is unable to fulfill its function.

Filaggrin Accessory proteins of intracellular localization, of primordial importance in keratinization.

Fontana-Masson staining Histotechnique based on the intracellular reduction of silver salts to metallic silver, with help of external agents.

Haptens Small antigenic determinants able to specifically combine to Ab, but which, unlike Ag, are unable to

E. Zappi, E.A. Zappi, *Dermatopathology*,
DOI 10.1007/978-1-4471-2894-6, © Springer-Verlag London 2013

induce Ab production unless they are coupled to a large molecule (carrier).

HLA system Genetic complex initially studied by tissue transplantation in mice, from where it received the name of "major histocompatibility complex" (MHC). This name, however, does not adequately describe this system's functions, which are not so much to determine the success or failure of a transplantation procedure, as to provide genetic individuality to individuals of human and animal species. For this reason, its name was replaced by human leukocyte antigen system, abbreviated as HLA. In the human species, the HLA system is located in the short arm of chromosome 6 and contains three regions, I, II, and III. Regions I and II produce class I and II Ag, respectively. Region III do not produce Ag but C components and other substances. Class I Ag are present virtually on the surface of every nucleated cell, whereas the presence of class II Ag is limited to the surface of immunocompetent cells, such as B cells, dendritic cells, and macrophages. The presence in a graft of class I Ag different from those of the recipient leads the immune system of the latter to recognize that graft as "non self" and to reject it. This is the reason for which class I Ag are called the "transplantation antigens."

Immunocomplexes (IC) Aggregates of Ag/Ab in variable proportions according to the circumstance under which they are formed. IC are usually liberated to the circulatory system, from where they are normally eliminated. Otherwise, they may be deposited onto inappropriate sites, giving rise to pathologic processes.

Immunoglobulins (Ig) Are tetrapeptide molecules formed by a pair of heavy chains to each of which a light chain is covalently attached. There are five classes of immunoglobulins, IgA, IgD, IgE, IgG, and IgM, each with its own class of heavy chain, designated by the Greek letters alpha, delta, epsilon, gamma, and mu, to which two classes of light chain, either kappa or lambda, are attached.

For the discussion of the general structure of the Ig, IgG can be taken as a model. IgG is a molecule with axial symmetry formed by two identical subunits. Each subunit is formed by a heavy G chain of 450 amino acids and a kappa or lambda chain of 212 amino acids. The heavy and the light chain, along with the two subunits, are joined to each other by disulphide bridges. In the case of the two subunits, the disulphide bridges are in the center of the molecule, in the area known as the "zone of the hinge." Both the heavy and the light chain have a variable and a constant zone: the former zone is found toward the N-end of the light or heavy chain and the constant one toward the C end of that chain.

By enzymatic action an IgG molecule may be split into two fractions, a Fab (fragment antibody binding) and other Fc (fragment crystalizable). The Fab contains the site for specific combination of the molecule with its corresponding Ag; in the Fc are localized binding sites, which, even if they are not able to combine to Ab, are of great biologic importance since they bind C fractions and macrophages, bringing them in close proximity to the target element.

IgG, IgE, and IgD are produced as monomers and exported into the circulation, except for IgD, which remains fixed to the surface of the cell which produces it. IgA, of predominant localization in the mucosae, is generated as a dimer, whose two parts are joined by a polypeptide, the J chain. An additional chain, the "secretory fraction," is attached to the IgA molecule, which facilitates its passage through the intestinal wall. IgM appears as a pentamer whose monomers are joined, as in the case of IgA, by J chains. IgM is also poured into circulation, except for a minor portion, which remains attached to the cell surface as IgD, where it intervenes in the Ag recognition process.

Immunoreactants Every humoral element active in an immunogenic reaction.

Laminin Extracellular accessory protein with a cruciform shape involved in the attachment of the PM to the LD.

Major histocompatibility system See HLA system, above.

Masson trichromic staining procedure Staining procedure used for the differentiation of mesenchymal tissues, in particular fibrous from muscular types. For this purpose, several stains are successively applied to the same tissue section.

Melanin/Perls staining procedure Combined procedure in which the successive application of the Fontana-Masson and the Perls staining procedure to a same tissue section allows the simultaneous detection of melanin and hemosiderin.

Metachromasia Development, at the end of a staining procedure, of a color different from that of the elements that were used in it. This phenomenon occurs when the agents used for the procedure have strong opposite charges. For this reason, when they are in contact, they react forming new substances, whose organoleptic properties – including color – are different from those of the original components.

Opsonization Is the process of attachment of C and Ab to the surface of a target element. This increases the attraction of macrophages to the target element, facilitating its eventual destruction.

PAS staining technique Histotechnique for carbohydrates detection consisting of treating tissues with periodic acid and then with Schiff reagent. Carbohydrates – eventually present in the tissue – under periodic acid attack liberate free aldehydes, which can be detected by the purple color they produce in contact with Schiff reagent.

Perls staining procedure Histotechnique for detection of iron in the form of hemosiderin. Tissues are treated with potassium ferrocyanide, which in the presence of hemosidering yields Prussian blue, of intense blue color.

Postcapillary venule The use of this term is only justified when specifically referring to venules with a high cylindrical epithelium entering into lymphatic glands. These venules allow the passage of lymphocytes from the blood into lymphatic circulation. Otherwise the term "postcapillary venules" is redundant, since every venule is postcapillary.

T cells (TC) Cells derived from the common lymphoid progenitors which differentiate within the thymus, where they acquire their antigenic receptors, being then transformed into T lymphocytes or T cells (TC). TC are liberated into the circulation, where basically two types of these may be recognized, T helper (T_H cell) and T cytotoxic (T_C cell). Other varieties of TC such as memory and supressor TC seem to be elements differentiated from either T_H or T_C cells.

Toluidine blue staining procedure Application of a metachromatic reaction (see above) for the detection of substances with a strong acid charge. In the particular case purported here, toluidine blue solution is applied onto tissue sections. A purple color develops on those structures where GAG is present.

Verhoeff/van Gieson Histotechnique for the staining of elastic fibers based on the use of iodine and ferric hematoxylin.

Bibliography

Dermatopathology

Graham JH, Johnson WC, Helwig EB, editors. Dermal pathology. Hagerstown: Harper & Row; 1972.

Lever WF, Schaumburg-Lever G. Histopathology of the skin. 7th ed. Philadelphia: J.B. Lippincott Co; 1990.

Mehregan AH, Hashimoto K, editors. Pinkus' guide to dermatohistopathology. 5th ed. Norwalk: Appleton & Lange; 1991.

Montagna W, Parakkal PF. The structure and function of skin. 3rd ed. New York: Academic; 1974.

Dermatology

Bologna JL, Jorizzo JL, Rapini RP. Dermatology. Edinburgh: Mosby; 2004.

Braun-Falco O, Plewig G, Wolff HH, Burgdorf WHC. Dermatology. 3rd ed. Berlin: Springer; 2008.

James WB, Berger TG, Elston DM, editors. Andrews' diseases of the skin. 10th ed. Philadelphia: W.B. Saunders; 2006.

Medicine

Braverman IM. Skin signs of systemic diseases. 3rd ed. Philadelphia: W.B. Saunders Company; 1998.

Dorland's illustrated medical dictionary (28th ed). Philadelphia: WH Saunders 1994.

Goldman L, Shafer AI, editors. Cecil textbook of medicine. 22nd ed. Philadelphia: W.B. Saunders; 2011.

Basic Sciences

Alberts B, et al., editors. Molecular biology of the cell. 4th ed. New York: Garland Science; 2002.

Fawcett DW, Jensh RP, editors. Bloom & Fawcett concise histology. New York: Chapman & Hall; 1997.

Goldsmith LA, editor. Physiology, biochemistry and molecular biology of the skin. (2nd ed. New York: Oxford University Press; 1991.

Hib J, editor. Histologia de Di Fiori. Buenos Aires: Editorial El Ateneo; 2001.

Male D. Immunology. An illustrated outline. 4th ed. Edinburgh: Mosby; 2004.

Mescher AL, editor. Junqueira's basic histology. 12tth ed. New York: McGraw Hill; 2010.

Roitt J, Brostoff J, Male D. Immunology. 5th ed. St.Louis: C.V. Mosby Company; 1985.

Pathology

Beutner EH, Chorzelski TP, Bean SB. Immunopathology of the skin. 2nd ed. New York: Wiley; 1979.

Enzinger F, Weiss SW. Soft tissue tumors. 5th ed. St.Louis: Mosby; 2008.

Florey HW, editor. General pathology. 4th ed. Philadelphia: W.B. Saunders Co; 1970.

Mooi WJ, Krausz T. Biopsy pathology of melanocytic disorders. London: Chapman & Hall Medical; 1992.

Kumar V, Abbas AK, Fausto N, Aster JC, editors. Robbins and Cotran pathologic basis of disease. 8th ed. Philadelphia: Saunders Elsevier; 2010.

Rosai J, editor. Atlas of tumor pathology, vol. 3. Washington, D.C.: Armed Forces Institute of Pathology; 1990/2002.

Rosai J. Rosai and Ackerman surgical pathology. 10th ed. Mosby: Edinburgh; 2008.

Willis RA. Pathology of tumors. 2nd ed. London: Butterworth & Co Ltd; 1953.

Index

E. Zappi, E.A. Zappi, *Dermatopathology*,
DOI 10.1007/978-1-4471-2894-6, © Springer-Verlag London 2013

MIX
Papier aus verantwortungsvollen Quellen
Paper from responsible sources
FSC® C105338

Printed by Books on Demand, Germany